INSTRUCTOR'S MANUAL FOR MAHAN AND ESCOTT-STUMP:

KRAUSE'S FOOD, NUTRITION, AND DIET THERAPY

NINTH EDITION

Sandra S. Witte, PhD, RD

Assistant Professor
Department of Enology, Food Science, and Nutrition
California State University
Fresno, California

W. B. SAUNDERS COMPANY
A Division of Harcourt Brace & Company
Philadelphia   London   Toronto
Montreal   Sydney   Tokyo

W. B. Saunders Company
A Division of Harcourt Brace & Company
The Curtis Center
Independence Square West
Philadelphia, Pennsylvania 19106-3399

Instructor's Manual for Mahan and Escott-Stump:
Krause's Food, Nutrition, and Diet Therapy,   ISBN 0-7216-5836-9
Ninth Edition

Portions of this work were published in previous editions.

Printed in the United States of America

Last digit is the print number: 9   8   7   6   5   4   3   2   1

CONTENTS

PART V—MEDICAL NUTRITION THERAPY

CHAPTER 1

DIGESTION, ABSORPTION, TRANSPORT, AND EXCRETION OF NUTRIENTS

OVERVIEW

The purpose of this chapter is to provide the foundation for an understanding of the relationship of diet to physiological and pathophysiological functions. The learner proceeds from ingestion of food, to the chemical and physical changes that remove nutrients from food and prepares them for absorption or excretion from the body, to absorption of nutrients, and finally, to mechanisms of transport from the gastrointestinal tract to the various body tissues.

LEARNING OBJECTIVES

This chapter will prepare the learner to be able to

1. List the functions of the alimentary tract.
2. Identify the organs of the alimentary tract and their functions.
3. Describe the chemical and physical changes that occur between ingestion of food and absorption and excretion of nutrients.
4. Describe absorption mechanisms and the anatomical characteristics of absorptive tissue.
5. Identify the enzymes involved in the digestive process for carbohydrate, fat, and protein; the site of synthesis; and the actions of these enzymes.
6. Describe the digestive and absorptive process for each of the major nutrients.
7. List the factors involved in food digestion.

CHAPTER OUTLINE

NOTES, TERMS, & TRANSPARENCY MASTERS

I. Alimentary System

Figure 1–1 (Handout) illustrates the anatomical structures that make up the the digestive system. Some secretions are indicated.

II. Digestion and Absorption

Table 1–1 summarizes enzymatic digestion and absorption. Illustrates the concept of enzyme + substrate = product   (E + S = P).

   A. Regulators of gastrointestinal activity

Key Concept: *Integration* of the digestive, nervous, and endocrine systems

1

1. Neural mechanisms	**Table 1–2** summarizes gastrointestinal neurotransmitters. **parietal cells**
2. Hormonal mechanisms	**Table 1–3** summarizes important functions of gastrointestinal hormones. Illustrates the concept of multiple factors influencing the digestive process. **gastrin, secretin, cholecystokinin, gastric inhibitory polypeptide (GIP)**

B. Digestive process
  1. Digestion in the mouth — **peristalsis**

  2. Digestion in the stomach — **chyme**
  3. Digestion in the small intestine

C. Absorptive mechanisms
  1. Small intestine — **Figure 1–2** illustrates the anatomical structure of the intestinal villi. **villi, microvilli, brush border**

  2. Diffusion and active transport — **Figure 1–3** illustrates the membrane absorption and transport mechanisms. **facilitated diffusion, passive diffusion, active transport**

D. Digestion and absorption of nutrients
  1. Carbohydrates — **Figure 1–4** is a simplified schematic illustration of starch (amylose) digestion; it does not include digestion of amylopectin (branched). **Figure 1–5** illustrates both digestion and absorption of carbohydrate. **Key concept:** Regardless of the form of carbohydrate ingested, the body will break it down to glucose or related hexoses, the useable form of carbohydrate. **amylase, sucrase, lactase, maltase**

  2. Proteins — **proteolytic enzymes**

  3. Lipids — **Figure 1–6** is a simplified illustration of digestion and absorption of lipid. **Key concept:** Chylomicrons are lipoproteins. **enterogastrone, pancreatic lipase, micelles**

  4. Other nutrients — **Figure 1-7 (Handout)** provides a summary of secretions (left side) and absorptive sites (right side), showing integration of the lymphatic and blood systems.

E. Factors affecting digestion
  1. Psychologic factors
  2. Bacterial action

  3. Effects of food processing

III. Role of the Large Intestine

Key concept: Certain species of bacteria normally inhabit the gut and are not pathogenic.

defecation

CASE STUDY INSIGHTS

Note: **Flatus** and **spastic colitis** are used in the case description but are not used in the chapter. Flatus is defined in Key Terms, Chapter 28. Spastic colitis is not discussed in the text, but can be defined as irritable bowel syndrome (IBS), also discussed in Chapter 28.

1. Why would a high-fiber diet be useful in managing spastic colitis?

Normal bowel function is dependent on sufficient stool bulk to stimulate defecation. In the absence of organic disorders, high-fiber diets are often effective as a means of increasing stool bulk and promoting normal bowel function. No information is given about the client's normal fiber intake. This should be determined as part of the dietary counseling.

2. Why is extra fluid needed with increased fiber intake?

One characteristic of dietary fiber is its hydration capacity. Wheat bran is particularly effective in absorbing water and results in an increase in stool bulk and softness. The addition of fluid along with fiber is necessary for maximizing the stool bulking effect of the dietary fiber. If insufficient fluid is ingested with increased fiber intakes, the stool will be hard and dry, increasing the risk of fecal impaction.

3. The diet recommends extra bran. Identify four ways in which extra whole bran could be added to Mary's daily diet. Include recipes with the case study for four foods that could be used with added bran.

A variety of answers are acceptable here. Emphasis should be on how dietary recommendations given in terms of nutrients can be carried out in terms of food eaten. Assist students in assessing whether their recommendations are likely to be palatable and, therefore, acceptable to the client.

SUGGESTED TEST QUESTIONS

1. Nutrients absorbed by the small intestine are transported to the liver by the
* a. portal vein.
  b. hepatic vein.
  c. inferior vena cava.
  d. mesenteric vein.

2. Following surgical removal of a large portion of the small intestine, problems likely to develop are a result of
  a. changes in dietary habits.
  b. impaired digestion.
* c. loss of absorptive tissue.
  d. elimination of dietary residue.

3. The greatest activity in carbohydrate digestion takes place primarily in the
   a. mouth.
   b. stomach.
   * c. small intestine.
   d. colon.

4. It is essential that a patient's stomach be empty prior to surgery to prevent vomiting and aspiration. Under normal circumstances, what is the maximum time it should take for the stomach to empty?
   a. 2 hour
   * b. 4 hours
   c. 6 hours
   d. 8 hours

5. The sight or smell of food produces vagal stimulation of the parietal cells of the gastric mucosa, resulting in increased production of
   a. insulin
   * b. hydrochloric acid
   c. cholecystokinin
   d. secretin

6. Malabsorption of fat resulting from an impaired ability to produce adequate bile salts for micellar formation may be improved by
   a. increasing short-chain fatty acids in the diet.
   * b. increasing medium-chain fatty acids in the diet.
   c. increasing long-chain fatty acids in the diet.
   d. restricting dietary intake of cholesterol.

7. Toxicity from dietary minerals is generally prevented by
   * a. the reserve capacity of protein carriers.
   b. the presence of non-specific protein carriers.
   c. an increased urinary output of minerals.
   d. an increased fecal output of minerals.

8. When assessing a patient for constipation, you would compare the patient's defecation pattern with the normal defecation pattern, which is defined as
   a. one soft B.M. each day.
   b. one B.M. every three days.
   c. a B.M. after each meal.
   * d. one that occurs with varying frequency.

9. Which of the following best describes the function of secretin?
   a. It stimulates gastric secretions and increases motility.
   b. It stimulates contraction of the gallbladder and the release of bile.
   * c. It stimulates the pancreas to secrete water and bicarbonate into the duodenum.
   d. It stimulates the parietal cells to secrete gastrin.

10. The intestinal hormone released in the presence of fat and glucose that results in the release of insulin is
    * a. gastric inhibitory peptide (GIP).
    b. cholecystokinin.
    c. gastrin.
    d. intestinal lipase.

11. Which of the following enzymes are released from the pancreas?
    a. insulin, trypsin, secretin
    b. lactase, isomaltase, dextrinase
    c. protease, pepsin, gastrin
    * d. trypsin, chymotrypsin, carboxypolypeptidase

12. Nutrients are normally digested in which order?
    a. carbohydrate, fat, protein
    b. protein, fat, carbohydrate
    * c. carbohydrate, protein, fat
    d. protein, carbohydrate, fat

13. Dietary fat is absorbed from the intestine as part of a
    a. chylomicron.
    * b. micelle.
    c. triglyceride.
    d. lipoprotein.

14. An advantage to medium chain triglycerides when fat malabsorption occurs is that they can
    * a. pass directly into the portal vein without esterification.
    b. pass directly into the lymphatic system without esterification.
    c. transport long chained triglycerides through the lymph.
    d. pass through the lymphatic system undigested.

15. Most vitamins are absorbed from the small intestines into the blood by
* a. passive diffusion.
  b. active diffusion.
  c. facilitative diffusion.
  d. passive osmosis.

16. The large intestine is the primary site of absorption for
  a. water and fats.
  b. carbohydrates.
  c. protein.
* d. water, bile salts, and some vitamins.

17. Enterohepatic circulation is particularly effective in
* a. conserving bile salts by recycling them back to the liver.
  b. conserving enzymes by recycling lactase, sucrase, and maltase back to the intestinal mucosa.
  c. regulation of lipoprotein levels in the blood stream.
  d. transport of chylomicrons via the lymphatics.

18. Cellulose and lignin are fibers that are
  a. converted into glucose prior to absorption.
  b. converted into glucose and absorbed by active transport.
* c. excreted in the feces unchanged.
  d. excreted in the feces as glucose.

CHAPTER 2

Energy

OVERVIEW

The purpose of this chapter is to lead the student through a logical progression of how energy needs for individuals and energy potential of foods are determined. The chapter begins with a discourse on the various demands the body has for energy, both as essential (metabolic activity and thermic effect of food) and conditional (physical activity). From here, the learner progresses to how energy needs for humans are measured and how the energy potential of foods is determined. This is followed by the more practical approach—calculation of human energy needs and food energy potential. The application of the Recommended Dietary Allowance for energy is also included.

LEARNING OBJECTIVES

This chapter will prepare the learner to be able to

1. Identify the body functions that contribute to total energy expenditure (TEE) and define each.
2. Compare and contrast basal energy expenditure (BEE) and resting energy expenditure (REE).
3. Explain how body size and composition relate to basal metabolic rate (BMR).
4. Illustrate how BMR varies in different stages of the life cycle and in the presence of some physiological and environmental influences.
5. Define thermic effect of food (TEF) and identify two types of thermogenesis that contribute to the TEF.
6. Compare the calorie, Calorie, kilocalorie (kcal), joule, and kilojoule (kJ).
7. Describe how energy expenditure is measured in humans.
8. Use a variety of methods to calculate the REE for an individual.
9. Use two different methods to calculate the TEE for an individual.
10. Determine the energy potential of foods and alcoholic beverages using the caloric value of carbohydrate, protein, fat, and alcohol.
11. Explain the method used to determine the RDA for energy.

CHAPTER OUTLINE	NOTES, TERMS, & TRANSPARENCY MASTERS
I. Components of Energy Expenditure	**resting energy expenditure (REE), thermic effect of food (TEF), total energy expenditure (TEE)**
A. Resting (or basal) metabolic rate	**Table 2-1** show how the REE is distributed among tissues and organs in the body for maintenance of normal function.

6

1. Measurement of metabolic rate

Figure 2-1 is a nomogram for estimating food allowance (caloric needs). Instructions for use are included. The determination requires a series of successive applications of new information.
basal energy expenditure (BEE), basal metabolic rate (BMR), resting metabolic rate (RMR)

2. Factors affecting metabolic rate

Figure 2-2 is a graphic illustration of the difference in BMR by gender.

B. Physical activity

Table 2-2 is a reference for energy required to sustain various activity levels based on multiples of the REE. Use of this reference requires that the duration of each activity is known and that all 24 hours (1440 minutes) per day are accounted for.
Table 2-3 is a reference for estimating TEE using a general activity level for the 24-hour period. This is also based on multiples of REE.
Table 2-4 provides estimates of energy expenditures (in kcal/min) for various of activities if the duration of each activity is known. Estimates are based on the person weighing 150 lbs. Recommended adjustments are given in the table footnotes.
Figures 2-3, 2-4, and 2-5 illustrate various types of physical activity.

C. Thermic effect of food

diet-induced thermogenesis, obligatory thermogenesis, adaptive (facultative) thermogenesis

II. Energy Measurements
A. Units of measurement

calorie, Calorie, kilocalorie (kcal), joule, and kilojoule (kJ)
Direct students' attention to Clinical Insight: The Joule.

B. Calorimetry
1. Direct calorimetry

direct calorimetry

2. Indirect calorimetry

Figure 2-6 is an illustration of how indirect calorimetry is done
indirect calorimetry, respiratory quotient (RQ)

3. Measuring food energy

Figure 2-7 compares the energy in carbohydrate, fat, and protein for gross energy (heat of combustion), digestible energy, and available energy.

III. Energy Calculations
   A. Calculating human energy requirements
      1. Resting energy expenditure

Table 2-5 provides several methods for determining REE. This is a good time to inform students of which method will be used in this class.

Key concept: There are limitations to each method, and all methods provide only an estimate of energy expenditure.

Table 2-6 provides a method for estimating REE using only body weight. Formulas using several factors, such as age, gender, height, and weight, generally provide a more accurate estimate.

      2. Physical activity
      3. Thermic effect of food
      4. Total energy expenditure

Table 2-7 presents two methods for determining the TEE. The first step requires determination of ideal body weight (IBW) (discussed in Chapter 21). This is a good time to tell students which method will be used in this class.

Table 2-8 provides an example of how TEE is determined for an individual. The two methods in Table 2-7 are both shown, and the differing results are explained.

   B. Calculating food energy

Key concept: Given the carbohydrate, protein, and fat content of a food, the energy potential in calories can be determined.

Appendix 41 contains nutrient values for selected foods. Direct students' attention to Clinical Insight: Calculation of Energy Content of Alcoholic Beverages.

IV. Recommended Energy Allowances

Table 2-9 lists the Recommended Dietary Allowances for energy. Both the REE and the average energy allowance are given.

CASE STUDY INSIGHTS

Note: The case study does not state the purpose of the client's appointment with the Dietetic Counselor except that he wants to start an exercise program.

1. What other information is needed to give Mr. Queue nutritional guidance?

Is weight status appropriate? If not, will weight change be a goal? Duration of proposed exercise periods is important. His normal dietary intake must be known.

2. What specific advice may be useful to Mr. Queue on days when he is more active?

If weight status is appropriate, maintenance of his current weight requires additional food to meet his increased energy needs. If weight is determined to be greater than his recommended weight for height, maintaining a consistent food intake on all days, whether active or inactive, will increase use of body stores of fat to meet increased energy needs. Maintenance of adequate fluid intake should be emphasized.

3. Mr. Queue thinks that he can now double his energy intake by this increase in activity. Calculate his normal needs and estimate for him the increases that will actually occur based on his planned activities.

Method 1 for Determining TEE (Table 2-5)

Before beginning exercise program:

a. Table 17-10 (Chapter 17) gives Mr. Queue's desirable body weight (IBW) as 136–151 lbs. The calculation is demonstrated using the midpoint of this range.
b. Basal needs = 1 kcal/kg IBW/hr × 24 hr
                = 1 kcal × 65 kg × 24 hr
                = 1560 kcal
c. Subtract for sleep (assume Mr. Queue sleeps 8 hr/day)
   Sleep   = 0.1 kcal/kg IBW/hr of sleep
                = 6.5 kcal × 8 hr
                = 52 kcal
   1560 kcal for basal needs – 52 kcal for sleep = 1508 kcal
d. Activity level for Mr. Queue is light to moderate. See Table 2-3.
   1508 kcal × 1.6 = 2413
e. Thermic effect of food (add 10% of BEE plus activity increment)
   0.10 × 2413 kcal = 241 kcal
   2413 kcal for BEE plus activity + 241 kcal for TEF = 2654 kcal

After beginning exercise program:

a. IBW remains at 136–151 lbs.
b. Basal needs remain at 1560 kcal.
c. Sleep remains the same at 52 kcal (BEE – sleep = 1508 kcal).
d. Activity level for Mr. Queue is not substantially changed, but is now considered moderate. See Table 2-3.
   1508 kcal × 1.7 = 2564 kcal
e. TEF increases to 256 kcal (BEE plus activity + TEF = 2820 kcal
   The estimated increase in energy needs for his exercise program is about 166 kcal/day.

SUGGESTED LEARNING ACTIVITIES

1. Provide students with a demonstration, followed by guided and independent practice of the calculations in the chapter. Students may also need to review conversion of standard measurements of weight (pounds and ounces) and height (inches), often used in the United States, to metric measurements which are required in the formulas.

    a. Calculation of REE and TEE:
    53-year-old male, height 5'10",
    weight 174 lbs
    40-year-old female, height 5'5",
    weight 137 lbs
    21-year-old male, height 6'1",
    weight 186 lbs
    75-year-old female, height 5'2",
    weight 117 lbs

    b. Calculation of potential energy of foods (See Appendix 1):
    4 oz of applesauce, unsweetened
    1 cup of whole milk
    1 slice of whole wheat bread (about 1 oz)
    3 oz of cooked roast beef
    1/2 cup of cooked sliced carrots

2. For each of the hypothetical individuals listed above, students can calculate REE and TEE using the various methods presented in the text, including the RDA. Have them compare the results obtained for an individual using different calculation methods.

3. a. Have students keep a food diary or provide a 24-hour recall and then determine the potential energy value of their food intake.
    b. Have students select one of the methods for calculating the TEE and apply their own individual information to the formula.
    c. Compare the results of the calculated energy intake and the calculated energy needs. Explain why the two can be different.

SUGGESTED TEST QUESTIONS

1. A patient is to have diagnostic tests performed to determine basal metabolic rate. Which of the following conditions are necessary for an accurate result?
    a. complete physical and mental rest
    b. 10–12 hours after last meal
    c. morning, after the subject has awakened
 * d. all of the above

2. Which of the following is *least* significant in determining RMR?
    a. body surface area
    b. lean body mass
 * c. age and sex
    d. total body weight

3. An elevation in body temperature with fever results in
    a. no change in the metabolic rate.
 * b. an increase in the metabolic rate of 7% per °F above normal.
    c. an increase in the metabolic rate of 13% per °F above normal.
    d. a decrease in the metabolic rate of 10% per °F above normal.

4. You have been assigned to care for a patient whose body temperature is 104.6°F. Calculate the patient's BMR at this high temperature compared to his normal BMR.
    a. 113% of normal
    b. 121% of normal
    c. 135% of normal
 * d. 142% of normal

5. For patients who drink coffee containing caffeine throughout the day (~1 cup every 2 hours), the effect on the TEF would be
 * a. an increase of 8–11%.
    b. an increase of 18–20%.
    c. a decrease of 10%.
    d. no change.

6. When determination of energy requirements must be accurate to ensure optimal treatment, the best method to use is
    a. indirect calorimetry.
    b. Harris-Benedict formula.
*   c. direct calorimetry.
    d. nomographic chart.

7. The basal metabolic rate is highest during
    a. digestion of a meal.
*   b. periods of rapid growth.
    c. periods of exercise.
    d. during sleep.

8. The principal regulators of metabolic rate are the hormones
*   a. thyroxine and norepinephrine.
    b. insulin and glucocorticoids.
    c. epinephrine and corticosteroids.
    d. glucagon and insulin.

9. The contribution of physical activity to total energy expenditure is best described as
    a. a predictable constant.
    b. slightly variable.
    c. most consistent during childhood.
*   d. highly variable.

10. Indirect calorimetry measures
    a. the amount of heat produced at rest.
    b. the energy potential of foods consumed.
*   c. the amount of oxygen consumed and carbon dioxide excreted, or respiratory quotient (RQ).
    d. the RMR.

11. The highest RQ is obtained when the diet is primarily
    a. mixed nutrients.
*   b. carbohydrate.
    c. fat.
    d. protein.

12. The thermic effect of food is.
    a. at a maximum 4 hours after eating.
*   b. at a maximum 1 hour after eating.
    c. usually still significant 10 hours after eating.
    d. only present for 30 minutes after eating.

13. Recent studies have shown that the RMR is determined primarily by
*   a. the extent of lean body mass.
    b. the extent of adipose tissue.
    c. age, gender, and health status.
    d. body weight.

14. Which of these best describes the change in the metabolic rate during pregnancy?
    a. It decreases as a result of a decrease in physical activity.
    b. It increases as a result of fetal growth.
*   c. It increases as a result of fetal growth and the mother's increased cardiac output.
    d. It decreases as a result of an increase in adipose tissue.

15. The energy required to digest, absorb, and metabolize nutrients is called
*   a. obligatory thermogenesis.
    b. adaptive thermogenesis.
    c. facultative thermogenesis.
    d. nutritive thermogenesis.

16. The energy values for carbohydrate, protein, and fat are
    a. 4 calories per gram
    b. 7 calories per gram
    c. 4, 7, and 4 calories per gram, respectively
*   d. 4, 4, and 9 calories per gram, respectively

17. The total daily energy requirement is calculated by which of these formulas?
    a. REE + TEF – SDA
    b. REE + activity – TEF
*   c. REE + activity – sleep + TEF
    d. REE × IBW

CARBOHYDRATES

OVERVIEW

The purpose of this chapter is to highlight the functions and metabolism of dietary carbohydrates. Important dietary carbohydrates and their sources are identified. In carbohydrate metabolism, the emphasis is on the continual provision of glucose as an energy substrate through various metabolic pathways (glycolysis, glycogenesis, glycogenolysis, Cori cycle, alanine cycle, and gluconeogenesis). The role of dietary fiber, its classifications, sources, and recommended intake are presented.

LEARNING OBJECTIVES

This chapter will prepare the learner to be able to

1. Describe the mechanism by which photosynthesis provides carbohydrate for energy to humans.
2. Identify the classifications of carbohydrates and list the characteristics of each class.
3. Explain how monosaccharides are interchanged in carbohydrate metabolism.
4. List the major metabolic pathways involved in carbohydrate metabolism.
5. Identify the hormones involved in maintenance of blood glucose levels and what the effect of each hormone is.
6. List the functions of carbohydrate.
7. Define dietary fiber, crude fiber, soluble fiber, and insoluble fiber.
8. State the physiological effects of fiber and how they relate to various diseases.
9. Identify sources of fiber in the diet.
10. State the recommended daily intake of fiber.
11. Describe changes in carbohydrate consumption in the United States.

CHAPTER OUTLINE ———————————— NOTES, TERMS, & TRANSPARENCY MASTERS

I. Definition and Composition

hexoses, pentoses

    A. Photosynthesis

Figure 3-1 is a simplistic illustration of the photosynthetic process. Emphasis should be on the sources of the chemical compounds involved in the reaction.

II. Classification

Key concept: monosaccharides are the simplest carbohydrate form. The disaccharides, oligosaccharides, and polysaccharides are made up of more than one monosaccharide.

12

A. Monosaccharides

B. Disaccharides

C. Polyhydroxy alcohols

D. Alternative sweeteners

E. Polysaccharides

III. Carbohydrate Metabolism
A. Monosaccharides

B. Gluconeogenesis

monosaccharide, disaccharide, oligosaccharide, polysaccharide
Figure 3-2 (Transparency) shows the Fischer projection and Haworth structural representations of glucose and fructose.
Table 3-1 lists the chemical forms of carbohydrate and carbohydrate derivatives along with food sources for each and end-products of digestion. The list extends beyond dietary carbohydrates and also includes indigestible forms.
Table 3-2 compares the degree of sweetness of sugars and artificial sweeteners.
glucose, dextrose, glycogen, fructose, galactose, mannose

sucrose, maltose, lactose, invert sugar, malt sugar, milk sugar

sorbitol, mannitol, xylitol

Key concept: Alternative sweeteners are also called artificial sweeteners. Their nutritive value is considered negligible.
Table 3-2 provides a list of artificial sweeteners and their current approval status in the U.S.

Figure 3-3 shows a simplified Haworth structural representation of glycogen, including both the linear α-1,4 bonds and the branching α-1,6 bonds.
starch, amylose, amylopectin, modified food starch, dextrins, glycogen, cellulose, hemicellulose, noncellulose polysaccharides, methyl cellulose, carboxymethylcellulose, pectin, gums, mucilages, algal polysaccharides

Figure 3-4 illustrates the interrelationship of the metabolism of glucose, fructose, and galactose in the liver. It shows how these three monosaccharides can be interchanged to meet metabolic demand.

Figure 3-5 (Transparency) illustrates glycolysis, glycogenolysis, and glycogenesis.
Key concept: In the absence of carbohydrate in the diet, the body's demand for glucose is met by taking the carbon skeletons of primarily lactic acid, amino acids, and glycerol to synthesize glucose, though this process is usually circuitous via glycogen.
gluconeogenesis

C. Regulation of blood sugar

Key concept: There are variations in the glucose levels of blood, but they remain relatively constant and predictable during the fed state, postabsorptive state, and starvation or fasting. The maintenance of normal blood sugar is a complex interaction of mechanisms that increase glucose in the blood and remove it from the blood.

Figure 3-6 (Transparency) shows two mechanisms by which glucose is recovered from muscle tissue. In the Cori cycle, glucose is metabolized in the muscle to lactate via pyruvate in glycolysis. The lactate is carried by the blood back to the liver where it is converted to pyruvate again. The pyruvate is then converted to glucose by gluconeogenesis. In the alanine cycle, the pyruvate resulting from glycolysis in the muscle is converted to the amino acid alanine and carried back to the liver. In the liver through gluconeogenesis, the alanine is converted back to pyruvate and then glucose.

Figure 3-7 illustrates maintenance of blood glucose. The left side shows how glucose is mobilized into the bloodstream, while the right side shows how glucose is removed from the bloodstream.

insulin, glucagon, epinephrine, glucocorticoids, thyroxine, growth hormone

IV. Functions of Carbohydrate in the Body

glucuronic acid

V. Dietary Fiber

A. Definition

Table 3-1 is referenced here for examples of fiber. **roughage, fiber**

B. Assay and food composition data

crude fiber, dietary fiber

C. Characteristics of fiber

1. Physical properties
   a. soluble fiber
   b. insoluble fiber

Table 3-3 summarizes soluble and insoluble fibers and their sources.

2. Physiological properties

Table 3-4 summarizes the various physiological effects of fiber, which can be individually related to the disease conditions presented (diseases of the colon, cardiovascular disease, diabetes, and obesity). **constipation**

D. Occurrence in food

Table 3-5 lists the fiber content of common portions of various foods. The food sources are all representative of plant sources. Degree of processing is also a factor.

E. Recommendations and intake

VI. Carbohydrate in the American Diet
   A. Recommended Dietary Allowance

ketosis

   B. Food sources of carbohydrate

Table 3-6 lists the carbohydrate content of specific foods (concentrated sweets, fruits, milk, grain products, and vegetables). Note that milk is the only animal source of carbohydrate on the list.

   C. Trends in consumption of carbohydrate

Table 3-7 shows the changes in carbohydrate consumption as a dietary component during the twentieth century.

Table 3-8 provides the changes in sources of carbohydrate consumed during the twentieth century.

Figure 3-8 shows a comparison of the amount of sugar consumed as sugar to the total amount of sugar available.

Key concept: A significant shift has occurred from the purchase and consumption of table sugar to the purchase and consumption of foods containing sugar added in processing.

CASE STUDY INSIGHTS

1. What changes would you suggest to Joe at this time?

While increased fermentation and gas production is expected with increased fiber intake, the increase for Joe K. may have occurred too rapidly for his intestinal tract to adjust to the increase. The amount of fiber Joe is now ingesting exceeds recommendations and may not be warranted.

Check Joe's diet for inclusion of foods known to be gas forming, particularly cruciferous vegetables and legumes. You could also suggest to Joe that he reduce his fiber intake to determine if his increased gas and flatulence decreases to a more acceptable level of comfort. Assure him that he will achieve the benefits of dietary fiber with intakes of 25–35 g daily. He should be encouraged to focus on five or more servings of fruits and vegetables and six or more servings of whole-grain breads, cereals, and legumes (if tolerated). Also emphasize the importance of adequate fluid intake.

2. Calculate the fiber content of your own diet for three days. How many grams of fiber did you eat? What guidelines would you follow to change your intake to the recommended intake of 25–35 g daily?

Responses will vary depending on individual diets.

SUGGESTED TEST QUESTIONS

1. The recommended minimum blood glucose
    level to ensure normal central nervous system
    function is
    * a.   70 mg/dL.
    b.   100 mg/dL.
    c.   180 mg/dL.
    d.   250 mg/dL.

2. Sorbitol, mannitol, and xylitol differ from arti-
    ficial sweeteners in that they
    a.   leave no aftertaste.
    b.   are absorbed rapidly.
    * c.   do have nutritive value.
    d.   cannot be used in cooking.

3. Mr. D. has been placed on a weight-reduction
    diet but is allowed to eat candies sweetened
    with sorbitol. Excessive consumption of the
    candy might be apparent by
    a.   the presence of constipation.
    * b.   the presence of diarrhea.
    c.   an increase in dental caries.
    d.   excessively high blood glucose levels.

4. Which of the following is appropriate to teach
    a patient who is using fructose as a sweetener?
    a.   Fructose is dependent on insulin for cellu-
    lar entry.
    b.   Fructose remains unchanged in the body
    and is excreted in the urine.
    * c.   Fructose can be converted to glucose and
    result in a rise in blood sugar if present in
    large amounts.
    d.   Fructose has no impact on serum glucose
    and can be ingested in unrestricted
    amounts.

5. Which of the following hormones results in a
    decrease in serum glucose levels?
    a.   epinephrine
    b.   glucagon
    c.   glucocorticoid
    * d.   insulin

6. Patients who are to increase the fiber in their
    diet should be taught that fiber from crucifer-
    ous vegetables also contributes indoles and
    phenols, which have been associated with
    a.   decreased blood pressure.
    b.   delay in skin aging.
    c.   increased serum glucose.
    * d.   a lower risk of colon cancer.

7. Research suggests that an increase in dietary
    fiber may be indicated for the treatment of dia-
    betics. Fiber delays gastric emptying and
    shortens intestinal transit time, both of which
    can lead to
    * a.   a hypoglycemic effect.
    b.   a hyperglycemic effect.
    c.   a decrease in ketone production.
    d.   an increase in glucose absorption.

8. The major end-product of digestion of dietary
    carbohydrate is
    a.   fructose.
    b.   sucrose.
    c.   mannose.
    * d.   glucose.

9. Under normal conditions, the central nervous
    system is dependent on which of these as an
    energy source?
    a.   ketone bodies
    * b.   glucose
    c.   fatty acids
    d.   amino acids

10. Individuals who lack sufficient levels of the
    enzyme lactase are unable to hydrolyze lactose
    adequately into
    a.   fructose and galactose.
    b.   sucrose.
    * c.   glucose and galactose.
    d.   mannose and glucose.

11. Glycogen can best be described as
    a. a carbohydrate that the body metabolizes the same as cellulose.
    b. a disaccharide derived from animal sources of carbohydrate.
    c. a monosaccharide obtained from the hydrolysis of starch in the diet.
*   d. the major storage form of glucose in animals.

12. When adequate glucose is not available, amino acids are converted to glucose through the process of
*   a. gluconeogenesis.
    b. glycolysis.
    c. glycogenesis.
    d. Cori cycle.

13. Insulin lowers blood sugar by stimulating
    a. gluconeogenesis and lipolysis.
*   b. cellular oxidation, lipogenesis, and glycogenesis.
    c. the secretion of glucagon.
    d. the release of glucose from glycogen.

14. The hormones that function to increase glucose in the blood are
*   a. epinephrine, glucagon, and growth hormone.
    b. glucagon and epinephrine.
    c. vasopressin and prostaglandin.
    d. insulin and GIP.

15. The disaccharide that remains in the intestine longer than the other disaccharides and thus encourages bacterial growth is
    a. sucrose.
    b. galactose.
    c. maltose.
*   d. lactose.

16. A diet that lacks at least 50–100 g of carbohydrate per day is likely to lead to
*   a. ketosis.
    b. glycogenesis.
    c. lipogenesis.
    d. unstable blood sugars.

17. The National Cancer Institute recommends a daily intake of how many grams of dietary fiber?
    a. 11–13 g
    b. 10–20 g
*   c. 25–35 g
    d. more than 40 g

CHAPTER

LIPIDS

OVERVIEW

The purpose of this chapter is to highlight the types, functions, and metabolism of dietary fat. Recent information on omega-3, omega-6 and trans-fatty acids is included, but digestion of dietary lipids is not. Lipid transport in the blood as lipoproteins is mentioned. Metabolism of fats, primarily β-oxidation and formation of ketone bodies, is presented. Comprehensive recommendations for intake of lipids are made.

LEARNING OBJECTIVES

This chapter will prepare the learner to be able to

1. Identify the major classification of lipids and the lipids in each class.
2. Compare the structures of saturated fatty acids, monounsaturated fatty acids, and polyunsaturated fatty acids.
3. State the importance of essential fatty acids, omega-3 fatty acids, and omega-6 fatty acids.
4. Define saponification, hydrogenation, and rancidity.
5. State the functions of lipids.
6. Define compound lipids, sterols, and synthetic lipids and give two examples of each.
7. State how dietary lipids are carried in the blood.
8. Explain β-oxidation, ketone body formation, and triglyceride synthesis.
9. Identify the hormones regulating lipid metabolism and state their action.
10. State the recommended daily intake of fat.
11. Identify sources of fat in the diet.
12. Describe changes in fat consumption in the United States.

CHAPTER OUTLINE ——————————— **NOTES, TERMS, & TRANSPARENCY MASTERS**

I. Classification, Composition, and Function

Table 4-1 lists significant lipids by classification (simple, compound, and miscellaneous).
Key concept: The most abundant lipids are triglycerides (triacylglycerols), accounting for about 95% of lipids in nature.
triglycerides, triacylglycerols

    A. Fatty acids

Table 4-2 lists common fatty acids, including the number of carbons, double bonds, and food sources.

18

Figure 4-1 (**Transparency**) illustrates the chemical formula, number, and position of double bonds of 18-carbon fatty acids.
phospholipid, omega-6 family, linoleic acid

1. Saturated fatty acids

saturated fatty acid (SFA)

2. Monounsaturated fatty acids

monounsaturated fatty acid (MUFA)

3. Polyunsaturated fatty acids

polyunsaturated fatty acid (PUFA), omega-3, omega-6

    a. essential fatty acids

Figure 4-2 illustrates the relationship of linoleic acid and α-linolenic acid to other biologically active fatty acids.
Figure 4-3 shows the effects of PUFAs on the immune, nervous, and vascular systems.
linoleic acid, α-linolenic acid, essential fatty acid (EFA), eicosanoids, prostaglandins, thromboxanes, leukotrienes

    b. omega-3 fatty acids
    c. trans-fatty acids

Figure 4-2 is also used here.

B. Triglycerides

Figure 4-4 (**Transparency**) shows a Fischer projection of the structures of the compounds involved in the synthesis of triglycerides.

1. Physical properties

2. Reactions
    a. saponification

saponification

    b. hydrogenation

Figure 4-5 simplistically illustrates how the addition of hydrogen to an unsaturated fat (with some double bonds) results in a saturated fat (with no double bonds)
hydrogenation

    c. rancidity

rancidity, butylated hydroxyanisole (BHA), butylated hydroxytoluene (BHT)

3. Functions
    a. energy
    b. Other functions

C. Compound lipids

1. Phospholipids

Figure 4-6 uses a Fischer projection to show the structure of the phospholipid lecithin.

Key concept: Compound lipids contain carbon, oxygen, hydrogen, and one or more other elements. Phospholipids contain phosphorus. Lecithin, a phospholipid, contains phosphorus and nitrogen.
phospholipid

    a. lecithin

Figure 4-6 is also referenced here.
lecithin, phosphatidycholine

    b. other phospholipids

cephalins, lipontols, sphingomyelins

  2. Glycolipids

cerebrosides, gangliosides

D. Sterols
  1. Classification and structure

Figure 4-7 is a Haworth structural representation of cholesterol, the most well known of the sterols. Emphasis is on the complexity of the compound.
cholesterol, ergosterol, β-sitosterol

  2. Cholesterol

Figure 4-7 shows cholesterol.
Key concept: Cholesterol is a sterol unique to animals and is not found in plants.

  3. Vitamin D activity

7-dehydrocholesterol, cholecalciferol

E. Synthetic lipids

Key concept: These lipids are made in the laboratory and are not naturally occurring.

  1. Medium-chained triglycerides

medium-chained triglyceride (MCT)

  2. Structured lipids

interesterification

  3. Fat substitutes

Table 4-3 lists the available fat substitutes and their chemical origins.
Key concept: Fat substitutes are not necessarily calorie free.

II. Lipid Transport and Storage

lymphatic system, chylomicron, apolipoprotein, lipoprotein lipase (LPL), lipoprotein

III. Lipid Metabolism
  A. Catabolism of fatty acids and triglycerides

Figure 4-8 shows the oxidation of a fatty acid. The breakdown of fatty acids results in acetyl CoA, which can enter a number of metabolic pathways, including the citric acid cycle.
glycerol, free fatty acid, hormone-sensitive lipase, β-oxidation, carnitine

B. Ketone bodies

**acetoacetic acid, β-hydroxybutyric acid, ace-
tone, ketone bodies, ketoacidosis, ketonuria**

C. Triglyceride synthesis
D. Hormonal regulation

lipogenesis, lipolysis

IV. Dietary Intakes
   A. Recommended intakes

Key concept: There is no RDA for fat. The recommendations for fat intake are based on a number of scientific studies that estimate the optimal fat intake to maintain health and prevent
disease. Of greatest concern for low fat intake
is adequate intake of essential fatty acids.

   B. Food sources of fat

Table 4-4 lists the fat content of common foods by
groups, ranging from a zero fat group to a
group with more than 25 g of fat.
Table 4-5 compares the fat content of beef, chick-
en, and milk, illustrating the variations for
each food.
Table 4-6 shows the variations in fatty acid groups
(SFA, MUFA, PUFA) in six food groups.

   C. Trends in fat and cholesterol consumption

Table 4-7 shows a decrease in fat intake in the
U.S. The table also shows that total fat intake
remains above the recommended intake.

CASE STUDY INSIGHTS

1. From what you have learned about lipids, what might his condition be?

A deficiency of essential fatty acids (EFAs), specifically linoleic acid, manifests with dermatitis and has
been reported with the use of parenteral nutrition support if lipid emulsions are not used with the parenteral
nutrition solutions.

2. What should you review about the tube feeding content?

The feeding is most likely deficient in fat. About 1–3% of total daily energy needs should be provided
by EFA to prevent deficiency. If the patient is receiving a parenteral feeding, assess the formulation to
determine if fat is given, how much, and the percentage of EFA in the lipid emulsion used. If the patient is
receiving a tube feeding, review the nutritional content of the feeding. Most likely another enteral formula
can be used the will provide sufficient EFA.

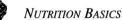

3. How will altering the lipid content of tube feeding impact the course of his recovery (e.g., weight, lipid levels)?

If lipid is added to his feedings without changing the carbohydrate or protein content, the result will be an increase in total caloric intake. If weight gain is a goal, this is appropriate. If not, the total caloric value of his intake should be adjusted to meet his needs for weight maintenance. Blood lipid levels will increase, and the EFA content of both blood cholesterol and phospholipid will increase with the addition of EFA to the diet.

4. What lab values should be reviewed to determine if lipid levels are changing?

Increased intakes of EFA would be reflected in an increase in the EFA content of blood cholesterol esters and phospholipids. Therefore, these two compounds can be used as indices of increased EFA.

SUGGESTED TEST QUESTIONS

1. Most natural fats contain
    a. short chain fatty acids.
    b. medium chain fatty acids.
    *   c. long chain fatty acids.
    d. essential fatty acids.

2. One of your patients asks you to explain the difference between saturated and unsaturated fats. You would say that saturated fatty acids
    a. contain no hydrogen.
    *   b. contain all the hydrogen they can hold, thus they are saturated with hydrogen.
    c. contain only double bonds and fewer carbon atoms.
    d. are usually those fats that are in liquid form.

3. The effect of insulin on fat metabolism is that it
    a. promotes breakdown of triglycerides from adipose tissue.
    b. promotes β-oxidation of fatty acids to acetyl CoA.
    *   c. promotes synthesis of triglycerides for storage in adipose tissue.
    d. increases production of ketone bodies from β-oxidation.

4. A patient receiving enteral feedings has an increase in fatty stools, and the physician suspects fat malabsorption. She orders medium chain triglycerides (MCTs) to be added to the feedings. The MCTs should improve the patient's condition because they are
    *   a. absorbed directly into the portal vein system.
    b. not absorbed and also reduce glucose absorption.
    c. absorbed very slowly and do not enter the lymphatics.
    d. a good source of fat-soluble vitamins.

5. The organ primarily responsible for the regulation of lipid levels in the body is the
    a. small intestine
    b. pancreas
    c. gallbladder
    *   d. liver

6. In teaching a patient to reduce the saturated fat in his diet, you would instruct him to avoid prepared foods containing
    a. olive and peanut oil.
    *   b. coconut and palm oil.
    c. safflower and corn oil.
    d. canola and cottonseed oil.

7. The teaching plan for a patient who is to reduce her total fat intake would usually include a recommendation to decrease her intake of food containing more SFA, such as
  * a. beef.
  b. pork.
  c. poultry.
  d. corn.

8. The best source of omega-3 fatty acids is
  a. corn and safflower oil
  b. coconut and palm oil
  c. soybean oil
  * d. fish oil

9. One of the major functions of omega-3 fatty acids is
  a. to decrease the clearance of chylomicrons from the plasma.
  * b. to increase the clearance of chylomicrons from the plasma.
  c. to decrease the synthesis of adipose tissue.
  d. to increase the synthesis of adipose tissue.

10. Essential fatty acids include
  a. linolenic acid and arachidonic acid.
  b. linoleic acid and arachidonic acid.
  * c. linoleic acid and linolenic acid.
  d. eicosapentaenoic acid and phosphatidyl-choline.

11. An adult on long-term fat-free intravenous feedings or parenteral feedings may develop
  a. ketosis.
  b. hypertriglyeridemia.
  c. hyponatremia.
  * d. eczema.

12. The storage life and stability of essential nutrients in fats and fat-containing foods are increased by the addition of
  * a. BHA and BHT.
  b. monoglycerides.
  c. disodium sulfate.
  d. emulsifiers.

13. Exposure of skin to ultraviolet light from the sun converts cholesterol to
  a. ergosterol.
  b. cholesterol esterase.
  * c. 7-dehydrocholesterol.
  d. prostaglandins.

14. Chylomicrons are removed from the blood a few hours after eating by the action of
  * a. lipoprotein lipase
  b. low-density lipoproteins
  c. carnitine
  d. adrenalcorticotropic hormone

15. The oxidation of long chain fatty acids requires the presence of
  a. only carnitine
  * b. carnitine and oxygen
  c. only magnesium
  d. magnesium and oxygen

16. When the body relies on stored fat for energy, the production of acetoacetic acid surpasses the oxidizing ability of the tissues. The end result is production and accumulation in the blood of
  a. glucose
  b. acetyl CoA
  c. lactic acid
  * d. ketone bodies

17. The recommended daily intake of fat in the diet is
  a. less than 50 g.
  b. 10% of total calories from MUFA and 15% from PUFA.
  * c. less than 30% of total calories.
  d. 75–100 g of fat.

18. The recommend daily intake of EFA to prevent EFA deficiency is
  a. 1–3 g.
  b. 1–3% of total caloric intake.
  c. 10 g.
  d. 10% of total caloric intake.

CHAPTER 5

PROTEINS

OVERVIEW

The purpose of this chapter is to highlight the importance of protein in the diet. A brief review of the structure and composition of protein is presented. The concept of amino acids as the essential elements in protein is emphasized. The metabolic fates of dietary protein in the body are reviewed. Methods for evaluation of the quality of protein are presented along with the concept of complementary proteins. The RDA for protein at various ages is included. Sources of protein and specific amino acids in foods are listed.

LEARNING OBJECTIVES

This chapter will prepare the learner to be able to

1. Identify the composition of proteins.
2. List the common chemical components of amino acids.
3. Identify the essential amino acids, conditionally essential amino acids, and nonessential amino acids.
4. State the metabolic fates of amino acids.
5. Describe how protein status is assessed.
6. List the hormones that regulate protein metabolism.
7. Describe the technique for evaluating the quality of dietary protein.
8. Define complementary protein and give an example of how it is used.
9. State the RDA for protein for adults.
10. Identify food sources of protein.
11. Define marasmus, kwashiorkor, and marasmic kwashiorkor and explain how they occur.

CHAPTER OUTLINE ———————————— **NOTES, TERMS, & TRANSPARENCY MASTERS**

I. Composition

Key concept: Protein is essential to human health in a different way than carbohydrate or fat. Note that its meaning is "of first importance."
nitrogen, nitrogen cycle

II. Structure and Composition

Figure 5-1 shows the basic structure of an amino acid and the common components, an amine group and a carboxy group.

24

Figure 5-2 (Transparency) shows the joining of two amino acids by a peptide bond to form a dipeptide. The carboxy carbon of one amino acid is joined to the nitrogen of a second amino acid to form the peptide bond.
amino acids, peptide bonds, polypeptides, primary structure, secondary structure, tertiary structure, globular proteins, simple proteins, conjugated proteins, nucleoproteins, mucoproteins, glycoproteins, lipoproteins, phosphoproteins, metalloproteins, derived proteins

III. Functions of Protein

anabolic process, energy source, structural role, antibodies, transportation, maintenance of homeostasis

IV. Amino Acids
   A. Essential and nonessential amino acids

Table 5-1 lists the 20 amino acids found in most proteins and classifies them as essential, conditionally essential, or nonessential.
Table 5-2 presents the estimated requirements for the essential amino acids for various age groups.
essential amino acids, nonessential amino acids, conditionally essential amino acids

   B. Metabolic pool of amino acids

Figure 5-3 illustrates the sources of amino acids coming into the amino acid pool and the destination of amino acids leaving the pool.

   C. Special functions of amino acids

Note that citrulline is related to the synthesis of urea. Citrulline is found in the body but is not commonly found in structural proteins such as those in the diet.

V. Protein Metabolism
   A. Amino acid catabolism

Figure 5-4 (Transparency) illustrates two mechanisms by which amino acids are catabolized or broken down: transamination and deamination. Both processes involve formation of α-keto acids, similar to amino acids without the nitrogen.
Figure 5-5 shows the role of ornithine in the urea cycle. Ornithine is found in the body but is not commonly found in structural proteins such as those in the diet.
oxidative deamination, alanine cycle, urea, ornithine cycle

   B. Protein synthesis

Figure 5-4 is referenced here for transamination.
transamination

C. Assessment of protein status

Key concept: Protein is about 16% nitrogen; thus, losses of nitrogen from the body can be equated with losses of protein, after accounting for dietary intake.

D. Hormonal regulation

growth hormone, insulin, testosterone, glucocorticoids, thyroxine

VI. Evaluation of Dietary Protein Quality
   A. Measurement techniques

Table 5-3 lists the digestibility of proteins in various foods for humans.

Table 5-4 compares the essential amino acid requirements at various ages with the essential amino acid content of various foods. Note that proteins from animal sources correlate closely with human requirements.

protein efficiency ratio (PER), biologic value (BV), net protein utilization (NPU), amino acid requirement pattern, amino acid score, limiting amino acid

   B. Complimentary proteins

Table 5-5 indicates which food groups in the diet provide adequate amounts of each essential amino acid.

complementary proteins

VII. Dietary Intakes
   A. Recommended Dietary Allowances

Table 5-6 shows the RDA for protein for various age groups by gender.

reference proteins

   B. Food sources of protein

Figure 5-6 illustrates the wide distribution of protein in foods and categorizes food by quantity of protein in common sized servings.

   C. Trends in consumption of protein

VIII. Protein Deficiency
   A. Protein-energy malnutrition

Figure 5-7 is a photograph of two boys of the same age, one with a protein-deficient diet and the other with a protein-sufficient diet. The difference in growth is significant.

Figure 5-8 shows two photographs of a child before and after treatment for kwashiorkor. On the left, the child is shown with severe edema associated with the deficiency. On the right, the child is shown after refeeding.

protein-energy malnutrition (PEM), marasmus, kwashiorkor, marasmic kwashiorkor

CASE STUDY INSIGHTS

1. What would you suggest for a breakfast or midmorning snack?

Determine the reason that Suzanne skips breakfast (e.g., no time, not hungry, nothing to eat). Suggestions should be based on this information. Hard-cooked eggs and string cheese are easy to transport (maintain safe temperatures). Peanut butter on toast or in a sandwich could also be a choice. Including a glass of milk in the morning is helpful to ensure that all amino acids are provided.

2. What suggestions would you make for weight gain?

Determine if foods consumed are of sufficient caloric density. High intake of fruits and vegetables can reduce appetite and lower total caloric intake. Second, determine if the quantity of food consumed is sufficient to meet needs. Depending on these factors, you can suggest an increase in quantity, such as eating more frequently or increasing portion sizes, or an increase in caloric density, such as eating more peanut butter, whole milk, and cheese.

3. Discuss the pros and cons of adding a multiple vitamin and mineral supplement to her diet.

Suzanne should be encouraged to meet her nutrient needs from her diet, not from supplementation. If her diet is balanced and contains a variety of foods, vitamin and mineral needs will be met.

4. Provide two vegetarian main dish recipes that would be acceptable for her diet plan.

A variety of recipes are available. Direct students to resources for vegetarian recipes, such as *Recipes for a Small Planet* by Frances Moore Lapie, *Laurel's Kitchen* (Nilgiri Press), and *The New American Diet* by Sonja Connor.

SUGGESTED TEST QUESTIONS

1. In the early stages of marasmus in a child, the most notable manifestation the caregiver would see is
*   a. reduced growth.
    b. muscle wasting.
    c. absence of subcutaneous fat.
    d. all of these.

2. Kwashiorkor is most likely to be seen in children at age
    a. newborn to 6 months.
    b. 6 months to 1 year.
*   c. 1–4 years.
    d. 5–8 years.

3. The recommended dietary allowance (RDA) for dietary protein for adults in the United States is

    a. 2.2 g/kg
    b. 1.5 g/kg
*   c. 0.8 g/kg
    d. 0.61 g/kg

4. High intakes of protein in the diet ($\geq$ 2 times the RDA) over a lifetime should be avoided because
    a. protein foods tend to be the most expensive in the diet.
*   b. renal damage and osteoporosis may result.
    c. nitrogen toxicity may result.
    d. people experience a bitter taste in their mouths.

5. For most people in the United States, the most common source of protein in the diet is
*   a. animal protein.
    b. legumes.
    c. cereals.
    d. fruits and vegetables.

6. The body's synthesis of niacin, a vitamin, and serotonin, a neurotransmitter, depends on the diet providing the amino acid
   a. lysine.
   * b. tryptophan.
   c. tyrosine.
   d. leucine.

7. Which of these groups are all essential amino acids?
   a. arginine, tryptophan, threonine, serine
   b. glycine, histidine, isoleucine, leucine
   c. valine, glutamine, asparagine, alanine
   * d. phenylalanine, threonine, histidine, leucine

8. The removal of the amine group from an amino acid prior to oxidation for energy is called
   a. preamination.
   b. β-oxidation.
   * c. deamination.
   d. reverse amination.

9. In the ornithine cycle, arginine is utilized for the synthesis of
   * a. urea.
   b. amino acids.
   c. protein.
   d. nonessential amino acids.

10. Marasmus in an adult caused by chronic semi-starvation is characterized by
    a. pitting edema.
    b. hypoalbuminemia and edema.
    c. enlarged fatty liver and hyperalbuminemia.
    * d. muscular wasting and absence of subcutaneous fat.

11. Marasmic kwashiorkor, a major nutritional problem in developing countries, is
    a. extreme calorie deprivation.
    b. loss of subcutaneous fat.
    c. extreme protein deprivation.
    * d. extreme protein deprivation in the presence of energy deficiency.

12. The percentage of absorbed nitrogen retained in the body for growth or maintenance is indicated by
    * a. the biological value (BV).
    b. the net protein utilization (NPU).
    c. the protein efficiency ratio (PER).
    d. the recommended dietary allowance (RDA).

13. During the life cycle, the grams per kilogram requirement for protein
    a. remains unchanged.
    b. continually increases.
    c. continually decreases.
    * d. continually decreases accept during pregnancy and lactation.

14. The limiting amino acid in legumes is
    * a. methionine.
    b. lysine.
    c. cysteine.
    d. histidine.

15. The hormones that stimulate protein synthesis include
    a. glucocorticoids, insulin, growth hormone.
    * b. growth hormone, insulin, testosterone.
    c. corticosteroids, insulin, thyroxine.
    d. glucagon, insulin, testosterone.

16. After 4–5 days of negative nitrogen balance, the body will
    a. increase urinary nitrogen output.
    b. develop a greater need for protein than before.
    * c. reestablish equilibrium at the lower level of protein intake.
    d. stop production of urea to conserve protein.

17. Vegetarian diets use the concept of complementary proteins to
    * a. combine plant foods so that all essential amino acids are present.
    b. increase the palatability of the diet.
    c. supplement the intake of dietary proteins.
    d. ensure variety in the diet.

18. Protein intake in the United States is most likely to be
    a. insufficient to meet needs.
    b. exactly what the RDA for protein is.
    * c. in excess of needs.
    d. of poor quality.

CHAPTER 6

VITAMINS

OVERVIEW

The purpose of this chapter is to examine the vitamins essential to human nutrition. Information presented for vitamins includes absorption, transport, storage, excretion, metabolism, functions, requirements, food sources, deficiencies, and toxicities. For vitamins having varied or complex methods of measurement, explanations and equivalents are given. The chapter concludes with a brief presentation of vitamin-like substances (choline and myo-inositol), antivitamins, vitamin antagonists, and antimetabolites.

LEARNING OBJECTIVES

This chapter will prepare the learner to be able to

1. Summarize the absorption, transport, storage, excretion, and metabolism of each vitamin.
2. Identify the major functions of each vitamin.
3. Identify the appropriate unit of measurement for assessing the requirement and food content for each vitamin.
4. State the Recommended Dietary Allowance (RDA) for each vitamin.
5. Identify a minimum of five food sources for each vitamin.
6. Identify the deficiency signs or conditions associated with each vitamin.
7. List potential causes of deficiencies other than a poor diet.
8. Identify the potential for toxicity of each vitamin.
9. Name two vitamin-like compounds.
10. Define antivitamin and give two examples.

CHAPTER OUTLINE ———————————— **NOTES, TERMS, & TRANSPARENCY MASTERS**

I. Fat-Soluble Vitamins
   A. Vitamin A (retinol)   **retinal, retinoic acid, carotenoids**

       1. Absorption, transport, and storage   **Figure 6-1 (Transparency)** is a flow chart illustrating how vitamin A enters the body with the diet and is subsequently delivered to target cells for metabolism.
                                            Note: Appendix 30 provides additional information on the retinol binding protein.
                                          retinyl esters, retinaldehyde, beta-carotene, retinol-binding protein (RBP)

29

2. Functions

3. Nutrient interactions

4. Measurement

opsin, rhodopsin, iodopsin

Table 6-1 (Transparency) provides the conversions needed for vitamin A measurement: RE, IU, retinol, beta-carotene, and pro-vitamin A
International Units (IU), retinol equivalents (RE)

5. Recommended Dietary Allowance

Table 6-2 provides the current RDA for vitamin A using RE.
Note: **Appendix 30** provides more information on the serum values of vitamin A and interpretation of results of laboratory measurement.

6. Sources

Table 6-3 lists food sources of both preformed vitamin A and beta-carotene.
Key concept: Preformed vitamin A occurs only in foods of animal origin.

7. Deficiency

keratinization, night blindness, corneal ulceration

   a. Night blindness

   nyctalopia

   b. Xerophthalmia

   xerosis conjunctivae

   c. Infection

   d. Cutaneous changes

   Figure 6-2 is a photograph of early follicular hyperkeratosis on the buttocks.
   follicular hyperkeratosis (phrynoderma)

   e. Prevention and treatment of avitaminosis A

8. Toxicity

Table 6-4 lists the signs of vitamin A toxicity.
Key concept: There is a difference between hypervitaminosis A and hypercarotenosis.
hypervitaminosis A, Accutane, teratogen, hypercarotenodermia

B. Vitamin D (calciferol)

Figure 6-3 (Transparency) is an integrated illustration of the metabolism of vitamin D with the associated functions.
Table 6-5 (Transparency) provides the terminology and equivalents associated with vitamin D.
7-dehydrocholesterol, ergosterol, cholecalciferol, prohormone, calcitriol, ercalcitriol

1. Absorption, transport, and storage

vitamin D plasma-binding protein (DBP)

2. Metabolism

cholecalciferol, 25-hydroxycholecalciferol (25-OH D$_3$), 1,25-dihydroxycholecalciferol (1,25-(OH)$_2$ D$_3$), parathyroid hormone (PTH)

3. Functions

keratocytes, alkaline phosphatase

4. Measurement

Note: Although vitamin D measurements continue to use IU, the preferred measure is micrograms (μg) of vitamin D$_3$. See Table 6-3.

5. Recommended Dietary Allowance

Table 6-6 provides the current RDA for vitamin D using μg.

6. Sources

Table 6-7 lists food sources of vitamin D. Note the role of fortification of milk.

7. Deficiency
    a. Rickets

Figure 6-4 is a photograph of two children with rickets-induced deformities.
Figure 6-5 is a photograph of a child with rachitic rosary and a pot belly, both associated with rickets.
hyperphosphatemic vitamin D refractory rickets, rachitic rosary, pigeon chest

    b. Osteomalacia

Key concept: Osteomalacia should not be confused with the more commonly discussed condition, osteoporosis.
osteitis fibrosa cystica of the bones

8. Toxicity

Table 6-8 lists the signs of vitamin D toxicity.
hypervitaminosis D

C. Vitamin E (tocopherol)
    1. Metabolism

tocopherols (alpha, beta, gamma, delta), tocotrienols

    2. Functions

glutathione peroxidase

    3. Measurement

Note: Although vitamin E measurements continue to use IU, by international agreement, the RDA is listed in milligrams (mg) of RRR-alpha- tocopherol or mg of alpha-tocopherol equivalents.
milligrams of RRR-alpha-tocopherol

    4. Recommended Dietary Allowance

Table 6-9 provides the current RDA for vitamin E using alpha-tocopherol equivalents.

    5. Sources

Table 6-10 lists food sources of vitamin E.

    6. Deficiency
    7. Toxicity

D. Vitamin K
  1. Chemical and physical properties   **phylloquinone, menaquinone, menadione**
  2. Absorption and transport
  3. Functions   **Figure 6-6** provides a schematic of the cascade theory of blood coagulation.
       gamma-carboxyglutamic acid (Gla), prothrombin, warfarin, dicumarol

  4. Measurement   **Note:** There is no standard unit for measurement of vitamin K.

  5. Recommended Dietary Allowance   **Table 6-11** provides the current RDA for vitamin K using micrograms (μg).

  6. Sources   **Table 6-12** lists food sources of vitamin K.

  7. Deficiency   **hemorrhagic disease of the newborn**
  8. Toxicity

II. Water-Soluble Vitamins   **B complex**

  A. Thiamin (vitamin B$_1$)   **pyrophospate (TPP), triphosphate (TTP)**

    1. History   **antineuritic vitamin**

    2. Chemical characteristics and stability   **thiaminase**
    3. Absorption, synthesis, and storage
    4. Functions
    5. Recommended Dietary Allowance   **Table 6-13** provides the current RDA for thiamin.

    6. Sources   **Table 6-14** lists food sources of thiamin.

    7. Deficiency   **Table 6-15** is a list of the clinical features of thiamin deficiency.
       Figure 6-7 is a photograph of the swelling of the legs and pitting edema associated with wet beriberi.
       beriberi, dry beriberi, wet beriberi, infantile beriberi

    8. Toxicity

  B. Riboflavin (vitamin B$_2$)   **flavin adenine dinucleotide (FAD), flavin adenine mononucleotide (FAM)**

    1. History
    2. Chemical characteristics and stability
    3. Absorption, transport, and excretion
    4. Functions   **flavokinase**

    5. Recommended Dietary Allowance   **Table 6-16** provides the current RDA for riboflavin.

6. Sources	**Table 6-17** lists food sources of riboflavin.
7. Deficiency	**Table 6-18** lists signs that may indicate a possible riboflavin deficiency. The signs are nonspecific for many conditions. **ariboflavinosis, cheilosis, angular stomatitis**
8. Toxicity	
C. Niacin	**nicotinamide, nicotinic acid, nicotinamide adenine dinucleotide (NAD), nicotinamide adenine dinucleotide phosphate (NADP)**
1. History	**pellagra**
2. Chemical characteristics and stability	
3. Absorption and storage	
4. Functions	
5. Clinical uses	
6. Recommended Dietary Allowance	**Table 6-19** provides the current RDA for niacin in niacin equivalents (NE). **Key concept:** Niacin can be synthesized from the amino acid tryptophan. The NE includes that potential source as well as preformed niacin. **niacin equivalents (NE)**
7. Sources	**Table 6-20** lists food sources of niacin in NE. Foods may be rich in niacin, tryptophan, or both.
8. Deficiency	**Figure 6-8** is a photograph of the pellagrous dermatitis associated with niacin deficiency. **pellagra**
9. Toxicity	
D. Vitamin B_6 (pyridoxine, pyridoxal, pyridoxamine)	**pyridoxal phosphate (PLP), pyridoxamine phosphate (PMP)** **Note:** The term *pyridoxine* or *vitamin B_6* is used to designate all of the complex of closely related chemical compounds.
1. History	
2. Chemical properties	
3. Absorption, transport, and excretion	
4. Functions	**phosphorylase, gamma-aminobutyric acid (GABA)**
5. Recommended Dietary Allowance	**Table 6-21** provides the current RDA for vitamin B_6.
6. Sources	**Table 6-22** lists food sources of pyridoxine.

7. Deficiency

8. Toxicity

E. Folate (folic acid, folacin, pteroylmono-
    glutamate)
    1. History
    2. Chemical and physical properties
    3. Absorption, metabolism, and storage

    4. Functions

    5. Recommended Dietary Allowance

    6. Sources

    7. Deficiency

    8. Toxicity

F. Vitamin B$_{12}$ (cobalamine)
    1. Chemical characteristics and stability

    2. Absorption, transport, and storage
    4. Functions
    5. Recommended Dietary Allowance

    6. Sources

    7. Deficiency
    8. Toxicity

G. Pantothenic acid
    1. Functions

    2. Estimated Safe and Adequate Daily
        Dietary Intake

Key concept: Deficiencies of pyridoxine are often associated with drug–nutrient interactions.

methyltetrahydrofolic acid, tetrahydrofolic acid (THFA), formyltetrahydrofolic acid, citrovorum factor

formiminoglutamic acid (FIGLU)

Table 6-23 provides the current RDA for folate.

Table 6-24 lists food sources of folic acid.

Figure 6-9 is a photograph of a tongue characterized by glossitis as a result of folic acid deficiency.
Key concept: Folate is particularly susceptible to drug–nutrient interactions. See Chapter 18.
megaloblastic anemia

cyanocobalamine

intrinsic factor, transcobalamin I and II

Table 6-25 provides the current RDA for vitamin B$_{12}$.

Table 6-26 lists food sources of vitamin B$_{12}$.
Key concept: Vitamin B$_{12}$ occurs only in foods of animal origin.

megaloblastic anemia

coenzyme A

Table 6-27 provides the current recommendations for pantothenic acid in terms of the Estimated Safe and Adequate Daily Intake.

3. Sources

    Table 6-28 lists the pantothenic acid content of various foods.
    Note: This nutrient is widespread in foods.

4. Deficiency and toxicity

H. Biotin
  1. History
  2. Chemical characteristics and stability
  3. Functions
  4. Absorption, transport, and excretion

biocytin

  5. Estimated Safe and Adequate Daily Dietary Intake

    Table 6-29 provides the current recommendations for biotin in terms of the Estimated Safe and Adequate Daily Intake.

  6. Sources

    Table 6-30 lists the biotin content of some foods.

  7. Deficiency
  8. Toxicity

avidin, carbamazepine, primidone

I. Ascorbic acid
  1. History
  2. Chemical characteristics
  3. Absorption and storage
  4. Functions

antiscorbutic factor, hexuronic acid

collagen

  5. Recommended Dietary Allowances

    Table 6-31 gives the RDA for vitamin C.

  6. Sources

    Key concept: The vitamin C content of food depends on several factors. Because the vitamin is easily oxidized, unstable in heat and alkaline conditions, and highly soluble in water, losses can occur through handling and preparation techniques.
    Table 6-32 lists the vitamin C content of selected foods.

    Table 6-33 is a summary of all of the vitamins presented in this chapter.

  7. Deficiency

    Figure 6-10 is a photograph of scorbutic gums associated with vitamin C deficiency.
    Clinical Insight: "Vitamin C and the Common Cold"
    scurvy

  8. Toxicity

hemolytic anemia

III. Factors Not Proven to be Vitamins
    A. Choline
        1. Functions   **lecithin (phosphatidyl choline)**
        2. Dietary intake
        3. Sources
        4. Deficiency

    B. Myo-inositol   **phytic acid**
        1. Functions
        2. Deficiency
        3. Toxicity

    C. Antivitamins (vitamin antagonists or antimetabolites)

CASE STUDY INSIGHTS

What recommendations do you have for her as her nutrition counselor?

1. About folacin?. What impact do oral contraceptives have on folacin levels?

Oral contraceptives have been shown to reduce absorption of folate. A folate deficiency during pregnancy has been shown to result in neural tube defect in the fetus. It is important that JoAnne improve her folate status before becoming pregnant and that she maintain the RDA for folate in pregnant women after conception. The combination of a folate and vitamin B_{12} deficiency has been associated with increased risk for cardiovascular disease.

2. About iron and vitamin C intakes?

JoAnne's low hemoglobin and hematocrit values may be an indicator of iron deficiency. This could result from poor dietary intake or blood loss related to her recent surgery. A diet history would help to determine the cause. Vitamin C enhances the absorption of iron and also blocks degradation of ferritin. Her vitamin C status and her intake of vitamin C should also be investigated.

3. About good sources of vitamin B_{12}?

Vitamin B_{12} is found only in animal foods. Beef liver, clams, oysters, and crab are particularly high in this vitamin, but other animal foods contain amounts sufficient to meet the RDA when included in the diet. At greatest risk for deficiency of vitamin B_{12} is the strict vegan who consumes no animal foods at all.

4. About the use of over-the-counter vitamin supplements after surgery?

If JoAnne's diet is well-balanced, it should provide adequate nutrients for her postoperative recovery. If she does take an over-the-counter vitamin supplement, it should not exceed the RDA for any of the vitamins.

SUGGESTED TEST QUESTIONS

1. Although costly, mortality from vitamin A deficiency in developing countries can be reduced by 30–70% through
   * a. massive intermittent dosing with 200,000 IU of vitamin A.
   b. increased availability of foods high in vitamin A.
   c. fortification of MSG with vitamin A.
   d. fortification of milk products with vitamin A.

2. A single dose of vitamin A greater than 660,000 IU can result in hypervitaminosis A, which includes symptoms of
   a. night blindness and increased susceptibility to infections.
   * b. nausea, vomiting, fatigue, and weakness.
   c. xerophthalmia, keratomalacia, and hyperkeratosis of conjunctiva.
   d. decreased numbers of T-lymphocytes, follicular hyperkeratosis, and phrynoderma.

3. When assessing a female patient with severe cystic acne, the use of Accutane would be contraindicated if
   * a. she is pregnant.
   b. she is hypercholesterolemia.
   c. she has gastroenteritis.
   d. she is hypertensive.

4. Which of the following individuals are at risk for a deficiency of vitamin D?
   a. dark-skinned individuals who work outside
   b. fair-skinned individuals who are exposed to the sun for only brief periods each day
   * c. individuals who are homebound and bedfast
   d. individuals who do not drink vitamin D fortified milk

5. While instructing a patient on dietary intake of vitamin D, he asks you if it matters if he uses butter or margarine. Which response would you give?

   a. Margarine is less likely to increase the risk of heart disease and is thus a better choice.
   b. Butter is more expensive than margarine, so margarine is the better choice.
   * c. Butter is a food of animal origin and margarine is of plant origin, making butter the better choice.
   d. Butter is a food of animal origin and margarine is of plant origin, making margarine the better choice.

6. Children most likely to be at risk for vitamin D deficiency include
   a. those who have had prolonged breast-feeding.
   b. those with malabsorption syndrome.
   c. those requiring long-term anticonvulsant therapy.
   * d. all of the above.

7. Visible symptoms of rickets, which results from a vitamin D deficiency, include
   a. emaciation.
   b. pot belly and beading of ribs.
   c. decreased size of wrists and ankles.
   * d. profuse sweating and restlessness.

8. Vitamin D deficiency in children manifests as rickets, while it manifests in adults as
   a. hypocalcemia.
   b. osteoporosis.
   * c. osteomalacia.
   d. hypophosphatemia.

9. The development of vitamin D toxicity is most often seen in
   * a. infants and small children given supplemental vitamin D.
   b. adolescents drinking large amounts of fortified milk.
   c. pregnant women taking prenatal vitamins.
   d. homebound elderly adults.

10. The continued use of antibiotic therapy can reduce bacterial flora in the gut and result in
   * a. a deficiency of vitamin K.
   b. a deficiency of vitamin C.
   c. toxicity of vitamin A.
   d. toxicity of vitamin B.

11. Hemorrhagic disease of the newborn can be easily prevented through administration of what vitamin shortly after birth?
    a. vitamin C
    b. vitamin B
    c. vitamin D
  * d. vitamin K

12. Normal bone development, epithelial cell formation, and visual pigment formation all depend on
    a. pyridoxine.
    b. vitamin D.
  * c. vitamin A.
    d. ascorbic acid.

13. A retinol equivalent (RE) represents the sum of
  * a. preformed vitamin A and carotenoids.
    b. niacin, thiamin, and riboflavin.
    c. vitamin D, calcium, and phosphorus.
    d. all the B vitamins.

14. Vitamins with increased susceptibility to oxidation are
    a. vitamin C and niacin.
    b. riboflavin and vitamin D.
  * c. vitamins A and C.
    d. thiamin and vitamin E.

15. The symptoms associated with vitamin A deficiency are
    a. abnormal blood clotting, peripheral neuropathy, and fever.
    b. muscular cramps, bone deformities, nerve damage.
    c. cheilosis, stomatitis, dermatitis.
  * d. keratinization, corneal ulcerations, loss of appetite.

16. The most common toxicities of fat-soluble vitamins appear to be for
  * a. vitamins A and D.
    b. vitamins D and E.
    c. vitamins E and K.
    d. vitamins A, D, and K.

17. The absorption of ingested vitamin D occurs along with the absorption of
    a. protein and lactose.
  * b. lipids.
    c. carbohydrate and niacin.
    d. thiamin and glucose.

18. Which form of vitamin D increases the uptake of calcium and phosphate and is produced by the kidneys?
    a. 7-dehydrocholesterol
    b. 25-hydroxycholecalciferol
    c. vitamin D_3
  * d. calcitriol

19. The permanent effect of rickets occurring in childhood is
  * a. malformation of bones due to deficient mineralization of the organic matrix.
    b. reddening and exfoliation of the skin.
    c. keratinization of the mucous membranes lining the respiratory tract.
    d. central nervous system abnormalities.

20. The functions of vitamin E are primarily a result of its
  * a. ability to act as an antioxidant.
    b. involvement in energy metabolism.
    c. involvement in blood clotting.
    d. ability to aid in the synthesis of protein.

21. Patients using anticoagulant drugs such as dicumarol are at risk for decreasing
    a. the peroxidation of polyunsaturated fatty acids.
  * b. vitamin K-dependent clotting factors.
    c. coenzymes vital to tissue respiration.
    d. the oxidation of glucose and fatty acids.

22. The role of water-soluble vitamins in energy production is shown by the tricarboxylic acid cycle's dependence on
    a. ascorbic acid, thiamin, riboflavin, and niacin.
    b. niacin, ascorbic acid, pantothenic acid, and thiamin.
    c. pyridoxine, niacin, thiamin, and riboflavin.
  * d. thiamin, niacin, riboflavin, and pantothenic acid.

23. A thiamin deficiency is most likely to manifest with which of these clinical signs?
*   a. mental confusion, muscular wasting, and peripheral neuropathy
    b. bone deformities, muscular cramping, and edema
    c. night blindness, loss of appetite, and dermatitis
    d. edema, dermatitis, and keratinization

24. Protein metabolism requiring transamination reactions is dependent on
    a. thiamin.
*   b. pyridoxine.
    c. riboflavin.
    d. niacin.

25. A folic acid deficiency will have widespread manifestations due to
    a. keratinization.
    b. skeletal deformities.
*   c. alteration of DNA metabolism.
    d. night blindness.

26. The role of vitamin C can best be described as
*   a. enhancing iron absorption and collagen formation.
    b. essential for calcium and phosphate absorption.
    c. serving as a structural component of cell membranes and necessary for hemoglobin formation.
    d. essential in bone development and calcium deposition.

27. A thiamin deficiency occurs most often in
    a. individuals who eat unenriched grains.
    b. infants.
    c. those who consume large amounts of freshwater fish.
*   d. alcoholics.

28. A diet that is poor in animal protein and includes a high intake of corn products may indicate that the patient is at risk for
*   a. niacin deficiency.
    b. vitamin C deficiency.
    c. hypervitaminosis A.
    d. vitamin E toxicity.

30. Vegetarians who avoid all animal products, including milk and eggs, may become deficient in
    a. vitamin C.
*   b. vitamin B_{12}.
    c. vitamin D.
    d. riboflavin.

CHAPTER 7

MINERALS

OVERVIEW

The purpose of this chapter is to examine the minerals essential to human nutrition. Information presented for macrominerals and trace elements includes absorption, excretion, metabolism, functions, requirements, food sources, deficiencies, and toxicities. Additional trace elements with undefined requirements, including silicon, vanadium, boron, tin, nickel, arsenic, bromine, and lead, are also presented.

LEARNING OBJECTIVES

This chapter will prepare the learner to be able to

1. State the functions of each of the macrominerals and trace elements.
2. State the Recommended Dietary Allowance (RDA) or the Estimated Safe and Adequate Daily Dietary Intake (ESADDI) for each of the macrominerals and trace elements.
3. Identify a minimum of three food sources for each of the macrominerals and trace elements.
4. Identify conditions associated with deficiencies of the macrominerals and trace elements.
5. Explain the interrelationship of calcium, phosphorus, magnesium, and vitamin D.
6. Explain the interrelationship of ascorbic acid and iron.
7. Explain the interrelationship of zinc, copper, and iron.

CHAPTER OUTLINE ——————————— NOTES, TERMS, & TRANSPARENCY MASTERS

I. Structure and Function
   A. Mineral composition of the body   **macrominerals, microminerals, trace elements, ultratrace elements, cation, anion**

   B. Functions of minerals

II. Macrominerals
   A. Calcium
      1. Skeletal calcium   **nonexchangeable pool, exchangeable pool, trabeculae, osteoclastic, osteoblastic, hydroxyapatite**

      2. Serum calcium   **free or ionized calcium, anion-complexed calcium, protein-bound calcium**

3. Functions
4. Absorption and utilization
    a. Factors that increase calcium absorption
    b. Factors that decrease calcium absorption | **oxalic acid, phytic acid**
5. Maintenance of serum calcium levels | **parathormone, calcitonin, glucocorticoids, thyroid hormone, estrogen**
6. Excretion
7. Recommended Dietary Allowance

Table 7-1 provides a list of the current RDA for calcium by age and gender.
Figure 7-1 (Handout) illustrates the patterns of calcium intake for males and females in the United States.

8. Sources and intake

Table 7-2 lists foods by their calcium content.
Figure 7-2 is an illustration of foods grouped by calcium content.

9. Deficiency
    a. Bone deformities | **osteomalacia, rickets**
    b. Tetany
    c. Hypertension
    d. Other diseases
10. Toxicity

B. Phosphorus
    1. Functions | **phosphorylation-dephosphorylation, phosphate buffer system, hydroxyapatite**
    2. Absorption
    3. Excretion
    4. Recommended Dietary Allowance

Table 7-3 lists the current RDA for phosphorus by age and gender.
phosvitin, calcium phosphorus ratio

    5. Sources

Table 7-4 provides the phosphorus content of food.
Key concept: Phosphorus is closely associated with protein in food. Note that foods high in calcium may also be high in phosphorus.

    6. Deficiency

C. Magnesium
    1. Functions
    2. Absorption and excretion
    3. Recommended Dietary Allowance

Figure 7-3 (Handout) is a graphic illustration of the patterns of magnesium intake for males and females in the United States.
Table 7-5 lists the current RDA for magnesium.

4. Sources and intakes

Table 7-6 provides the magnesium content of select foods.
Key concept: Magnesium is part of the chlorophyll molecule found in green plants.

5. Deficiency
6. Magnesium and disease

D. Sulfur

aconitase, glutathione, heparin, chondroitin sulfate

E. Sodium, chloride, and potassium

III. Trace Elements

See **Table 7-23** for Estimated Safe and Adequate Daily Dietary Intakes for copper, manganese, fluoride, chromium, and molybdenum.

A. General characteristics
 1. Functions
 2. Sources

B. Iron
 1. Functions

Figure 7-4 (Transparency) illustrates iron metabolism in adults.
Table 7-7 lists the compounds in the body that contain iron and their functions.
hemoglobin, heme, myoglobin, cytochromes, cytochrome P-450 system, transferrin, lactoferrin

 2. Absorption and transport

heme iron, nonheme iron, mobilferrin, apoferritin, ferritin, total iron-binding capacity (TIBC)

   a. Efficiency of absorption
   b. Factors affecting absorption

meat, fish, and poultry (MFP) factor, intrinsic factor, phytate, tannins

 3. Storage

ferritin, hemosiderin, hemosiderosis, hemochromatosis

 4. Excretion
 5. Recommended Dietary Allowance

Table 7-8 lists the current RDA for iron.

 6. Sources and intake

Table 7-9 lists the iron content of selected foods.
Figure 7-5 (Handout) illustrates the absorbed iron requirements in males and females of various ages.

 7. Deficiency

hypochromic, microcytic anemia

 8. Iron overload

hereditary hemochromatosis, transferrin overload

C. Zinc
  1. Functions — **metallothionein**

  2. Absorption — **Figure 7-6 (Transparency)** illustrates the absorption of zinc the relationship between metallothionein and cysteine-rich intestinal protein (CRIP).
    albumin, transferrin, alpha-2 macroglobulin

    a. Inhibiting factors
    b. Enhancing factors
  3. Excretion
  4. Recommended Dietary Allowance — **Table 7-10** lists the current RDA for zinc.

  5. Sources and intakes — **Table 7-11** lists the zinc content for some foods.

  6. Deficiency — See **Clinical Insight: "Zinc in Children's Diets."**
    Table 7-12 summarizes the clinical manifestations of zinc deficiency.
    hypogonadism, hypogeusia, alopecia, acrodermatitis enteropathica

  7. Toxicity

D. Copper
  1. Functions
  2. Absorption, Transport, and Excretion — **ceruloplasmin**
  3. Metabolism
  4. Estimated Safe and Adequate Daily Dietary Intake — **Table 7-13** lists the current ESADDI for copper.

  5. Sources and intakes — **Table 7-14** lists the zinc content of selected foods.

  6. Deficiency — **microcytic hemochromic anemia, neutropenia, leukopenia, cone demineralization, Menkes' disease**

  7. Toxicity — **Wilson's disease**

E. Iodine
  1. Absorption and excretion — **triiodothyronine (T$_3$), thyroxine (T$_4$)**

  2. Recommended Dietary Allowance — **Table 7-15** lists the current RDA for iodine.

  3. Dietary sources — **Table 7-16** lists the iodine content of some foods.

  4. Deficiency — **Figure 7-7** is a photograph of a goiter caused by iodine deficiency.
    Figure 7-8 is a photograph of an infant with cretinism caused by iodine deficiency.
    mental cretinism, goiter, goitrogens, *Escherichia coli*

5. Toxicity

F. Fluoride
   1. Functions   **fluorapatite**

   2. Estimated Safe and Adequate Daily Dietary Intake   **Table 7-17** provides the current ESADDI for fluoride.

   3. Sources and intakes   **Key concept:** The major dietary source of fluoride is drinking water. The issue of fluoridated versus nonfluoridated water is of interest here.

   4. Toxicity   **fluorosis**

G. Chromium
   1. Functions   **glucose tolerance factor**
   2. Absorption and excretion
   3. Estimated Safe and Adequate Daily Dietary Intake   **Table 7-18** provides the current ESADDI for chromium.
   4. Sources and intakes
   5. Deficiency

H. Cobalt
   1. Functions
   2. Absorption and excretion
   3. Recommended intakes
   4. Sources and intakes
   5. Deficiency
   6. Toxicity

I. Selenium   **glutathione peroxidase, cellular glutathione peroxidase, extracellular glutathione peroxidase, Type I iodothyronine 5'-diodinase, selenprotein P**

   1. Functions
   2. Absorption and excretion
   3. Recommended Dietary Allowance   **Table 7-19** provides the current RDA for selenium.
     Note: The current (1989) RDA was the first time that selenium was included.

   4. Sources and intakes   **Table 7-20** lists the selenium content of selected foods. See **Appendix 30** for more information.

   5. Deficiency   **Keshan disease, Kashin-Beck disease**
   6. Toxicity

J. Manganese
   1. Functions
                             glutamine synthetase, pyruvate carboxylase, superoxide dismutase

   2. Absorption and excretion
                             transmanganin

   3. Estimated Safe and Adequate Daily Dietary Intake
                             Table 7-21 provides the current ESADDI for manganese.

   4. Sources and intakes
   5. Deficiency
   6. Toxicity

K. Molybdenum
                             xanthine oxidase, aldehyde oxidase, sulfite oxidase

   1. Estimated Safe and Adequate Daily Dietary Intake
                             Table 7-22 provides the current ESADDI for molybdenum.
   2. Sources and intakes

L. Summary table
                             Table 7-23 summarizes all the minerals known to be required for maintenance of human health.

IV. Trace Elements: Requirements Undefined
   A. Silicon
                             organosilicon compounds
   B. Vanadium
   C. Boron
   D. Tin
   E. Nickel
   F. Additional trace elements
                             Figure 7-9 is a flow chart of the procedure used by the FDA to determine if there is significant scientific agreement on a health claim.

CASE STUDY INSIGHTS

1. What concerns do you have about Miles' intake of iodine since he is avoiding table salt? In what other foods might he consume iodine?

You are not given information about where Miles lives. There is a possibility that he is in a goiter region, but it is not too likely. He can meet his iodine needs with a well-balanced diet that includes both saltwater and freshwater fish, meat, milk, and eggs from animals fed a diet containing iodine, fruits, and vegetables grown in iodine-rich soil and numerous processed foods for which iodine is part of additives.

2. His usual diet, which is low in fruits and vegetables, could be low in which minerals? What suggestions do you have for increasing the intake of these minerals?

A person whose diet does not include adequate fruits and vegetables could be at risk for deficiencies of several minerals that are found most amply in these foods. The potential deficiencies include potassium, calcium, magnesium, iron, and zinc. Since other foods also provide these minerals, a thorough diet history would be recommended if there is a concern.

Of most concern regarding Miles' mineral intake would be potassium. He is taking a potassium-depleting diuretic for control of his blood pressure. Fruits and vegetables are good sources of potassium. The most appropriate thing for this patient is to increase his intake of fruits and vegetables. If this is not possible, determine by diet history whether there is a risk for deficiency of any mineral, potassium in particular. Supplementation is a choice, but not necessarily the best one.

3.   He drinks very little milk. What would you recommend for including more calcium in his diet?

Vegetables can provide appreciable amounts of calcium. Those containing oxalate (chard, spinach, rhubarb, and beet greens) would not be good sources. If Miles begins to eat more fruits and vegetables as recommended, it would also provide him with more calcium. Another alternative is for him to drink calcium-fortified orange juice, which would increase both his calcium and potassium intakes.

4.   Fluoridated water is not available. Does this concern you?

The fluoridation of water has a significant effect on increasing the intake of fluoride. However, fluoride deficiency is not usually a concern when the diet is well-balanced and adequate in other nutrients. Rich sources include tea, fish, and foods cooked in Teflon-coated pans. Beef liver is a rich source, but it is also high in cholesterol and may be inconsistent with recommendations for managing his hypercholesterolemia.

SUGGESTED TEST QUESTIONS

1.   The richest food source of iodine in the diet is
*   a.   saltwater fish.
   b.   freshwater fish.
   c.   cow's milk.
   d.   eggs.

2.   The physical sign of adult iodine deficiency that can be described as an enlarged neck is
   a.   muscle spasms.
*   b.   simple goiter.
   c.   hypertension.
   d.   diarrhea.

3.   Individuals most often at greatest risk for iron deficiency are
   a.   infants under 2 years of age.
   b.   the elderly.
   c.   menstruating women.
*   d.   pregnant teenagers.

4.   Which of these is the best description of calcium?
   a.   It is the least abundant mineral in the body and aids iron absorption.
*   b.   It is the most abundant mineral in the body and functions in nerve transmission and heartbeat regulation.
   c.   It is the most abundant mineral in the body and aids in the absorption of zinc.
   d.   It is the least abundant mineral in the body and is absorbed with manganese.

5.   In response to an elevated serum calcium, the body will
   a.   increase secretion of parathyroid hormone to slow down calcium absorption.
   b.   increase calcitriol secretion to inhibit calcium mobilization and absorption.
*   c.   secrete calcitonin to lower serum calcium by inhibiting further bone resorption.
   d.   secrete calcitonin to lower serum calcium by mobilizing calcium from the bone.

6. When a patient experiences muscle spasms such as leg cramps and irritability of the nerve fibers, it may be an indication of calcium deficiency clinically known as
   * a. tetany.
   b. osteomalacia.
   c. rickets.
   d. osteoporosis.

7. Magnesium, an intracellular cation, is found in abundance in
   a. refined foods and dairy products.
   b. milk and fruits.
   c. fish and meat.
   * d. seeds, nuts, and legumes.

8. Sulfur in the diet occurs primarily as part if the amino acids
   * a. cystine, cysteine, and methionine.
   b. cystine, phenylalanine, and threonine.
   c. valine, leucine, and isoleucine.
   d. methionine, tryptophan, and cysteine.

9. The serum protein transferrin is responsible for
   a. transporting phosphorus to the bone.
   * b. transporting iron in the blood for use in heme synthesis.
   c. transporting phosphorus from the bone to the tissues.
   d. transporting calcium to the bone.

10. The absorption of iron in foods is improved by the presence of
   a. ascorbic acid and vitamin D.
   b. an alkaline environment.
   * c. ascorbic acid and an acidic environment.
   d. an acidic environment.

11. A patient diagnosed with a zinc deficiency may exhibit
   * a. hypogeusia, delayed wound healing, and alopecia.
   b. hypergeusia, skeletal deformities, and anemia.
   c. diminished hearing, tinnitus, and alopecia.
   d. fatty liver, edema, and hyperlipidemia.

12. Wilson's disease occurs when the patient has a genetic deficiency in the liver's ability to synthesize
   * a. ceruloplasmin.
   b. cholesterol.
   c. albumin.
   d. transferrin.

13. Goitrogens, which inhibit the absorption or utilization of iodine, are found in
   a. fish, chicken, and beef.
   b. milk, cheese, and yogurt.
   c. apples, peaches, and pears.
   * d. cabbage, turnips, and peanuts.

14. The function of selenium and tocopherol is to protect cell membranes from
   a. fatty infiltration.
   b. calcium deposits.
   * c. oxidation damage.
   d. protein breakdown.

15. Glucose tolerance factor, which has been proposed to have a role in carbohydrate, protein, and lipid metabolism, contains the mineral
   a. zinc.
   * b. chromium.
   c. phosphate.
   d. iron.

16. The iron-containing protein that serves as a reservoir for oxygen in the muscle is
   * a. myoglobin.
   b. hemoglobin.
   c. hemosiderin.
   d. cytochrome.

17. The most abundant nonenzyme protein that contains zinc is
   a. hemosiderin.
   * b. metallothionein.
   c. ceruloplasmin.
   d. albumin.

18. The synthesis of thyroxine is dependent on the mineral
   a. copper.
   b. zinc.
   c. sulfur.
   * d. iodine.

19. The infant of a mother who had an iodine deficiency during pregnancy is at risk for
    a. goiter.
    b. hemosiderosis.
*   c. cretinism.
    d. tetany.

20. Fluoride can improve resistance to dental caries, but in excess can cause
*   a. fluorosis, mottling of the teeth.
    b. osteomalacia, softening of the bones.
    c. fluoride toxicity.
    d. iron-deficiency anemia.

21. A beverage considered to be one of the richest sources of manganese is
*   a. tea.
    b. coffee.
    c. milk.
    d. fruit juice.

22. Vitamin B_{12} contains the mineral
    a. molybdenum.
    b. silicon.
    c. tin.
*   d. cobalt.

23. The mineral essential in the oxidation of iron is
    a. zinc.
*   b. copper.
    c. vanadium.
    d. lead.

CHAPTER 8

WATER, ELECTROLYTES, AND ACID–BASE BALANCE

OVERVIEW

The purpose of this chapter is to provide the student with a basic understanding of the factors influencing water and electrolyte balance and acid–base balance in the body. The mechanisms of normal fluid balance are summarized. The major intracellular, extracellular, and intercellular ions are included. Factors controlling fluid intake and loss are presented, and the conditions of acidosis and alkalosis are reviewed. The chapter concludes with methods for compensation in disturbances of acid–base balance.

LEARNING OBJECTIVES

This chapter will prepare the learner to be able to

1. List the functions of water in the body.
2. Define intracellular, extracellular, and intercellular water.
3. Identify the major intracellular and extracellular cations.
4. Describe how fluid balance is achieved for the normal individual, identifying sources of intake and routes of excretion.
5. State the recommended intake of fluid.
6. Define metabolic acidosis, metabolic alkalosis, respiratory acidosis, and respiratory alkalosis.
7. Compare metabolic acidosis and respiratory acidosis.
8. Compare metabolic alkalosis and respiratory alkalosis.
9. State how the body can compensate for disturbances in acid–base balance.

CHAPTER OUTLINE

I. Body Water

    A. Functions of water

    B. Distribution of body water

NOTES, TERMS, & TRANSPARENCY MASTERS

Figure 8-1 (Transparency) shows the distribution of body water as a percentage of body weight from infancy to adulthood.

Figure 8-2 summarizes the effects of a loss of increasing amounts of body water.

intracellular water (ICW), extracellular water (ECW), intercellular (interstitial), edema

49

C. Water balance
  1. Water intake

Table 8-1 summarizes water balance, including mechanisms of intake and output under varying conditions.
antidiuretic hormone (ADH), metabolic water

  2. Water elimination

water loss, sensible, insensible, water intoxication

  3. Requirements for water

Table 8-2 lists the water content (as a percentage) of some common foods.
thirst

II. Electrolytes

Table 8-3 lists the normal electrolyte concentrations of serum, both cations and anions.

A. Sodium
  1. Functions
  2. Absorption and excretion
  3. Recommended intake
  4. Sources

renin-aldosterone system, aldosterone

B. Chloride
  1. Functions
  2. Absorption and excretion
  3. Sources
  4. Recommended intake

Table 8-4 lists the current Estimated Safe and Adequate Daily Dietary Intake (ESADDI) for sodium, chloride, and potassium.

C. Potassium
  1. Functions
  2. Absorption and excretion
  3. Sources
  4. Recommended intake

III. Acid–Base Balance

Table 8-5 classifies the four major acid–base imbalances and the conditions leading to these imbalances.

A. Acid generation
B. Regulation

Figure 8-3 (Transparency) illustrates the generation of $NaHCO_3$ and the subsequent buffering of the resulting H^+ ions.
buffer systems

C. Acid–base disorders

Table 8-6 lists the normal arterial blood gas (ABG) values.

  1. Metabolic acidosis
  2. Metabolic alkalosis
  3. Respiratory acidosis
  4. Respiratory alkalosis

anion gap

adult respiratory distress syndrome (ADRS)

D. Compensation

Table 8-7 summarizes the body's attempts to compensate for changes in acid–base balance and restore normal pH.

CASE STUDY INSIGHTS

1. How valid are weights in the Intensive Care Unit (ICU)?

   Any weight measurement is only as valid as the method used to obtain it. This patient's medical condition is most likely serious enough to require use of a bed scale to weigh him. His medical condition is also causing his fluid status to change rapidly. Provided the weights are measured accurately and consistently, the differences observed should be reliable enough to make decision on his fluid status. His I and O (intake and output) should also be measured and used along with the weights.
   (This is a good opportunity to discuss with students the ICU environment, patient to nurse ratios, and prioritizing of medical needs.)

2. What serum lab values should you evaluate during Jake's stay in the ICU?

   As Jake's medical course proceeds, he will experience hypovolemia. In this situation, serum lab values are elevated due to hemoconcentration. The intravenous fluids are being used to replenish lost fluids (fluid resuscitation). In the event he becomes overhydrated, serum lab values may become depressed, indicating hemodilution. Of significance in maintenance of fluid balance is the serum albumin and serum sodium. These two values are particularly important to monitor.

3. If his lungs were affected, which type of acidosis might occur?

   If his respiratory function is compromised, respiratory acidosis could occur. In this condition, the lungs are unable to excrete CO_2 at an adequate rate, thus resulting in a buildup of carbonic acid (H_2CO_3). The result is acidosis.

4. If his kidneys were affected, which type of acidosis might occur?

   If his renal function is compromised, metabolic acidosis could result. In this condition, the kidneys excrete excess bicarbonate, (HCO_3^-). The bicarbonate is necessary to buffer the H^+ ions produced in metabolic reactions. The excess H^+ ions result in acidosis.

5. What other concerns do you have about Jake's electrolyte imbalance?

   At this time, Jake's medical condition is not well described. You should proceed conservatively, not omitting any possible abnormalities. The following should be monitored continually until he is stable: weight, intake and output, and serum lab values.

6. At what point does weight loss indicate loss of lean body mass and not fluid?

   Thie is difficult to be specific with this patient. He will be experiencing fluid imbalance for at least the first 24–48 hours posttrauma. Depending on the nature of the injury, the fluid losses could be extensive. When lean body mass is lost, nitrogen balance can be determined using urinary nitrogen excretion. However, the traumatized patient is hypermetabolic due to injury and will be in negative nitrogen balance for a period of time. Increased losses of potassium, magnesium, phosphorus, and zinc occur with losses of lean body mass.

SUGGESTED TEST QUESTIONS

1. A person who is ill or injured is at risk for dehydration because of a decreased mechanism for
   a. swallowing.
   b. renal perfusion.
   c. renin-angiotensin-aldosterone.
   * d. thirst.

2. Increasing intake of dietary potassium can be easily accomplished with the inclusion of
   * a. fruits and vegetables
   b. saltwater fish
   c. grains
   d. cereals

3. The effect of excess aldosterone on maintaining fluid and electrolyte balance is a disturbance in the maintenance of
   a. sodium balance
   b. potassium balance
   c. chloride balance
   * d. all of the above

4. Water intoxication can be particularly dangerous if the result is
   * a. an increase in the volume of the brain cells.
   b. hypertension.
   c. decreased circulating blood volume.
   d. an increase in urinary output.

5. Fluid needs for most adults can be met by an intake of
   a. 1000 mL/day.
   b. 1500 mL/day.
   c. 2000 mL/day.
   * d. 2500 mL/day.

6. The distribution of total body water as a percentage of body weight
   * a. decreases significantly with age and is higher in athletes than in nonathletes.
   b. decreases significantly with age and is lower in athletes than in nonathletes.
   c. increases significantly with age.
   d. increases significantly with age and is lower in athletes than in nonathletes.

7. Interstitial water is the water that is found
   a. within body cells and the lymphatic system.
   b. within body cells.
   * c. between and around body cells.
   d. in the blood and the lymphatic system.

8. Thirst is stimulated in the hypothalamus gland as a result of
   * a. an increase in serum osmolality.
   b. a decrease in serum osmolality.
   c. an increase in serum osmolality and an increase in extracellular volume.
   d. a decrease in serum osmolality and an increase in extracellular volume.

9. The kidney can compensate for a loss of body water by excreting
   a. additional fluid and electrolytes.
   b. additional electrolytes.
   * c. a more concentrated urine.
   d. a less concentrated urine.

10. When fluid intake is determined by caloric intake, the recommended amount is
    a. 2 mL/kcal for adults and 3 mL/kcal for infants.
    b. 0.5 mL/kcal for both adults and infants.
    c. 2 mL/kcal for adults and 1 mL/kcal for infants.
    * d. 1 mL/kcal for adults and 1.5 mL/kcal for infants.

11. Reabsorption from the tubules of the kidney is stimulated by the mineralcorticoid secreted by the adrenal cortex known as
    * a. aldosterone.
    b. vasopressin.
    c. calcitonin.
    d. antidiuretic hormone.

12. For a normal, healthy adult, fluid balance is achieved when the amount of water taken in is
    a. half the amount of water that is lost.
    * b. about equal to the amount of water lost.
    c. twice the amount of water lost.
    d. unrelated to the amount of water lost.

13. The effect of dehydration on the specific gravity of urine is
 * a. an increase above normal.
   b. no change.
   c. a decrease below normal.
   d. a three-fold increase.

14. The difference in fluid requirements of infants and adults is most influenced by
   a. the lower percentage of body water in infants.
 * b. the higher percentage of body water in infants.
   c. the smaller surface area per unit body weight of infants.
   d. the smaller amount of adipose tissue in infants.

15. When sodium is ingested in large amounts in a short time, the result can be
   a. hypotension.
   b. muscular cramps.
 * c. edema and hypertension.
   d. increased urinary output of potassium.

16. The intracellular fluid is dominated by the cation
   a. sodium.
   b. calcium.
   c. magnesium.
 * d. potassium.

17. The extracellular fluid is dominated by the cation within the
   a. body cells.
 * b. extracellular fluid.
   c. interstitial fluid.
   d. intracellular fluid.

18. The maintenance of acid-base balance by the regulation of hydrogen ions is the function of the
   a. lungs.
   b. liver.
 * c. kidney.
   d. adrenal glands.

19. A major source of hydrogen ions generated in the body is
 * a. normal tissue metabolism.
   b. ingestion of highly acidic foods.
   c. oxidation-reduction reactions.
   d. reabsorption of bicarbonate.

20. Metabolic acidosis results from
   a. an accumulation of bicarbonate.
   b. decreased ventilation and retention of carbon dioxide.
 * c. an accumulation of acids from abnormal metabolism.
   d. excessive loss of carbon dioxide from the lungs.

CHAPTER 9

NUTRITION DURING PREGNANCY AND LACTATION

OVERVIEW

The purpose of this chapter is to present the nutritional requirements and concerns that affect women during pregnancy and lactation. The chapter begins with identifying the outcome of pregnancy as it relates to both preconception and prenatal nutritional status. Physiological changes during pregnancy, recommended nutrient intakes, guidelines for meal planning, and concerns about alcohol, caffeine, and artificial sweeteners are presented. The complications of pregnancy are reviewed with appropriate recommendations for nutritional management. Nutritional needs during lactation are reviewed. Techniques for breastfeeding and management of common problems associated with breastfeeding are included. The chapter concludes with a perspective of nutrition as it relates to fertility and conception.

LEARNING OBJECTIVES

This chapter will prepare the learner to be able to

1. State the nutrition-related factors influencing the outcome of pregnancy.
2. Explain the relationship of maternal weight gain to infant birth weight and outcome of pregnancy.
3. List the recommendations for maternal weight gain during pregnancy for a variety of maternal characteristics.
4. Describe the physiological changes associated with pregnancy and the nutritional concerns related to the changes.
5. State the Recommended Dietary Allowances (RDA) for the pregnant woman.
6. State the recommendations for use of sodium, alcohol, caffeine, and artificial sweeteners during pregnancy.
7. State the recommendations for the number of servings from the six major food groups (breads and cereals, vegetables, fruits, diary products, meat/meat substitutes, and fats and sweets) for the pregnant woman.
8. Identify the nutrition-related complications associated with pregnancy and the recommended management of the complications.
9. Explain the implications of cultural beliefs and customs practiced during pregnancy.
10. State the Recommended Dietary Allowances (RDA) for the lactating woman.
11. Explain the effect of maternal diet on the nutritional composition of human milk.
12. Describe the technique for breastfeeding an infant, including maternal preparation, frequency and length of feedings, and positioning of infant.
13. Identify the complications associated with breastfeeding and recommendations for management of the problems.
14. State the relationship between nutrition and fertility.

54

CHAPTER OUTLINE	NOTES, TERMS, & TRANSPARENCY MASTERS

CHAPTER OUTLINE

NOTES, TERMS, & TRANSPARENCY MASTERS

I. Pregnancy

A. Effect of nutritional status on pregnancy outcome

   1. Historical perspective

miscarriages, abortions, stillbirths, neonatal deaths, malformations

   2. Relationship of perinatal mortality and birth weight

low birth weight

     a. Maternal size

     b. Maternal weight gain during pregnancy

Key concept: Adequate weight gain is a critical factor in the outcome of pregnancy. The recommendations vary depending on preconception weight and nutritional status.

Figure 9-1 shows the composition of weight gain of a healthy, well-fed Northern European woman and a poor, underfed woman from India.

Figure 9-2 illustrates the perinatal mortality rates related to weight gain of the mother during pregnancy.

Table 9-1 summarizes the recommended weight gain during pregnancy based on prepregnancy BMI. The BMI calculation uses Quetelet's Index.

Figure 9-3 is a graphic illustration of recommended weight gain patterns based on prepregnancy weight.

nulliparous

     c. Obesity

     d. Adolescence

     e. Multiple births

B. Nutritional supplementation during pregnancy

C. Physiologic changes of pregnancy

   1. Blood volume and composition

   2. Cardiovascular and pulmonary

   3. Gastrointestinal

   4. Renal

   5. Placenta

USDA Special Supplemental Food Program for Women, Infants, and Children (WIC)

D. Nutritional requirements

   1. Energy

     a. Recommended intake

     b. Exercise

     c. Consequences of energy restriction

2. Protein
3. Vitamins
   a. Folic acid
   b. Vitamin B$_6$ See **Focus On: "Premenstrual Syndrome."**
   c. Ascorbic acid
   d. Vitamin A   **Teratogen Society**
   e. Vitamin D
   f. Vitamin E
   g. Vitamin K
4. Minerals
   a. Calcium
   b. Phosphorus
   c. Iron   **maternal anemia**
   d. Zinc
   e. Copper
   f. Sodium   **Key concept:** Aggressive restriction of sodium is
                                         unwarranted in pregnancy and daily consump-
                                         tion of sodium should not fall below 2–3 g.

   g. Magnesium
   h. Fluoride   **Table 9-2** summarizes the current RDA for all 19
                                         nutrients for pregnant and lactating women.

E. Guide for eating during pregnancy   **Table 9-3** provides a daily food pattern for preg-
                                         nancy. Both nonvegetarian and vegetarian
                                         meal patterns are given.

   1. Recommended food intake   **Table 9-4** gives a sample menu for a pregnant
                                         woman based on the food patterns in Table 9-3.
                                         Figure 9-4 is a photograph of a dietitian providing
                                         dietary counseling for a pregnant woman.

   2. Alcohol   **Figure 9-5** shows two photographs of an infant
                                         with fetal alcohol syndrome, one at birth and
                                         one at age 1 year.
                                         Figure 9-6 (Handout) illustrates the transfer of
                                         substances across the placental membrane sep-
                                         arating the mother and fetus.
                                         fetal alcohol syndrome, fetal alcohol effects

   3. Non-nutritive substances in foods
      a. Caffeine
      b. Artificial sweeteners   **phenylketonuria (PKU)**
      c. Contaminants
   4. Beliefs, avoidances, cravings, and   **food avoidances, cravings, aversions**
      aversions
      a. Pica

                                         Table 9-5 summarizes the recommendations for
                                         nutritional care for the pregnant woman.
                                         geophagia, amylophagia

F. Diet-related complications of pregnancy
   1. Nausea and vomiting   **hyperemesis gravidarum**
   2. Heartburn
   3. Constipation and hemorrhoids
   4. Edema
   5. Diabetes mellitus   **gestational diabetes, macrosomia**

   6. Pregnancy-induced hypertension (PIT)   **preeclampsia, eclampsia**

II. Lactation   **Table 9-6** is a list of the advantages of breastfeed-
                                        ing. The list is limited to those advantages
                                        afforded the infant. There are also advantages
                                        for the mother.

A. Physiology of lactation   **Figure 9-7** illustrates the structure of the mamma-
                                        ry glands. The relationship of structure to lac-
                                        tation is highlighted.
                                        Figure 9-8 illustrates how the sucking action of
                                        the infant stimulates milk production and
                                        secretion via the hypothalamus and pituitary
                                        glands.
                                        prolactin, oxytocin, let-down

   1. Nutritional requirements of lactation
       a. Energy
       b. Protein
       c. Lipid
       d. Vitamins and minerals

B. Breastfeeding an infant
   1. Preparation
   2. The technique   **Figure 9-9** is a photograph of a mother nursing
   3. Duration of breastfeeding   her infant.
                                        colostrum, rooting reflex

   4. Exercise and breastfeeding
   5. Common problems   **Table 9-7** lists common problems of breastfeeding
       a. Engorged breasts   and the recommended methods for managing
       b. Sore nipples   the problems.
       c. Inverted (retracted) and flat
           nipples
       d. Plugged ducts
       e. Infection
       f. Leaking
       g. Failure to thrive in the breast   **Figure 9-10** is a flow chart that identifies the
           feeding infant   causes and outcomes of failure to thrive for an
                                        infant.

   6. Relactation and induced lactation
   7. Breast pumping and milk storage

III. Nutrition, Fertility, and Conception   **amenorrhea, dysmenorrhea**

CASE STUDY INSIGHTS

1. What would you recommend to improve the baby's position during nursing? How will this improve the nursing experience?

Both mother and baby need to be in a comfortable position. The baby's head, back, and buttocks should be fully supported. Holding the baby close also helps reduce pulling on the nipple and subsequent soreness.

2. What advice would you give Ms. Lopez about her fatigue?

It is not uncommon for a new mother to experience fatigue. She needs to work with the baby's schedule, making sure she gets adequate rest. She also needs to eat regular, well-balanced meals.

3. How would you design an eating plan for Ms. Lopez that she can follow?

Answers will vary. Students should be reminded that before developing an eating plan, they need to obtain a diet history, a description of daily routine and activities, and the client's own eating preferences.

STUDENT ACTIVITY

1. Invite a speaker who works with breastfeeding mothers, such as someone from Le Leche League, a Lactation Specialist, or a nurse practitioner. Ask the guest to include recommendations on diet that are given to the nursing mothers, as well as general information.

SUGGESTED TEST QUESTIONS

1. Leg cramps associated with pregnancy may be improved by
    a. an increase in milk products and an increase in activity level.
    b. an increase in milk products and a decrease in activity level.
    * c. a decrease in milk products and addition of nonphosphate calcium supplements.
    d. a decrease in milk products and addition of magnesium-based antacid.

2. Edema in the feet and lower legs experienced during pregnancy can usually be considered
    * a. normal unless accompanied by proteinuria and hypertension.
    b. normal and requiring only a mild diuretic.
    c. abnormal and requiring a low sodium diet.
    d. abnormal and requiring hospitalization.

3. According to the National Academy of Sciences, women with normal preconception weight should gain how much during pregnancy?
    a. 10-15 lb
    b. 20-25 lb
    * c. 25-35 lb
    d. 35-45 lb

4. A normal physiological adaptation during pregnancy is an increase in blood volume and a decrease in the kidney's ability to excrete water, both of which can result in
    * a. edema.
    b. proteinuria.
    c. hypoglycemia.
    d. constipation.

5. The risk of a neural tube defect occurring *in utero* can be reduced by
* a. an increase in folic acid intake throughout the child-bearing years.
 b. ensuring an adequate intake of niacin during the first six weeks of pregnancy.
 c. providing an adequate protein intake throughout pregnancy.
 d. increasing intake of vitamin C during the first trimester.

6. A pregnant patient with lactose intolerance can increase her calcium intake by increasing consumption of
 a. milk and ice cream.
 b. cheese and ice cream.
* c. yogurt and cheese.
 d. ice cream.

7. When counseling a newly pregnant patient about alcohol consumption, the most appropriate recommendation is to
 a. avoid alcohol for the first trimester, then no more than 1 oz of alcohol per day.
* b. avoid alcohol completely throughout the pregnancy.
 c. limit consumption to 1 oz. of alcohol per day.
 d. limit consumption to 2 oz. of alcohol per day.

8. When managing pregnancy-induced hypertension, the patient should be instructed to
* a. ensure adequate protein intake.
 b. decrease the use of calcium supplementation.
 c. use diuretics to control symptoms.
 d. limit the intake of sodium.

9. The difference between the diet of the breast-feeding mother and the diet of the pregnant woman is that
 a. intake of all nutrients is the same as pre-conception for the lactating mother.
 b. the energy level during lactation should be severely restricted to promote weigh loss.
 c. fluids are forced for the pregnant woman and limited during lactation.
* d. intake of all nutrients are increased during lactation.

10. The typical feeding pattern of a breast-fed infant is influenced by the digestibility of breast milk, and the infant is more likely to
 a. have more frequent stools.
* b. want to be fed more often than a formula-fed baby.
 c. be able to go 4–5 hours between feedings.
 d. adjust more rapidly to a set schedule.

11. A common complaint during pregnancy is constipation caused by
* a. an increase in the level of progesterone.
 b. a decrease in the level of progesterone.
 c. an increase in the level of estrogen.
 d. a decrease in the level of estrogen.

12. The 1989 RDA for energy intake in the second and third trimesters is the sum of the energy requirement for the nonpregnant woman and a daily addition of
 a. 100 kcal.
 b. 200 kcal.
* c. 300 kcal.
 d. 400 kcal.

13. The 1989 RDA for protein in the second and third trimesters is the sum of the protein requirement for the nonpregnant woman and a daily addition of
 a. 5-10 g.
* b. 10-16 g.
 c. 15-25 g.
 d. 25-45 g.

14. To ensure the maintenance of health during pregnancy, vitamin intake requirements increase for
 a. vitamins A and C.
* b. folic acid and vitamins B and C.
 c. vitamins C, D, and K.
 d. vitamins A, D,and K.

15. One symptom of a decline in serum calcium due to an imbalance between calcium and phosphorus is
* a. leg cramps.
 b. nausea.
 c. hypertension.
 d. hypotension.

16. Iron supplementation during pregnancy is
    a. rarely needed.
    b. only needed if the woman has a poor diet.
* c. often acknowledged as necessary to prevent iron-deficiency anemia.
    d. only prescribed if the woman becomes anemic.

17. During pregnancy, a diagnosis of maternal anemia can be made with which of these biochemical indices?
    a. a hematocrit of >45%; a hemoglobin of >30 g/dL.
    b. a hematocrit of >40%; a hemoglobin of >20 g/dL.
    c. a hematocrit of <40%; a hemoglobin of <15 g/dL.
* d. a hematocrit of <32%; a hemoglobin of <11 g/dL.

18. The most frequently given recommendation about sodium for pregnant women is
    a. aggressive restriction is warranted.
* b. aggressive restriction is unwarranted.
    c. sodium intake should not exceed 1 g per day.
    d. sodium intake should not exceed 2 g per day.

19. For the pregnant woman who consumed caffeine-containing beverages before pregnancy, the most appropriate advice is
    a. restriction is unnecessary.
    b. eliminate all sources from the diet.
* c. do not consume unnecessary caffeine.
    d. limit caffeine to that provided by weakly brewed tea.

20. Pregnant women having the condition of pica have a compulsion for persistent ingestion of
    a. sweet and starchy foods.
* b. unsuitable substances having little or no nutritional value.
    c. salty foods.
    d. fatty foods.

21. When a pregnant woman complains of nausea and vomiting during the early months of her pregnancy, relief may come from consuming
    a. liquids with meals and having small, frequent feedings.
    b. high fat foods and including liquids with meals.
* c. small, frequent meals low in fat and limiting liquids to between meals.
    d. three regular meals per day with liquids taken with meals.

22. The occurrence of pregnancy-induced hypertension (PIH) is manifested by
* a. hypertension, proteinuria, and edema.
    b. hypotension, hyperalbuminemia, and excessive urine output.
    c. abdominal cramping and weight loss.
    d. weight loss, edema, and hypertension.

23. When a lactating woman develops a breast infection, the most appropriate advice is to
    a. stop nursing at once.
    b. offer milk only from the noninfected breast.
* c. continue nursing, offering the infected breast first.
    d. continue nursing, offering the noninfected breast first.

24. For the first 6 months of lactation, the RDA for energy is
    a. 200 kcal less than the RDA for pregnant women.
* b. 500 kcal more than the RDA for nonpregnant women.
    c. 100 kcal more than the RDA for pregnant women.
    d. the same as the RDA for pregnant women.

CHAPTER

NUTRITION IN INFANCY

OVERVIEW

The purpose of this chapter is to provide the student with information about the normal growth and development of an infant in order to lay the foundation for identifying and planning nutrient needs. A comparison of human breast milk and commercial infant formulas it given. Recommendations for introduction of juice, semi-solid, and solid foods are provided. The developmental landmarks and the associated uses of appropriate foods in the diet is reviewed. Guidelines for what, where, how much, and when infants and children should be fed are presented.

LEARNING OBJECTIVES

This chapter will prepare the learner to be able to

1. Summarize the normal growth patterns of infants and children.
2. Identify the nutritional needs of infants for all nutrients included in the Recommended Dietary Allowances (RDA) and for fluid.
3. Compare the nutrient composition of human breast milk and commercial infant formulas.
4. State the properties of human milk that are not found in commercial infant formulas.
5. State the recommended timing of the introduction of juice, semi-solid, and solid foods to the diet of an infant.
6. Explain how it is determined whether an infant is getting enough to eat.
7. Identify the cause of baby bottle tooth decay and state how it can be avoided.
8. State the recommendations for determining portion sizes for young children and creating an appropriate feeding environment.

CHAPTER OUTLINE ———————————— NOTES, TERMS, & TRANSPARENCY MASTERS

I. Physiological Development

Figure 10-1 includes a photograph of two girls at age 20 months born 1 month apart and having a 1-lb difference in birth weight. The figure also shows the growth of the two girls plotted on the NCHS Growth Charts. The emphasis is on the differences in growth patterns.

61

II. Nutrient Needs of Infants

   A. Energy

   B. Protein

   C. Lipid
   D. Carbohydrate

   E. Water

   F. Minerals
     1. Calcium
     2. Iron
     3. Zinc
     4. Fluoride
   G. Vitamins

III. Milk for Infants

   A. Composition of human and cow's milk
   B. Antiinfective factors

   C. Formulas
   D. Whole cow's milk
   E. Formula preparation

IV. Foods for Infants

V. Feeding the Infant
   A. Early feeding patterns

   B. Baby bottle tooth decay
   C. Development of feeding skills

Table 10-1 lists the current RDA for infants and children from birth to 3 years of age.

catch-up, lag down

Key concept: The need for protein during infancy is greater than at any other time during the life cycle. Although the total amount of protein required for an adult exceeds that required for an infant or child, the requirement based on grams of protein per kilogram of body weight is much greater.

Clostridium botulinum

Table 10-2 lists the water requirements for infants and children.
Key concept: The fluid requirements for infants and children is greater than that for adults. Though the total amount of fluid required for an adult exceeds that required for an infant or child, the requirement based on milliliters of fluid per kilogram of body weight is greater.

hemorrhagic disease of the newborn

Table 10-3 provides a reference for the nutrient composition of human milk and the variety of commercial infant formulas.
renal solute load

Lactobacillus bifidus

See **Table 10-3.**

Table 10-4 summarizes the procedures for home-prepared infant foods.

Table 10-5 lists the indicators of infant satiety during the first year of life.
colostrum

D. Addition of semi-solid foods

Table 10-6 provides a reference for matching developmental landmarks, changes in food characteristics, and examples of appropriate foods for the first 2 years of life.

Figure 10-2 is a photograph of a grandparent feeding an infant.

Table 10-7 provides recommendations for the introduction of juice, semi-solid foods, and table foods for the first year of life.

Figure 10-3 is a series of four photographs illustrating various feeding skills observed in infants and children ages 7 months to 2 years.

E. Feeding the older infant
F. Size of servings
G. Types of food
H. Forced feeding
I. Where the child should eat

CASE STUDY INSIGHTS

1. To get an accurate assessment of this infant's intake, what additional information is needed?

The information as provided is vague. It would be helpful to determine the frequency and amount of solid foods being eaten. Also you need to determine if other liquids such as fruit juice are being used.

2. Is Baby M growing appropriately? Explain your answer.

Infants vary in how long after birth before their growth channel is established. In the case of Baby M, she is in the same growth channel for both height and weight and has stayed in the same growth channel since birth. Given this information, it would appear that the baby is growing normally.

3. What is Baby M's estimated energy intake? Is this appropriate?

Using 20 kcal/oz and an intake of six 8-oz bottles of formula daily, her intake from formula alone is 960 kcal (20 kcal/oz × 48 oz). The mother has indicated that the baby is also eating some solids. To determine the energy intake with more accuracy, you also need to know the frequency and amount of solid foods.

Using 15 lbs (6.8 kg) as the median weight for a 3-month-old infant in the 95th percentile, the RDA for energy during the first 6 months is 108 kcal/kg. This gives an estimated requirement of 734 kcal/day (6.8 kg × 108 kcal/kg). There is a difference of 226 kcal per day, which could be explained by inaccuracy in the diet history. It does appear that the mother is mixing the formula correctly.

4. Would you guess that this infant is ready for semi-solid foods? What would you look for in a feeding evaluation?

The infant is younger that expected for being ready for semi-solid foods. There is insufficient information to determine if the infant is developmentally ready. Discuss with students the indicators for developmental readiness, as well as other factors that may motivate a mother to begin feeding solids.

SUGGESTED TEST QUESTIONS

1. In summarizing the growth expectations of most normal infants, new parents could be told that
   a. the birth weight is usually regained by the end of the first month.
   b. infants will triple their birth weight by 6 months of age.
   * c. infants will double their birth weight by 4–6 months of age.
   d. infants will triple their length by 3 years of age.

2. To meet the fluoride needs of a breast-fed infant, parents should be instructed to
   a. begin giving fluoride supplements immediately following birth.
   b. supplement the mother's diet with fluoride.
   * c. not be concerned about fluoride until tooth eruption begins, then give fluoridated water several times per day.
   d. not be concerned about fluoride until the infant is eating solid foods, then the foods will provide sufficient fluoride.

3. The *least* significant source of iron in an infant's diet is
   a. dry cereals.
   b. cereal and fruit mixtures.
   * c. strained fruits and vegetables.
   d. strained meats.

5. The risk of using honey or corn syrup in home-prepared formulas for infants is that
   a. the added sweetener will cause the infant to crave sweets.
   b. the sugars present cannot be digested by the infant.
   c. the honey and corn syrup will settle out in the formula and cause a curdled appearance.
   * d. the infant has no immunity to the botulism spore that may be present.

5. Infants are particularly susceptible to developing dehydration because
   a. their mass to surface area ratio is low.
   b. their insulation is poor, resulting in increased water loss.
   * c. their renal concentrating ability is less than that of older children.
   d. the increased liquidity of the stools results in greater fluid loss.

6. The addition of iron to the diet of both formula-fed and breast-fed infants should begin by
   a. 6 weeks.
   * b. 4-6 months.
   c. 6-9 months.
   d. 1 year.

7. Breast milk does not provide the infant with adequate amounts of
   a. vitamin C.
   b. niacin.
   * c. vitamin D.
   d. vitamin A.

8. The introduction of semi-solid and strained foods to the infant's diet is recommended at
   a. 6-8 weeks.
   b. 2-4 months.
   * c. 4-6 months.
   d. 6-8 months.

9. The appropriate serving size for foods offered to a small child is
   a. a teaspoon for each year of age.
   * b. a tablespoon for each year of age.
   c. one-half cup of each food served.
   d. one cup total.

10. The digestion of starch requires pancreatic amylase, which is known to reach adult levels
    a. at 28-32 weeks of gestation.
    b. at birth.
    c. after 4 weeks of age.
    * d. after 6 months of age.

11. Using only cow's milk to feed infants is contraindicated because it is
    a. too low in fat and protein.
    b. too high in fat and protein.
 * c. hard to digest and increases the renal solute load.
    d. hard to digest and decreases the renal solute load.

12. The nutrients requiring earliest supplementation in the breast-fed infant are
 * a. fluoride and vitamin D.
    b. iron and magnesium.
    c. vitamin C.
    d. all fat-soluble vitamins.

13. The reduced incidence of infections seen in breast-fed infants occurs because
    a. human milk is higher in fat.
 * b. human milk has antiinfective factors.
    c. commercial infant formula is higher in iron.
    d. commercial infant formula is higher in fat.

14. The infant's protein requirements are
    a. lower on a per kilogram basis than those of the older child.
    b. lower on a per kilogram basis than those of the adult.
 * c. higher on a per kilogram basis than those of the adult.
    d. the same on a per kilogram basis as those of the adult.

15. What is the recommendation for vitamin supplementation of infants fed commercially prepared formula?
 * a. It is rarely needed.
    b. Supplement all vitamins.
    c. Only water-soluble vitamins should be supplemented.
    d. Only fat-soluble vitamins should be supplemented.

16. Compared to mature human milk, colostrum has
    a. more fat and carbohydrate but less protein.
 * b. less fat and carbohydrate but more protein.
    c. more fat but less carbohydrate and protein.
    d. less fat but more carbohydrate and protein.

17. To reduce the risk of choking in an infant receiving solid foods, the caregiver should avoid feeding him
    a. cheese and pudding.
 * b. grapes and hot dogs.
    c. graham crackers and cheese.
    d. macaronia and cheese.

18. The use of low fat and nonfat milk for infants is
    a. appropriate for the overweight infant during the first year.
    b. appropriate for all infants during the first year.
 * c. inappropriate for infants during the first year.
    d. in appropriate for ill infants during the first 3 months of life.

19. To avoid the development of tooth decay in infants, the mother of a bottle-fed infant should be told to
    a. give the infant a bottle with fruit juice at bedtime.
    b. give the infant a bottle with milk at bedtime.
 * c. put the infant to bed without a bottle.
    d. give the infant a bottle with milk at bedtime if the infant is fussy.

CHAPTER

11

NUTRITION IN THE CARE OF THE LOW-BIRTH-WEIGHT INFANT

OVERVIEW

The purpose of this chapter is to provide an understanding of the complex needs of the infant born prematurely. The specific physiological problems related to immaturity and their resulting nutritional implications are presented. The chapter provides an in-depth review of the use of parenteral nutrition in the feeding of premature infants. The transition to feeding enterally is discussed, and the use of a variety of enteral feeding methods is included. The chapter concludes with the growth and nutritional assessment techniques recommended for premature infants.

LEARNING OBJECTIVES

This chapter will prepare the learner to be able to

1. Define low birth weight (LBW), very low birth weight (VLBW), extremely low birth weight (ELBW), small for gestational age (SGA), premature, postterm, intrauterine growth retardation (IUGR), appropriate for gestational age (AGA), and large for gestational age (LGA).
2. Identify the metabolic concerns for the premature infant.
3. Explain the rationale for using parenteral nutrition in the premature infant.
4. State the nutritional guidelines for fluid, energy, glucose, amino acids, lipid, vitamins, minerals, electrolytes, and trace elements for parenteral feeding of premature infants.
5. Explain the criteria for making the transition from parenteral feedings to enteral feedings.
6. State the nutritional guidelines for energy, protein, lipid, carbohydrate, and vitamins and minerals for enteral feeding of premature infants.
7. Describe the methods of delivering an enteral feeding to the premature infant.
8. Identify appropriate volume and composition of enteral feedings for premature infants.
9. Identify the appropriate references for growth and nutritional assessment of the premature infant.

| CHAPTER OUTLINE | NOTES, TERMS, & TRANSPARENCY MASTERS |

CHAPTER OUTLINE

NOTES, TERMS, & TRANSPARENCY MASTERS

I. Characteristics of Low-Birth-Weight Infants
   A. Gestational age and size

Figure 11-1 (Handout) illustrates the criteria for classification of newborns based on maturity and intrauterine growth.
low-birth-weight (LBW), very low birth weight (VLBW), extremely low birth weight (ELBW), small for gestational age (SGA), premature, postterm, intrauterine growth retardation (IUGR), appropriate for gestational age (AGA), large for gestational age (LGA)

   B. Infant mortality
   C. Problems of immaturity

Figure 11-2 is a photograph of an infant born at 27 weeks gestation weighing 870 g. The picture shows the complex medical support given to these infants.
Table 11-1 is a list of the problems commonly seen in premature infants.

II. Smaller Metabolic Reserves

Table 11-2 lists the expected length of survival for infants in starvation and semi-starvation based on birth weight.

III. Parenteral Nutrition
   A. Fluid

necrotizing enterocolitis, bronchopulmonary dysplasia, intraventricular hemorrhage, patent ductus arteriosus (PDA)

   B. Energy

Table 11-3 shows a comparison of the energy needs of premature infants on parenteral and enteral feedings.

   C. Glucose

Table 11-4 lists the guidelines and gives the formula for determining glucose load for premature infants.
glucose load

   D. Amino acids

Table 11-5 provides the guidelines for using of parenteral amino acids for premature infants.
metabolic acidosis, hyperammonaemia, azotemia

   E. Lipid

Table 11-6 provides the guidelines for using parenteral lipids for premature infants.
kernicterus, carnitine

   F. Electrolytes

Table 11-7 provides the guidelines for using parenteral electrolytes for premature infants.

G. Minerals

Table 11-8 provides guidelines for using parenteral minerals for premature infants.
osteopenia of prematurity

H. Trace elements

Table 11-9 provides guidelines for the use of parenteral trace elements for premature infants.

I. Vitamins

Table 11-10 provides guidelines for the use of parenteral vitamins for premature infants.
inositol

IV. Transition from Parenteral to Enteral Nutrition

V. Enteral Nutrition

Table 11-11 summarizes indications for initiating or advancing enteral feedings by category and associated factors.

A. Requirements
    1. Energy

Table 11-12 lists the energy estimates for enterally fed premature infants.

    2. Protein
        a. amount
        b. type

whey protein, taurine

    3. Lipid
        a. amount
        b. type

linoleic acid, linolenic acid, arachidonic acid

medium-chain triglycerides

    4. Carbohydrate
        a. amount
        b. type

lactose, sucrose, glucose polymers, glucosidase enzymes

    5. Minerals and vitamins

Table 11-13 summarizes the recommendations for vitamin use in enterally fed premature infants.

        a. calcium and phosphorus
        b. vitamin D
        c. vitamin E
        d. iron
        e. folic acid
        f. sodium

osteopenia of prematurity

hemolytic anemia

B. Methods of feeding
    1. Gastric gavage
    2. Transpyloric feeding
    3. Nipple feeding
    4. Breastfeeding

oral gavage, nasal gastric gavage

C. Volume of feedings

D. Tolerance of feedings   **abdominal distention, gastric residuals**

E. Composition of feedings
    1. Human milk   **human milk fortifiers**

    2. Premature infant formulas   **Table 11-14** provides a comparison of human milk
                                                  and standard and premature commercial infant
                                                  formulas for several nutrients.

F. Selection of feeding
G. Formula manipulation
    1. Concentration of formulas
    2. Caloric supplements

VI. Growth and Nutritional Assessment
    A. Growth rates and charts   **Figure 11-3** shows the Hall Growth Chart, com-
                                                  monly used to assess weight progress of a pre-
                                                  mature infant during the first 40 days of life.
                                                  Figure 11-4 shows a growth chart having a built-
                                                  in correction factor for prematurity. It provides
                                                  for 1 year of life based on corrected age.
                                                  Table 11-15 presents a method for adjusting
                                                  growth charts to accommodate prematurity in
                                                  the infant being assessed.
                                                  Figure 11-5 shows the use of the NCHS Growth
                                                  Charts to assess growth of a premature child
                                                  up through age 10 years.

    B. Laboratory indices

VII.   Discharge Care

VIII.   Neurodevelopmental Outcome   **Figure 11-6** includes two photographs of the child
                                                 whose growth was assessed in Figure 11-5.
                                                 The pictures were taken at ages 3-1/2 and 10
                                                 years of age.

CASE STUDY INSIGHTS

1. *On day 2 of life, this infant's intravenous fluid should volume be*
    a. *increased because the infant requires more calories.*
*   b. *decreased because the infant is over-hydrated.*
    c. *changed to enteral feedings because the infant is clinically stable.*

    The infant's intravenous fluid volume should be decreased because the infant is overhydrated (choice b).
The weight gain and poor urine output are indicators that the fluid may need to be restricted. Also, the
diagnosis is made that the baby has patent ductus arteriosus, another indicator for fluid reduction.

2. Intravenous fat should be provided to this premature infant
    a. using a 10% emulsion.
    b. using a 20% emulsion.
    c. using a 24-hour infusion.
*   d. both b and c.

Intravenous fat should be provided by using a 20% emulsion and a 24-hour infusion (choice d). The use of 20% lipid emulsions has been shown to have less risk of increasing plasma triglycerides, phospholipids, and cholesterol than do 10% lipid emulsions. Using a 24-hour infusion prevents an elevation in triglycerides and free fatty acids.

3. Milk from this premature infant's mother may be inadequate in
    a. fat.
*   b. calcium.
    c. anti-infective factors.
    d. taurine.

Calcium may be inadequate (choice b). The premature infant has increased requirements for calcium and phosphorus for bone mineralization. The normal calcium content of human milk does not meet this increased need sufficiently.

4. What nutritional supplementation should be added to this mother's milk?
    a. None, since human milk is nutritionally adequate for this premature infant.
    b. Human milk fortifier.
    c. Iron.
*   d. Human milk fortifier and iron.

Human milk fortifier and iron should be added (choice d). Since the infant is premature, calcium needs are increased (see question #3) and iron stores are inadequate. The frequent blood draws for biochemical analyses also contribute to a decrease in iron. Using a human milk fortifier with iron provides the infant with the necessary nutrients that are not provided by breast milk.

SUGGESTED TEST QUESTIONS

1. In caring for the low-birth-weight (LBW) infant, which of these is a preventable route of fluid loss?
    a. increased insensible water loss due to increased permeability of the skin
*   b. increased insensible water loss due to radiant warmers
    c. decreased ability of the kidneys to concentrate urine
    d. larger surface area relative to body weight

2. The initial fluid intake for the first day of life of an LBW infant is
    a. 50-100 mL/kg/day.
*   b. 80-105 mL/kg/day.
    c. 500 mL/day.
    d. 1000 mL/day.

3. Additional fluid may be lost in the premature infant who has also developed
    a. hypoglycemia.
    b. hypercholesterolemia.
*   c. hyperglycemia.
    d. hypovolemia.

4. Compared to the premature infant fed enterally, the premature infant fed parenterally
* a. requires less energy per kg body weight.
   b. requires an equal amount of energy per kg body weight.
   c. requires more energy per kg body weight.
   d. has very erratic energy requirements.

5. Enteral feedings for the LBW infant are important and should be initiated as soon as possible because enteral feedings
* a. promote bile flow.
   b. can always meet needs within 2 weeks.
   c. increase small villous growth in the small intestine.
   d. decrease intestinal enzymatic activity.

6. A possible complication of using large amounts of fat (60% or greater) in the feedings for LBW infants is
* a. ketosis.
   b. hypoglycemia.
   c. hypercholesterolemia.
   d. hypernatremia.

7. As the preterm infant is able to tolerate increasing amounts of fat and iron preparations, there is a concurrent increase in the need for
   a. vitamin A.
   b. vitamin C.
   c. vitamin D.
* d. vitamin E.

8. The preterm infant's renal immaturity and decreased ability to concentrate urine make it necessary to monitor sodium concentration in
   a. the stool and urine.
* b. the urine or serum.
   c. the urine.
   d. the serum.

9. In the preterm infant with an oral gastric gavage using the intermittent bolus technique, gastric distention may lead to vagal nerve stimulation, which can increase the incidence of
   a. hypertension.
   b. tachypnea.
* c. bradycardia.
   d. tachycardia.

10. Low-birth-weight infants receiving enteral feedings who are observed to have vomited should be evaluated for
   a. a too rapid increase in feeding volume.
   b. excessive feeding volume for their size and maturity.
   c. possible systemic illness.
* d. all of the above.

11. The abdominal circumference of the infant can be measured to help detect
* a. abdominal distention.
   b. portal vein hypertension.
   c. hepatomegaly.
   d. bowel activity.

12. The LBW infant receiving an enteral feeding by bolus technique should have gastric residuals checked
   a. 1 hour after each feeding.
* b. before each feeding.
   c. once each day at the same time.
   d. before an increase in feeding volume is initiated.

13. Low birth weight (LBW) is defined as a baby weighing
* a. <2500 g at birth.
   b. <1500 g at birth.
   c. <2500 g at 3 months after birth.
   d. <1500 g at 3 months after birth.

14. The recommended energy intake for an enterally fed LBW infant is
   a. 100 kcal/kg/day.
   b. 50-60 kcal/kg/day.
   c. 90-120 kcal/kg/day.
* d. 120-130 kcal/kg/day.

15. The risk of hyperglycemia associated with giving glucose in the parenteral nutrition formula can be reduced by administering glucose
* a. with amino acids.
   b. alone.
   c. with fat.
   d. with amino acids and fat.

16. As the LBW infant is transitioned from par-
    enteral to enteral feedings, the procedure is to
    a. advance it as quickly as possible.
    b. begin full volume enteral feeding.
    c. stop parenteral feeding, then begin enteral
        feeding.
*   d. maintain parenteral feeding until enteral
        feeding is well established.

17. The osteopenia of prematurity is most likely to
    occur in preterm infants being fed human milk
    not supplemented with
    a. protein.
*   b. calcium and phosphorus.
    c. vitamins A and D.
    d. the fat soluble vitamins.

18. The premature baby may have a high intrinsic
    need for folic acid because she
*   a. grows at a more rapid rate then the term
        infant.
    b. stores less folic acid than the term infant.
    c. grows at a slower rate then the term infant.
    d. cannot store folic acid.

19. The energy needs of parenterally fed LBW
    infants are less than those fed enterally because
*   a. absorptive loss does not occur when nutri-
        tional intake bypasses the intestinal tract.
    b. absorptive loss is less when nutritional
        intake bypasses the intestinal tract.
    c. the liver has better access to nutrients
        delivered parenterally .
    d. the liver has less access to nutrients
        delivered parenterally.

20. The IV fat emulsion being administered to an
    LBW infant should
    a. exceed 40% of total calories.
*   b. not exceed 40% of total calories.
    c. comprise 10-15% of total calories.
    d. comprise 5% of total calories.

21. The supplemental use of carnitine is currently
    under investigation because of its role in
    a. surfactant synthesis.
*   b. fatty acid transport into the mitochondria
        for oxidation.
    c. prevention of hyperbilirubinemia.
    d. preventing metabolic acidosis.

CHAPTER 12

NUTRITION IN CHILDHOOD

OVERVIEW

The purpose of this chapter is to extend the foundation set in previous chapters for nutritional support of normal growth and development. In addition to identifying nutrient requirements, the chapter also provides information on the evolving skills of the child and how these relate to food and food intake. The relationship of childhood diets to development of disease is included. The chapter concludes with a presentation of the problems common in the early childhood years that have a nutrition-related concern.

LEARNING OBJECTIVES

This chapter will prepare the learner to be able to

1. Identify normal growth patterns for children.
2. Explain how children respond to delays in normal growth and development.
3. State the recommended methods for assessing growth in children.
4. Identify the nutritional needs of children for all nutrients included in the Recommended Dietary Allowances (RDA).
5. Identify the nutrients most likely to be deficient in a child's diet and explain why.
6. Describe how the eating habits of children are likely to change as they grow older.
7. Explain how a child's eating habits are influenced by family environment, societal trends, media, peer influences, and the presence of illness or disease.
8. Identify how the diets of children can relate to the development of diseases in adulthood.

CHAPTER OUTLINE ——————————— **NOTES, TERMS, & TRANSPARENCY MASTERS**

I. Growth and Development
   A. Physical growth   **adiposity rebound**
      1. Catch-up growth
      2. Assessing growth   **Figure 12-1** shows the growth pattern of a boy who had an excessive weight gain at age 8 years and a girl who had a significant weight loss at age 2 years. Both patterns are illustrated on the NCHS Growth Charts.

II. Nutrient Needs
    A. Energy

Table 12-1 lists the current RDA for protein and energy for children ages 1 through 10 years.

    B. Protein

See **Table 12-1.**

    C. Minerals and vitamins

Refer to **Table 16-1** in Chapter 16 for the RDA for minerals and vitamins.
Figure 12-2 is a photograph of a preschool child drinking milk.

       1. Vitamin and mineral supplements

III. Providing an Adequate Diet

Table 12-2 is a summary of Piaget's theory of cognitive development and how it specifically relates to feeding and nutrition. It recognizes developmental periods and cognitive characteristics.

    A. Patterns of intake

    B. Factors influencing food intake
       1. Family environment

Figure 12-3 is a set of photographs of a Chinese family eating together. The importance of making mealtime a family event is emphasized.

       2. Societal trends
       3. Media messages
       4. Peer influence
       5. Illness or disease

    C. Feeding the preschool child

Table 12-3 presents a feeding guide for preschool children from ages 2 through 6 years. The guide includes recommended foods, portion sizes, and number of total servings per day.

       1. Group feeding

Figure 12-4 is a photograph of several young children eating together.

    D. Feeding the School-Age Child

Figure 12-5 is a photograph of three elementary school children preparing their own snack after school.
Figure 12-6 is a photograph showing a variety of nutritious snacks for school-aged children.

IV. Preventing Chronic Disease

National Cholesterol Education Program (NCEP)

V. Nutritional Concerns

    A. Obesity

Key concept: Obesity management in children must maintain a primary objective of meeting needs for normal growth and development.

B. Underweight and failure to thrive
C. Iron deficiency
D. Dental caries
E. Allergies
F. Attention-deficit hyperactivity disorder

Key concept: The role of salicylates, artificial flavorings and colorings, and sugar in the development of hyperactivity has not been validated. However, a diet with reduced intakes of these compounds would not be harmful if parents choose to implement such a diet.
attention-deficit hyperactivity disorder (ADHD)

VI. Nutrition Education

CASE STUDY INSIGHTS

1. What recommendations should be made to prevent relapse for BJ?

BJ has been making good progress. He should be monitored for continued weight loss. The goal for BJ should be to slow or eliminate weight gain while allowing time for an increase in height. If his behavior changes are continued, he should be able to avoid a relapse. He is now playing soccer but will need to have other activities when the soccer season is over. Plans for summer childcare should also be made with his needs in minds. Additional concerns are whether he has made friends and whether psychological counseling may be of use due to the divorce.

2. What other activities can BJ try to reduce the tendency to overeat?

Answers will vary. If he has made friends, there are a number of activities that he could do, such as bicycling and roller blading. Any similar activities typical for his age should be encouraged. He could also walk or ride his bike to school and to after-school activities.

3. How can his mother alter some favorite recipes to lower fat (e.g., his favorite meal is fried chicken with gravy, french fries, and pecan pie)?

There are many resources available for lower fat recipes. His favorite meal could be changed to baked chicken, gravy made with broth instead of pan drippings, and oven-browned potatoes instead of french fries. It will be difficult to reduce the fat in the pecan pie given its normal ingredients. Perhaps it could be a special treat that is allowed occasionally. BJ needs to learn how to deal with all types of foods in all settings.

SUGGESTED TEST QUESTIONS

1. To assess the growth of a child, appropriate general guidelines for measurements include which of these?
   a. Growth measurements should be made at 1, 4, and 10 years.
   b. Once the child's channel on the growth charts has been determined, it is not necessary to reevaluate on a regular basis.
   * c. Growth measurements of height, weight, and weight for height should be measured at regular intervals.
   d. Once the growth pattern is established, it will not vary until adolescence.

2. Children in the United States are not likely to suffer from protein deficiency because
   a. their protein needs are minimal.
   b. most parents are well educated about protein sources in the diet.
   c. the body can provide protein when the diet does not.
   * d. there is a cultural emphasis on protein foods in the diet.

3. A preschool child aged 1 to 3 years may be at risk for a deficiency of
   * a. iron.
   b. vitamin E.
   c. vitamin B.
   d. vitamin D.

4. The recommendations from the American Academy of Pediatrics on the use of supplements for children are that
   a. routine multiple vitamin and mineral supplements should be given.
   * b. no routine supplementation is needed except for fluoride in nonfluoridated areas.
   c. maximal doses of vitamins and minerals should be given because it is uncertain that children will eat enough of the nutrients in food.
   d. supplements should not be restricted because they are growing so rapidly that overdosing is unlikely.

5. Children between 1 and 3 years of age are likely to
   a. increase their milk consumption.
   * b. decrease vegetable consumption and increase consumption of sweets.
   c. stop eating meat such as ground beef and hot dogs.
   d. decrease their intake of starches.

6. The most successful method of feeding a preschool child is to
   a. provide three meals at scheduled intervals with an evening snack.
   b. provide the largest meal at breakfast and two other small meals.
   c. avoid scheduled meals and make preferred food available when the child is hungry.
   * d. provide small servings several times a day at scheduled meals and at snacks.

7. A child drinking large amounts of apple or pear juice throughout the day and limited amounts of water or milk may be at risk for
   * a. diarrhea.
   b. hypervitaminosis A.
   c. overhydration.
   d. constipation.

8. The outcome of a zinc deficiency in a child's diet may be
   a. increased fat stores.
   * b. short stature.
   c. chronic diarrhea.
   d. mental retardation.

9. During the nutritional assessment of a preschool child, an iron deficiency may be suspected if it is discovered that the child
   * a. continues to drink large quantities of milk.
   b. has a decreased appetite noted after the first birthday.
   c. shows a preference for meat.
   d. is consuming small amounts of food several times a day.

10. Appropriate dietary modification for reducing the development of dental caries in children includes
   a. eliminating all sucrose from their diets.
 * b. providing sucrose-containing foods along with protein foods.
   c. allowing sweets as desired but following each snack with dental hygiene.
   d. restricting children to three balanced meals per day.

11. The risk of an inadequate protein intake increases for children who
   a. are underweight.
   b. follow lacto-ovovegetarian diets.
   c. have low energy needs.
 * d. follow strict vegan diets and have limited food selection.

12. Carbohydrate malabsorption and chronic non-specific diarrhea in healthy children have been linked to the ingestion of
   a. sweet and salty snacks.
   b. fruits and vegetables.
   c. milk and milk products.
 * d. excessive amounts of fruit juices, particularly pear and apple.

13. To enhance the absorbability of nonheme iron sources, meals should contain
 * a. an increase in ascorbic acid, meat, fish, and poultry.
   b. a decrease in ascorbic acid, meat, and fish.
   c. an increase in milk and eggs.
   d. an increase in fruits and eggs.

14. Scientific research using controlled double-blind studies to validate the Feingold hypothesis has
   a. supported the theory that sugar causes hyperactivity.
 * b. not supported the theory that hyperactivity results from sensitivity to artificial colors and flavors in most children.
   c. supported the theory that additives cause hyperactivity.
   d. supported the theory that artificial colors and flavors can cause hyperactivity.

15. Children at risk for having a zinc intake lower than the recommended level are those who
 * a. do not like many meats or seafoods.
   b. do not receive zinc supplements.
   c. drink too much milk.
   d. do not like many vegetables.

16. The most accurate method for determining the energy requirements of a child is based on
   a. growth rates.
   b. age and height.
   c. age.
 * d. calories per kilograms or per centimeters of height.

CHAPTER

NUTRITION IN ADOLESCENCE

OVERVIEW

The purpose of this chapter is to provide the basic nutritional guidelines and concerns unique to the adolescent. The normal physiological changes associated with puberty are presented, along with the role of psychological factors. The Recommended Dietary Allowances (RDA) for ages 11 through 24 years are presented, as well as suggestions for numbers of servings from the basic food groups. The nutrients most likely to be deficient are identified. The nutrition-related concerns of adolescence, including eating disorders, acne, and behavioral problems, are reviewed.

LEARNING OBJECTIVES

This chapter will prepare the learner to be able to

1. Identify the normal physiological changes associated with adolescence.
2. Describe the methods appropriate for assessment of growth.
3. Explain the role of sexual maturity in assessing the growth of adolescents.
4. Identify the normal psychological changes associated with adolescence.
5. Identify the nutritional needs of adolescents for all nutrients included in the RDA.
6. List the nutrients most likely to be deficient in the diet of an adolescent.
7. State the most common nutrition-related problems of adolescence and the recommended management for each.

CHAPTER OUTLINE

NOTES, TERMS, & TRANSPARENCY MASTERS

I. Growth and Development
   A. Physiological changes

       1. Assessment of growth
       2. Sexual maturity rating

Figure 13-1 is a graphic illustration of the velocity of growth in height for boys and girls from age 1 to 18 years.

Figure 13-2 represents a time line that shows the height spurt in relation to other events at puberty. Both boys and girls are represented.

Table 13-1 lists five stages of physical indicators of sexual maturity. The stages are given for both boys and girls.

B. Psychological changes

   1. Body image

II. Nutritional Requirements
  A. Recommendations to support growth

   1. Energy

   2. Protein
   3. Minerals

   4. Vitamins

  B. Potential nutritional inadequacies

III. Food Habits

IV. Situations with Specialized Needs
  A. Pregnancy
  B. Eating disorders
   1. Anorexia nervosa
   2. Bulimia nervosa
   3. Obesity

  C. Hyperlipidemias
  D. Behavioral problems and delinquency
  E. Acne

V. Strategies for Improving Nutritional Well-Being
  A. Nutritional assessment
  B. Prerequisites for change

Table 13-2 lists the developmental tasks associated with age during adolescence.
tasks of adolescence

Figure 13-3 is a photograph of an older adolescent lifting weights.

Table 13-3 lists the current RDA for protein and energy for adolescent females and males, ages 11 through 24 years.

Figure 13-4 is a photograph of adolescent boys playing basketball.

calcium, iron, zinc, magnesium, iodine, phosphorus, copper, chromium, cobalt, fluoride

thiamin, riboflavin, niacin, vitamin D, vitamin A, vitamin E, vitamin C, vitamin B$_6$, folic acid

vitamin A, vitamin B$_6$, folate, riboflavin, iron, calcium, zinc, magnesium, copper, manganese, saturated fat, protein, sodium

Figure 13-5 is a photograph of an adolescent boy eating a hot dog.

Table 13-4 presents the recommended cut-off values for adolescents who are overweight or at risk for becoming overweight. The values are based on BMI using Quetelet's Index.

Table 13-5 is a list of the recommendations for daily eating for adolescents. The recommendations are based on four food groups and limited use of fats and sweets.

CASE STUDY 1 INSIGHTS: MALE ADOLESCENT

1. What suggestions would you make about Joe's breakfast and lunch meals?

Joe may not be receiving sufficient calories to support his daily activities. His breakfast and lunch are high in simple sugar. He should be encouraged to include more protein in his breakfast and lunch. He may want to plan healthy snacks, particularly before athletic events. He should be discouraged from skipping meals prior to wrestling events.

2. How much calcium does he need at age 17? If he drinks only one glass of milk each day, what percentage of his daily requirements is he missing?

At age 17, Joe requires 1200 mg of calcium per day. One cup of milk contains about 300 mg of calcium. If his diet is completely void of all other sources of calcium, this would create a 75% deficit. Students may need to be reminded about other sources of calcium.

3. What other nutrients might be low in Joe's diet? How can he change his diet to include the proper types of foods that he needs at this age?

Very little information is given about his dinner meal. More information is needed to assess adequacy. When making recommendations for changes to his diet, it is important that Joe be an active participant in the planning and that he realize his responsibility.

CASE STUDY 2 INSIGHTS: FEMALE ADOLESCENT

1. List at least four questions you would include in your assessment session with CR. Why would you include these questions?

Student responses will vary. One direction that questions may take is toward determining if an eating disorder is present or if CR is at risk for an eating disorder. According to the NCHS growth chart, she is on the 10th percentile for both height and weight for 14 years of age. A review of her growth history may be helpful. Other questions to ask may be related to her knowledge of food and nutrient content.

2. What are the particular nutritional requirements for a teenage girl in Tanner stage 1?

The nutritional requirements for a teenage girl in Tanner stage 1 correspond to the RDA for 11–14 years of age.

3. How would you address this girl's concern about meat and her desire to be a vegetarian?

You need to explain to CR the occurrence of fat in meat and other foods. If she is careful about her meat selections, she can still maintain a low-fat diet. She will also need to understand that excess calories contribute to weight gain, not just fat in the diet. She does not need to be discouraged from eating a vegetarian diet. However, she should be instructed on how to combine vegetable proteins to achieve nutritional adequacy.

4. How would you counsel this young person about her desire not to get fat?

Eating a well-balanced and varied diet along with regular exercise will allow her to maintain a healthy weight. It is important that she does not think that excess leanness is healthy and that she can correctly identify a normal weight.

5. What advice would you give this teen's parents on their interactions related to food?

This issue is related to the psychological factors associated with adolescence. Disagreeing with parents and asserting independence is common behavior for this age group. If C. R.'s parents are inclined to nag her or make her eating a major issue, she could respond with defiance, thus eating worse than she is now.

SUGGESTED TEST QUESTIONS

1. The growth experienced by a child during adolescence represents
   a. 50% of the adult height and 20% of the adult weight.
   b. 30% of the adult height and 30% of the adult weight.
   * c. 20% of the adult height and 50% of the adult weight.
   d. 10% of the adult height and 20% of the adult weight.

2. The greatest increase in height during puberty occurs
   * a. over the 18-24 month "growth spurt" period.
   b. continuously over the entire period.
   c. during the first year of puberty.
   d. primarily toward the end of puberty.

3. Based on the typical development of the 11- to 16-year-old child, during this period you can expect
   a. development of social intelligence and commitment to responsible citizenship.
   b. preparation for marriage and family.
   * c. development of conceptual and problem-solving, decision-making skills.
   d. selection of a vocation and preparing for that career.

4. Adolescents are most often at greatest risk for deficiency of
   a. vitamin D.
   * b. iron.
   c. vitamin C.
   d. potassium.

5. When assessing the pregnant adolescent, the concern for supplying enough nutrients to support the mother's own growth along with the growing fetus is valid for those who
   a. were well nourished prior to conception.
   b. sought medical care during pregnancy.
   * c. are of the lowest gynecological age.
   d. are below the desirable weight for age and height.

6. The weight status of most patients who are being treated for bulimia nervosa is
   a. greater than 20% below the desired weight for age and height.
   * b. close to that desired for age and height.
   c. usually well above the desired for age and height.
   d. generally not important in the assessment process.

7. A nutritional factor found to have the potential to exacerbate acne in the adolescent is
   a. excessive intake of chocolates.
   b. a diet high in fat.
   c. vitamin A deficiency.
   * d. zinc deficiency.

8. In assessing the nutritional status of adolescents, it must be kept in mind that
   * a. interpretation of data must be done using an age-specific data base.
   b. since there is relatively no risk for cardiovascular disease, this issue does not need to be addressed.
   c. they may be poor historians for supplying data.
   d. they will be interested in their nutritional status and eager to improve it.

9. The velocity of growth in height during adolescence compares with that of
   a. the first year of life.
   * b. the second year of life.
   c. the first 6 months of life.
   d. the fourth year of life.

10. To determine if weight is appropriate for height at a given age for a given gender, the data plotted on the NCHS Growth Charts should lie between the
   * a. 25th and 75th percentile.
   b. 10th and 30th percentile.
   c. 75th and 95th percentile.
   d. 5th and 25th percentile.

11. A condition dramatically characterized by binges and vomiting is
   a. anorexia nervosa.
   * b. bulimia nervosa.
   c. hyperemesis.
   d. hypermotility of the gastrointestinal tract.

12. In attempting to identify a relationship between the ingestion of food and the appearance of acne, scientific research has shown
   a. a strong correlation.
   * b. no correlation.
   c. a weak correlation.
   d. a strong correlation with certain foods.

13. When the medication Accutane is used in the treatment of acne, an expected side effect is
   a. weight loss.
   b. weight gain.
   * c. an increase in serum triglycerides and total cholesterol.
   d. a decrease in total cholesterol.

14. During the prepubertal period, the proportion of fat to muscle is
   * a. similar in males and females.
   b. greater in males than in females.
   c. less in females than in males.
   d. less in males than in females.

15. The correct interpretation of a low skinfold measurement in an adolescent whose weight is above the 75th percentile would be
   a. a state of overfat.
   * b. a state of overweight but not overfat.
   c. recent malnutrition.
   d. chronic malnutrition.

16. The effect of an adolescent's drive toward independence may be
   a. anorexia nervosa.
   b. a significant decline in dietary intake.
   c. a temporary rejection of family dietary patterns.
   * d. a significant increase in dietary intake.

17. The contribution of protein to an adolescent's diet of should be about what percentage of the total energy consumed?
   * a. 15–20%
   b. 7–8%
   c. 45%
   d. 20–30%

18. For the child who maintains a short stature during adolescence, the cause is most likely
   a. a poor intake of calories.
   b. a poor intake of calories and protein.
   * c. a genetically late initiation of puberty.
   d. the presence of anorexia nervosa.

NUTRITION IN AGING

LEARNING OBJECTIVES

This chapter will prepare the learner to be able to

1. Describe the concepts of longevity, life span, and life expectancy and the theories of aging.
2. Identify the physiological and psychological changes associated with the aging process.
3. Identify the nutritional needs of the elderly for all nutrients included in the Recommended Dietary Allowances (RDA).
4. State the principles of dietary planning for the elderly.
5. Describe community nutrition programs that are intended to provide nutritional support to the elderly.
6. Describe nutritional needs during prolonged illness in the elderly.
7. Identify the nutritional needs and concerns of the elderly who are institutionalized.
8. Explain the purpose and function of the Nutrition Screening Initiative.

CHAPTER OUTLINE ———————————— **NOTES, TERMS, & TRANSPARENCY MASTERS**

I. Longevity

                                               Figure 14-1 (Transparency) illustrates how the number of people age 65 years and older has increased since 1900 and is expected to continue to increase through the year 2030.

                                               elderly, life span, life expectancy

    A. Life span (maximum life span potential)

    B. Life expectancy

                                               Figure 14-2 is a photograph of an elderly man using a treadmill.

C. Theories of aging

program theory, error theories, cellular theories, free radicals, nutritional model

II. The Aging Process
  A. Sensory

Table 14-1 provides a list of the medical conditions that can alter the sense of taste.

  B. Oral health status

xerostomia

  C. Gastrointestinal

hypochlorhydria

  D. Metabolic
  E. Cardiovascular
  F. Renal
  G. Musculoskeletal

Table 14-2 is a reference for the interpretation of height and weight for people age 65–94 years.
sarcopenia

  H. Neurological
  I. Immunocompetence
  J. Psychological

III. Nutritional Requirements and Nutritional Status of the Elderly
  A. Energy
  B. Protein
  C. Carbohydrate
  D. Fat
  E. Minerals

Table 14-3 lists the current RDAs for people age 51 years and older.

  F. Vitamins

Key concept: The RDA currently does not differentiate nutritional needs after the first five decades of life.

  G. Water
  H. Nutritional status

Table 14-4 lists possible explanations for the undernutrition often seen in the elderly.

IV. Nutritional Care of the Elderly
  A. Dietary planning

Figure 14-3 is a photograph of a group of elderly people preparing a meal.

  B. Community nutrition programs

Title III of the Older Americans Act, Congregate and Home-Delivered Nutrition Programs for the Elderly, Meals on Wheels

  C. Nutritional needs during prolonged illness

V. Nutritional Care in Institutionalized Settings

Table 14-5 lists the issues that govern the regulation of nursing homes, as taken from the Omnibus Budget Reconciliation Act (OBRA) of 1987.

Table 14-6 is an overview of the multidisciplinary approach to assessing the geriatric individual in a nursing home.

Figure 14-4 is a photograph of several older people eating in an institutional setting.

VI. The Nutrition Screening Initiative

A. The six intervention areas

Healthy People 2000

Key concept: The six interdisciplinary interventions were identified by the Interventions Roundtable convened by the Nutritional Screening Initiative in 1992.

CASE STUDY INSIGHTS

1. *What recommendations do you have for monitoring Marion's diet, which influences her disease control so carefully?*

At home, Marion was able to select her own diet and meet the dietary recommendations for management of her medical condition. In the long-term care facility, her dietary needs should be given consideration by the dietitian; her diet prescription can also be met. Monitoring her medical condition (FBS, HgbA$_{1c}$, BUN, GFR, and BP) will be helpful in determining if her diet is successful.

2. *Since fluids are now a problem for her to swallow, what changes should be made to her trays sent to the facility dining room?*

The extent of her swallowing difficulties should be assessed by a feeding evaluation. Depending on the outcome of the evaluation, foods of appropriate consistency can be provided.

3. *Marion needs a snack in the afternoon and at bedtime to keep her blood sugars at the proper level. What are some suggestions that consider the need for thickened liquids, no added salt, no concentrated sweets, and a controlled protein diet?*

Finding foods that are consistent with the protein restriction is most challenging. Marion could have foods sweetened with artificial sweeteners, but the snacks need to have nutritive value for her diabetes control. A commercial adult formula may be the best alternative if blood glucose can be controlled.

SUGGESTED TEST QUESTIONS

1. Among the ten leading causes of death, the majority are closely associated with
 * a. diet or alcohol consumption.
   b. nondietary related malignancies.
   c. trauma.
   d. genetically determined bodily aging.

2. Effects of reducing weight to what is desirable for age, gender, and height may include a reduced risk of
   a. hypertension.
   b. cardiovascular disease.
   c. non-insulin-dependent diabetes mellitus.
 * d. all of the above.

3. In the normal aging process, changes that may adversely affect the patients' ability to take oral medications or follow prescribed diets are
   a. loss of hypoglossal control.
 * b. diminished sensitivity to sweet and salty taste.
   c. increased olfactory sense.
   d. increased salivation.

4. The atrophic gastritis of the stomach associated with aging may lead to
   a. decreased calcium and nonheme iron absorption.
 * b. increased absorption of vitamin B_{12}.
   c. decreased absorption of carbohydrates.
   d. increased transit time through the intestine.

5. Side effects reported by patients who are taking certain medications, such as for hypertension, may include
   a. increased hydrochloric acid production.
   b. decreased iron absorption.
 * c. xerostomia and decreased ability to masticate.
   d. decreased production of the intrinsic factor.

6. A dietary habit that may promote the decreasing kidney function associated with aging is
   a. increased vitamin C intake.
   b. decreased calcium intake.
   c. excessive intake of sucrose.
 * d. protein overnutrition.

7. Older adults are most likely to respond poorly to attempts to increase their protein intake when the protein is provided by
   a. legumes.
   b. red meats.
 * c. dairy products.
   d. fish.

8. The anemia seen in the elderly is most often a result of
   a. iron deficiency.
   b. poor dentition.
   c. decreased absorption of heme iron.
 * d. blood loss from the GI tract.

9. If a patient's signs and symptoms include impaired immune function, anorexia, delayed wound healing, dysgeusia, and pressure ulcers, you would suspect a deficiency of
   a. vitamin C.
 * b. zinc.
   c. potassium.
   d. vitamin B_{12}.

10. Population groups that have extended life spans also have which of these factors in common?
    a. nutrition and exercise
  * b. genetic factors and continued exercise
    c. nutrition and housing
    d. low fat diets and exercise

11. In the very old, the loss of endogenous opioids and exaggerated effects of cholecystokinin can result in
    a. weight loss.
    b. weight gain.
    c. decreased absorption of vitamin D.
  * d. anorexia.

12. The hypochlorhydria associated with the aging process can lead to
  * a. decreases in the absorption of calcium.
    b. increases in the absorption of calcium and heme iron.
    c. decreases in the absorption of fat.
    d. decreases in the absorption of the water-soluble vitamins.

13. A common complain in the elderly is constipation, which is often the result of
    a. increased motility in the small intestine.
    b. decreased motility in the small intestine.
  * c. decreased motility in the large intestine.
    d. increased motility in the large intestine.

14. In additional to decreased activity, the total energy needs of an individual between 30 and 90 years of age are affected by a 20% decrease in the basal metabolic rate because of a
  * a. decrease in lean body mass.
    b. increase in lean body mass.
    c. decrease in lean body mass and adipose tissue.
    d. increase in lean body mass and adipose tissue.

15. For an elderly person experiencing insulin sensitivity, improvement may occur by
    a. strictly adhering to a set number of food exchanges.
  * b. limiting the use of sugar and increasing complex carbohydrate and soluble fiber in the diet.
    c. decreasing the amount of carbohydrate and soluble fiber in the diet.
    d. carefully controlling total calorie intake.

16. Folate deficiency may be seen in the elderly in the absence of alcohol abuse because of
  * a. a diet lacking unprocessed, fresh, and nutrient-dense foods.
    b. drug-nutrient interactions.
    c. an increased intake of foods high in carbohydrate.
    d. chronic disease.

17. The current recommendation for adequate water intake in the elderly is
  * a. 30–35 mL/kg ideal body weight.
    b. 10–20 mL/kg ideal body weight.
    c. 40–50 mL/kg ideal body weight.
    d. 50–60 mL/kg ideal body weight.

NUTRITION IN THE COMMUNITY

OVERVIEW

The purpose of this chapter is to provide an expansive view of the role of the federal government and its agencies in meeting the food and nutritional needs of the nation. The chapter begins with identifying the sources of dietary and nutritional information available and how the information is used. The various nationally directed dietary recommendations that have evolved during the twentieth century are presented. The food and nutrition relief/support programs available to supplement needy individuals and families are covered next. The chapter concludes with an in-depth look at the issues related to providing a safe and adequate food supply.

LEARNING OBJECTIVES

This chapter will prepare the learner to be able to

1. Identify a variety of surveys used to monitor the nutritional status of the U.S. population.
2. List the major sets of dietary guidelines that have been developed and state their intent.
3. Identify the food assistance programs available for people otherwise unable to obtain adequate food.
4. Explain how the safety of the U.S. food supply is maintained.
5. Identify the regulatory agencies that are responsible for maintaining the safety of the food supply.
6. List the factors related to food safety that require monitoring.
7. Explain how agricultural residues are regulated in the food supply.

CHAPTER OUTLINE ———————————— NOTES, TERMS, & TRANSPARENCY MASTERS

I. Nutrition Food and Nutrition Data Sources

    A. National Health and Nutritional Examination Surveys

Table 15-1 is a summary of the recent food, nutrition, and health surveys, including the names of the surveys, timing, agencies, and purposes.

Figure 15-1 is a schematic drawing of the interrelationships of nutrition policy making, research, and monitoring.

NHANES, NHANES II, Hispanic HANES, NHANES III

    B. Nationwide Food Consumption Survey   **NFCS**

C. Continuing Survey of Food Intake of
    Individuals

Figure 15-2 (Transparency) compares the energy
    provided by carbohydrate, protein, and fat in
    the average American diet in 1977 and in 1985.
Focus On: Canadian Dietary Studies describes
    both methods and results of dietary data col-
    lection in Canada.
CSFII

D. National Nutrition Monitoring and Related
    Research Act

NNMRRA

E. Nutrition Screening Initiative

NSI

F. National Nutrient Data Bank

II. National Nutrition Guidelines and Goals

Table 15-2 is a historical list of the dietary recom-
    mendations for the U.S. public.

Table 15-3 lists the recommendations of the Sur-
    geon General's Report on Nutrition and Health.
**Food for Young Children; A Daily Food Guide;
    Food Guide Pyramid; Recommended
    Dietary Allowances; Dietary Guidelines for
    the United States; Dietary Guidelines for
    Americans; National Cholesterol Education
    Program (NCEP); Diet, Nutrition, and
    Cancer; Dietary Guidelines for Cancer
    Prevention; 5-A-Day Program for Better
    Health; Healthy People; Promoting
    Health/Preventing Disease: Objectives for
    the Nation; The Surgeon General's Report
    on Nutrition and Health**

A. *Healthy People 2000*

Key concept: *Healthy People 2000* provides spe-
    cific health directives intended to be complet-
    ed by the year 2000. This section provides
    examples of specific nutritional directives.

III. Food Assistance and Nutrition Programs

Table 15-4 is a list of the food programs adminis-
    tered by the USDA. The program and year ini-
    tiated, eligible individuals or groups, objec-
    tives of the program, and components of the
    program are given.

A. National School Lunch Program

School Breakfast Programs

B. Special Supplemental Food Program for
    Women, Infants, and Children
C. Food Stamp Program
D. Food Distribution and Nutritional
    Programs for Families and the Elderly

**Title III Elderly Nutrition Program of the
    Older Americans Act, Nutrition Education
    and Training Act (NET), Expanded Food
    and Nutrition Education Program (EFNEP)**

IV. Food Safety: Laws, Regulations, and Issues
  A. Technology and food safety

  B. Regulatory agencies

  C. Safety concerns

    1. Microbial contamination

    2. Natural toxins in food

    3. Intentional additives

      a. Approval procedure

      b. Foods Generally Recognized
         as Safe

      c. The Delaney Clause

      d. Food irradiation
      e. Nutraceuticals and functional
         foods
      f. Health claims
      g. Public attitudes
    4. Agricultural residues
      a. Pesticides

      b. Antibiotics
      c. Hormones

Table 15-5 is a historical list of the laws and rules that regulate U.S. food safety and quality.

Food and Drug Administration (FDA), Environmental Protection Agency (EPA), U.S. Department of Agriculture (USDA), Federal Trade Commission (FTC), Federal Communications Commission (FCC)

Table 15-6 lists toxic compounds found in naturally occurring substances, mostly foods, and their primary toxic effects.

Figure 15-3 illustrates the most common bacterial causes of foodborne illness.
Salmonella, Clostridium botulinum, Shigella, Staphylococcus, Campylobacter, Listeria moncytogenes, S. enteritidis, E. coli

safrole, solanine, aflatoxin

Table 15-7 is a list of the function of common food additives and their uses. Examples of foods containing such additives are given.

1985 Food Additives Amendment to the Food, Drug, and Cosmetic Act

GRAS

Delaney Clause of the Food Additives Amendment, doctrine of de minimis

1990 Nutrition Labeling and Education Act

Figure 15-4 is a photograph of an FDA employee monitoring residue levels of pesticides.
Table 15-8 presents the intake of selected pesticides found in diets in 1987.
acceptable daily intakes

estrogen diethylstilbestrol (DES), somatotropin, gonadotropin

CASE STUDY INSIGHTS

1. What suggestions do you have for Mrs. Ex as she reads labels and shops for her mother, whose income is limited?

Consideration should be given to being certain that Mrs. Ex understands the concept of nutrient density, how a nutrition label can be used to assess nutrient density, and other information would be helpful to her. She should be encouraged to avoided presweetened cereals. The use of frozen foods will need to be reviewed with her. They provide convenience, but they may not be affordable on a limited income and must be chosen with care for nutritional value.

2. Select a recipe for meatloaf and alter it slightly to add nutrient density. Test the recipe for flavor, appearance, and texture.

Nutrient density can be increased by using an egg and/or nonfat dried milk solids in the meatloaf and by using uncooked oatmeal in place of bread crumbs. Evaluation of the modified recipe should focus on nutrient value and palatability.

SUGGESTED TEST QUESTIONS

1. While *Salmonella, Shigella,* and *Staphylococcus* have long been recognized as major causes of food poisoning, the most frequent cause of bacterial diarrhea is
   a. *E. coli.*
   * b. *Campylobacter.*
   c. *Listeria.*
   d. *Clostridium botulinum.*

2. The process of irradiation of food has been introduced for the purpose of
   a. adding vitamin D.
   b. improving the flavor.
   c. removing the presence of insecticides and fumigants.
   * d. destroying insects and microorganisms.

3. The major function of the FDA in monitoring the food supply is for
   a. domestic food only.
   b. imported food only .
   * c. both domestic and imported food.
   d. farm produce only.

4. A patient concerned about the effect of growth hormone given to cattle in cooked meat should be told that

   * a. growth hormone from another species is not active in humans.
   b. growth hormone for cattle is not retained in the tissue.
   c. there is no evidence that bovine growth hormone absorbed by the intestine is harmful to humans.
   d. past experiments on bovine growth hormone have shown that it is not a benefit to meat or milk production.

5. Two antibiotics used in cattle to promote growth that are also used in humans to fight disease are
   a. cephalosporin and aminoglycoside.
   b. lincosamide and erythromycin.
   * c. tetracycline and penicillin.
   d. quinolone and aminoglycoside.

6. Information on nutrient intake and health status is made available through
   a. the National Nutrient Data Bank.
   * b. the National Health and Nutrition Examination Survey.
   c. the Nationwide Food Consumption Survey.
   d. the Continuing Survey of Food Intake of Individuals.

7. To qualify for federal cash reimbursement and food donations under the National School Lunch Program, a school must be
   a. located in a low income urban area.
   b. located in a low income rural area.
   * c. serving a lunch meeting specified nutritional requirements.
   d. serving at least 200 meals per day five days each week.

8. The organization responsible for regulating food and nutrition labeling is the
   a. USDA.
   b. FTC.
   * c. FDA.
   d. HHS.

9. Safrole, a flavoring agent from the sassafras root, cannot be used as a food additive because research has shown that is may be associated with
   a. food poisoning.
   b. bacterial infections.
   * c. liver cancer.
   d. food allergies.

10. The primary function of the Delaney Clause of the Food Additive Amendment is to prohibit the use of any substance shown to cause
    a. food allergies.
    b. cancer in animals.
    c. cancer in humans.
    * d. cancer in animals or humans.

11. The technology of microwave cooking poses safety concerns about
    * a. inadequate pathogen destruction because of irregular heating.
    b. exposure to the energy source.
    c. high energy usage involved.
    d. very high temperatures reached at the center of the food.

12. Food additives being used when the Food Additives Amendment was enacted and not required to be tested are classified as
    a. unintentional additives.
    * b. generally recognized as safe (GRAS).
    c. residues.
    d. incidental additives.

13. The use of hormones in cattle feed to promote growth is generally considered safe as long as residues do not occur
    * a. in meat and milk as they arrive at the marketplace.
    b. as they arrive at the packaging plant.
    c. at any time.
    d. in meat and milk after processing.

14. The most current nutritional recommendations from the USDA for daily dietary intake are presented in the
    a. Daily Good Guide.
    b. 5-A-Day Program for Better Health.
    * c. Food Guide Pyramid.
    d. Recommended Dietary Allowances.

15. The 1964 program that allows needy individuals and families to purchase reduced-price groceries is the
    a. Special Supplemental Food Program of Women, Infants, and Children.
    b. National School Lunch Program.
    * c. Food Stamp Program.
    d. Special Milk Program.

16. The use of health claims on product labels is regulated by the
    * a. 1990 Nutrition Labeling and Education Act.
    b. Federal Trade Commission.
    c. Federal Communication Commission.
    d. 1985 Fair Marketing Act.

17. An acceptable daily intake (ADI) is defined as
    a. amounts of vitamins and minerals believed to be safe but not included in the RDA.
    * b. the acceptable daily intake of a chemical that, if ingested over a lifetime, appears to be without appreciable risk.
    c. being similar to the GRAS list but not used in the same quantities.
    d. those food additives that can be added to foods without regulation.

CHAPTER 16

GUIDELINES FOR DIETARY PLANNING

OVERVIEW

The purpose of this chapter is to present both quantitative and qualitative requirements for nutrients for consumer and practitioner use. The Recommended Dietary Allowances (RDA) are the most quantitative of the references, although they include recommendations for only 19 nutrients. An additional 6 nutrients have Estimated Safe and Adequate Daily Dietary Intakes established. The Basic Four Food Groups and the Food Guide Pyramid are included along with an example of a modified Food Guide Pyramid for the Mediterranean diet. Additional cultural and religious dietary practices are presented. The chapter ends with the current nutrition labeling requirements and terminology.

LEARNING OBJECTIVES

This chapter will prepare the learner to be able to

1. Name the organizations responsible for the determination of nutrient needs.
2. Describe the evolution of the RDAs.
3. Describe the intent of the RDAs.
4. Define Estimated Safe and Adequate Daily Dietary Intakes.
5. State the difference between food consumption surveys and food monitoring reports.
6. Identify the food components that are public health issues.
7. Identify the diet- and alcohol-related causes of death.
8. Summarize the national guidelines for diet planning.
9. List the food groups in the Food Guide Pyramid and the recommended number of servings from each group.
10. Summarize the cultural and religious influences on dietary planning.
11. Identify foods required to have a nutrition label.
12. Define standard portion size.
13. Explain the criteria for making special dietary claims on product labels.

CHAPTER OUTLINE

I. Determining Nutrient Needs

   A. Recommended Dietary Allowances

     1. Definition

     2. Nature of Target Population
     3. Age–Sex Groups
     4. Reference Men and Women

   B. Estimated Safe and Adequate Daily Dietary Intakes

     1. Appropriate Use

     2. Future of the RDAs

II. Nutritional Status of Americans
   A. Food and nutrient intake data

   B. Status report from monitoring surveys
     1. 1987–1988 Nationwide Food Consumption Survey

NOTES, TERMS, & TRANSPARENCY MASTERS

Food and Agriculture Organization of the World Health Organization of the United Nations

Table 16-1 presents the 1989 RDAs, the most current at this time.
Table 16-2 is a summary of the evolution of the RDAs from 1941 to 1989.
RDA, Food and Nutrition Board (FNB) of the Institute of Medicine/National Academy of Sciences (IOM/NAS)

Key concept: The RDAs were developed for groups of people, not individuals. The recommended levels are intended to meet the known needs of practically all healthy people in the group.

Table 16-3 presents the median heights, weights, and recommended energy intake for individuals from birth to adulthood, including pregnancy and lactation.

Table 16-4 provides the six nutrients that the FNB makes recommendations for Estimated Safe and Adequate Daily Dietary Intakes (ESADDI).
Table 16-5 provides the recommendations for minimum estimated requirements of sodium, potassium, and chloride.

Table 16-6 provides the Recommended Nutrient Intakes (RNIs) for Canada. These are similar to the RDAs in the United States.

NFCS, NHANES

Department of Health and Human Services (DHHS), U.S. Department of Agriculture (USDA), Expert Panel on Nutrition Monitoring, Life Sciences Research Office

of the Federation of American Societies for Experimental Biology (FASEB), Continuing Survey of Food Intake of Individuals (CSII)

2. Nutrition Monitoring Report
   a. Food components constituting current public health issues
   b. Food components considered to be potential public health issues
   c. Nutrients not considered to be potential public health issues

III. National Guidelines for Diet Planning
   A. Current health issues

Table 16-7 lists the ten leading causes of death in the United States in 1991, including deaths related to diet and excessive intake of alcohol.

   B. Current guidelines for the United States and Canada

Table 16-8 summarizes of the most significant dietary guidelines that have been issued from 1977 to 1989.

IV. Implementing the Guidelines

Table 16-9 shows the guidelines in Table 16-8 as a composite to illustrate how the recommendations overlap.
Figure 16-1 (Handout) shows the Food Guide Pyramid developed by the USDA.
Figure 16-2 (Handout) shows an adaptation of the Food Guide Pyramid for application to the healthy Mediterranean diet.

V. Cultural Aspects of Dietary Planning
   A. Dietary patterns of southeast Asians

Table 16-10 summarizes the foods and preparation methods of Cambodian, Laotian, and Vietnamese diets.

   B. Dietary restrictions and patterns of religious groups
   1. Jewish food customs and dietary laws
   2. Muslim religious dietary code
   3. Dietary patterns from Oriental nations

Table 16-11 summarizes the foods and preparation methods of Chinese and Japanese diets.

   4. Hispanic dietary patterns

Table 16-12 summarizes the foods and preparation methods of Cuban and Spanish-American-Mexican diets.

   5. Mediterranean dietary patterns

Table 16-13 summarizes the food and preparation methods of Greek diets.

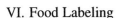

VI. Food Labeling

Figure 16-3 (Handout) illustrates the current food label format.

Table 16-14 provides a glossary of food labeling terminology.

Table 16-15 lists the Daily Reference Values (DRVs) used in food labeling.

Table 16-16 lists the Reference Daily Intakes (RDIs) used in food labeling.

A. Food products covered by new food label

B. Standardized serving sizes

C. Nutritional value and how food fits into the total diet   **Daily Value (DV)**

D. Standardized terms for nutrient content   **reduced sodium fat-free, low-calorie, healthy, lean, extra lean**

E. Appropriate health claims   **Key concept:** Health claims cannot appear on any foods that provide more than 20% of the Daily Value for fat.

CASE STUDY INSIGHTS

1. Discuss a dietary plan, following strict Kosher protocols, that would meet Marty's daily needs for calcium and magnesium without supplemental capsules.

The inclusion of a supplement of calcium and magnesium is not necessary if Marty's diet is well balanced. If he is not including milk and dairy foods in his diet, his diet must be carefully planned to include foods that do provide absorbable calcium. His intake of vegetables should provide adequate intakes of magnesium.

2. What suggestions would you offer him about dietary guidelines for a healthy heart?

A vegetarian diet tends to be naturally low in fat and saturated fat. This is more significant in the avoidance of cardiovascular disease, along with maintaining a normal weight. In developing a diet plan, emphasis should be on low-fat foods. If he is including eggs in his diet, he may be consuming appreciable amounts of cholesterol. A serum cholesterol should be determined (total, LDL-C, and HDL-C) and a history obtained to assess Marty's risk for disease.

3. What special requirements does an athlete need, and do they conflict with a Kosher dietary plan?

An athlete's nutritional needs are determined by the type of exercise performed, including intensity and duration. He needs to ensure adequate intake of calories and protein, along with B vitamins related to energy metabolism. If the weather is hot or he experiences excess sweating, minerals should be evaluated. There would be no conflict with his Kosher practices.

4. What impact does a vegetarian life-style have on a person following Kosher guidelines? Are there any special considerations?

A vegetarian diet can actually make following a Kosher diet easier. The dietary law forbidding the eating of meat and milk in the same meal or prepared with the same utensils would be easily met with the exclusion of meat from the diet.   ·

5. Discuss the new food label requirements as related to your client's dietary plan.

Marty is concerned about calcium intake. He can use food labels to help him determine calcium content of foods. He can also use the labels to determine fat content, a recommendation for decreasing risk of cardiovascular disease.

SUGGESTED TEST QUESTIONS

1. The RDAs are best described as
* a. the recommendations for the average amounts of nutrients that should be consumed daily by healthy people.
   b. the guidelines for individuals who may have experienced a period of inadequate intake.
   c. the minimum amounts that must be ingested on a daily basis to prevent malnutrition.
   d. the recommendations that have been calculated to be adequate in all states of health.

2. Nutritional labeling is intended to be used by consumers to make wise food choices and can be found on
* a. most all foods except ready-to-eat.
   b. foods that the manufacturer chooses to put them on.
   c. foods to which nutrients such as vitamins and minerals have been added.
   d. foods imported from others countries.

3. When evaluating purchased foods, the consumer should know that
   a. every nutrient in the prepared food must be listed.
   b. only protein, carbohydrates, and vitamins must be listed.

   c. information about sodium, cholesterol, and saturation of fat may be included at the option of the manufacturer.
* d. nutrition information on raw foods remains voluntary.

4. The RDAs should be used to assess the average amounts of nutrients that should be consumed
* a. daily over a period of time by healthy people.
   b. weekly by healthy people.
   c. daily over a period of time by healthy and ill people.
   d. weekly by healthy and ill people.

5. The consumer can rely on most of the RDAs to be
   a. estimated averages based on data from surveillance studies.
   b. actual measurements obtained from WHO studies.
   c. actual measurements obtained from the Ten State Survey.
* d. established at levels exceeding the requirements of most individuals.

6. Data collected from dietary surveys in general reveal that most energy intakes
   a. exceed recommendations.
   * b. do not exceed recommendations.
   c. are significantly higher than recommendations.
   d. are significantly lower than recommendations.

7. The data from surveys monitoring eating patterns of consumers in the United States suggest that most individuals are
   a. not interested in making changes.
   b. eating more saturated fat and cholesterol.
   * c. making an effort to eat less saturated fat and cholesterol.
   d. unaware of suggested dietary changes.

8. The most widespread nutrient deficiency observed in this country is lack of
   a. protein.
   b. calcium.
   * c. iron.
   d. vitamin C.

9. The Dietary Guidelines for Americans were developed by the
   a. FDA.
   b. WHO.
   * c. USDA and USDHHS.
   d. NCI.

10. To reduce the risk of cancer, the NCI Cancer Guidelines suggest that individuals consume a diet with a total fat intake of
    * a. 30% of calories or less.
    b. 10% of calories or less.
    c. 20% of calories or less.
    d. 40–45% of calories.

11. According to the Food Guide Pyramid, the recommended daily intake of bread, cereal, rice, and pasta is
    a. 4 or more servings.
    b. 4–6 servings.
    * c. 6–11 servings.
    d. 8–12 servings.

12. For nutrients known to be essential but for which evidence is insufficient to determine an RDA, guidelines have been developed called
    a. Recommended Daily Intakes.
    * b. Estimated Safe and Adequate Daily Dietary Intakes.
    c. Minimum Daily Intake.
    d. Estimated Dietary Minimums.

13. Among the ten leading causes of death, at least how many are related to diet or excessive intake of alcohol?
    a. two
    b. four
    * c. six
    d. eight

14. The main staple in the diet of southeast Asians is
    a. potatoes.
    b. wheat.
    c. legumes.
    * d. rice.

15. The traditional process of "koshering" meat and poultry is done to
    * a. remove all blood before cooking.
    b. season the meat or poultry with traditional Jewish herbs.
    c. bless the animal before slaughter.
    d. age the meat or poultry to increase tenderness.

16. Muslims who follow traditional dietary laws
    a. drink alcoholic beverages only on religious holidays.
    b. avoid all beef, lamb, veal, and pork.
    * c. fast during three days of every month.
    d. eat to capacity in preparation for a fast.

17. The current labeling regulations require
    * a. serving sizes of products be based on commonly consumed amounts.
    b. serving sizes of products be determined by the total number of calories present.
    c. foods without added nutrients must have a warning label.
    d. foods can be labeled fat free only if absolutely no fat is present.

CHAPTER 17

THE ASSESSMENT OF NUTRITIONAL STATUS

OVERVIEW

The purpose of this chapter is to introduce the student to the method for determining the state of nutritional health. This will also become the first component of the nutrition care process (Chapter 19). The chapter begins with a brief review of how nutritional deficiencies develop. This is followed by presentation of the elements of nutritional assessment. Discussion of assessment elements includes methods, interpretation, application, and usefulness.

LEARNING OBJECTIVES

This chapter will prepare the learner to be able to

1. Summarize the concept of nutritional balance using factors affecting nutrient intake and nutrient utilization.
2. Identify the two phases of nutritional assessment and state their purpose.
3. State the goals of nutritional assessment.
4. Identify five basic areas for data collection in nutritional assessment.
5. State the significance of the medical and social histories.
6. Compare the methods for collecting dietary intake data.
7. List the significant anthropometric measurements in nutritional assessment and what they indicate.
8. Calculate body mass index (BMI) and explain its interpretation and application.
9. Determine triceps skinfold thickness (TSF), mid-arm circumference (MAC), and arm muscle area (AMA).
10. Explain clinical evaluation and how it is significant to nutritional assessment.
11. Recognize the significance of drug–nutrient interactions on nutritional status.
12. Describe how biochemical indices are used to assess nutritional status.
13. Determine nitrogen balance.
14. Identify the components of the documentation of nutritional assessment.

CHAPTER OUTLINE

I. Development of Nutritional Deficiency

II. Nutritional Assessment

    A. Screening

NOTES, TERMS, & TRANSPARENCY MASTERS

Key concepts: Nutritional health can be compromised by either a deficiency or an excess of one or more nutrients. In both cases, the process is gradual, with no acute onset.

Figure 17-1 (Transparency) illustrates the balance needed in achieving optimal nutritional status. The concept is that many factors affect intake and utilization.

Figure 17-2 illustrates the process by which a nutrient deficiency occurs. The cause of the deficiency is not limited to poor dietary intake.

Key concept: Nutrition assessment involves two phases: screening and assessment.

Key concept: The purpose of screening is to determine who is at nutritional risk and thus requires a more thorough assessment of needs.

Table 17-1 is an example of a screening tool used in a clinic setting to determine nutritional risk of a patient.

Table 17-2 is an example of a screening tool used in an elderly congregate feeding program to determine nutritional risk of a patient.

Table 17-3 is an example of screening a patient that is not suspected of being at nutritional risk. This is not a tool but an actual sample documentation such as that found in a medical record.

Figure 17-3 is an example of screening a patient that is suspected of being at nutritional risk. This is both a tool and a documentation that would be entered into the medical record.

Table 17-4 shows how a hospitalized patient's status can be differentiated as high or moderate risk based on information found in the medical record.

Figure 17-4 is an example of a screening tool for a pediatric patient that is suspected of being at nutritional risk. This is both a tool and a documentation that would be entered into the medical record.

Table 17-5 is an example of a screening tool used for a healthy population. The tool can be completed by the client in most cases. The evaluation is based on a rating system, shown in **Table 17-6**.

B. Assessment

III. Components of Nutritional Assessment
   A. Histories
      1. Medical
      2. Social
      3. Dietary intake

Table 17-7 provides a list of the information included in the diet history.
diet history, nutritional history

   B. Nutrient intake analysis

nutrient intake analysis (NIA)

   C. 7-Day food record
   D. Retrospective data
      1. Food frequency

Table 17-8 is an example of a food frequency tool, which can be adapted for a specific population or to reflect specific nutrients.

      2. 24-hour recall

Table 17-9 is an example of a 24-hour recall. Note that the form also includes the method of assessment.
cross-check, validity, reliability

   E. Anthropometry

Note: The term *anthropometry* may need to be defined for the students.
anthropometric data
Figure 17-5 shows how the length (height) of an infant is measured.
See **Clinical Insight:** "Measurement of Height and Weight."

   F. Interpretation of height and weight

See **Appendices 6** through **15** for reference standards for infants, children, and adolescents (0-17 years of age). The use of growth charts should be demonstrated to the students.

      1. Reference standards

Note: Reference standards refer to adults only, as does body mass index (BMI).
Table 17-10 and **Appendix 16** illustrate a common height-weight chart used for interpretation of weights of adults (Metropolitan Life Insurance Tables). The limitations (that they reflect average weights of people who the insurance company considers good risks, that frame size determination may not be accurate, and that weight of clothing is estimation only) should be pointed out to students.

      2. Body mass index (BMI)

Note: Demonstrate calculation of BMI to students.
Appendix 18 provides tables for interpretation of BMI.

G. Body Composition
    1. Subcutaneous fat (skinfold thickness)

Figure 17-6 is a theoretical view of what is actually being measured when using the subcutaneous fat technique.

Figure 17-7 shows the position of the triceps skinfold thickness (TSF) measurement.

Figure 17-8 shows the position of the subscapular skinfold thickness measurement.

Appendices 20 through **23** show the reference standards for interpretation of TSF and subscapular skinfold thickness measurements. The interpretation is based on percentiles that may require explanation to the students.

triceps, subscapular

H. Circumference measurements
    1. Waist to hip circumference ratio (WHR)

Appendix 19 provides a nomogram for determining WHR. Some students may require assistance in use of nomograms.

    2. Mid-upper arm circumference (MAC)

Figure 17-9 illustrates the process for determining the MAC.

Appendices 24 through **27** provide standards for use in interpreting the MAC.

Figure 17-10 demonstrates the calculation of the bone-free arm muscle circumference using the TSF and the MAC.

acromion, olecranon

    3. Head circumference
    4. Calf circumference

I. Clinical examination

Table 17-11 is a detailed list of the physical signs associated with malnutrition. Some attention should be given to differential diagnoses (nonnutritional) associated with the physical signs.

Appendix 28 provides information on clinical and physical signs associated with malnutrition.

    1. Skin testing
    2. Drug–nutrient interactions

Chapter 18 covers the topic of drug–nutrient interactions.

J. Biochemical analysis

Table 17-12 lists the laboratory determinations commonly used to assess nutritional status. Some attention should be given to differential diagnoses.

Appendix 30 provides information on biochemical indices and their interpretation.

Note: Establishing the normal range depends on the method used for assay and thus may vary from lab to lab.

K. Nitrogen balance

Note: Determining nitrogen balance usually requires demonstration and opportunities for practice when first introduced to students. **Appendix 30** provides more information on nitrogen balance calculation.

IV. Documentation and Care Planning

Figure 17-11 is an example of a discharge summary. This is usually completed when the patient's nutritional problems are resolved or when she is discharged from the hospital.

STUDENT ACTIVITIES

1. Assign each student to work with a partner. Each student should complete the following anthropometric measurements on their partner: height, weight, frame size, TSF, and MAC. Using their partner's data, they should complete the following:
    a. Compare weight with the Metropolitan Life Insurance tables. Determine the percent reference weight.
    b. Determine the BMR. Determine the score and interpret according to health risk.
    c. Compare the TSF and MAC to reference standards.
    d. Use the TSF and MAC to determine the AMA. Compare the AMA with reference standards.

2. Assign each student to work with a partner. Each student should complete the following using their partner as the patient:
    a. food frequency
    b. 24-hour recall

3. Assign students to keep a food record of their own eating for a designated period of time (e.g., three days, with one day being a weekend day). Have the students complete a nutritional analysis and determine an average daily intake. Compare the average daily intake with the appropriate RDA.

CASE STUDY INSIGHTS

(This Case Study is not in the textbook.)

TR is a 45-year-old male patient presenting with complaints of feeling tired, having no appetite, loss of weight, dark blood in the stools, and pain in the region of the stomach. He is employed as a marketing director for a major manufacturing firm. He has been worried lately by a significant drop in sales. He is married and has two teenage children. His parents are both alive and well. He usually skips breakfast, eats lunch at a restaurant, and has dinner at home. He may have one or two alcoholic beverages two or three times per week. He is taking no medications, although he does use aspirin for shoulder pain that usually occurs after playing golf. His weight today is 180 lbs, and his usual weight is 190 lbs. He is 6 feet tall with a medium build. Lab data provided at this time are shown in the table at the top of the next page.

Hemoglobin	*13 g/dL*
Hematocrit	*37%*
Serum B$_{12}$	*800 pg/ml*
Total lymphocyte count	*3000 cell/mm^3*
Albumin	*4.4 gm/dL*
Glucose	*90 mg/dL*
Cholesterol	*220 mg/dL*

1.   *Assess TR's weight status using the adapted Metropolitan Life Insurance tables and BMI. Compare the results. Determine TR's percent weight loss.*

According to the adapted Metropolitan Life Insurance Company tables, TR should weigh within the range of 158–175 lbs. His current weight (180 lbs) is within 2% of the range for desirable weight. However, of significance here is the 10-lb weight loss. His usual weight is 8–9% above desirable weight. His BMI is 24.5. Both of these assessment parameters suggest that weight/body composition is within normal limits.

2.   *For each of the laboratory results provided, indicate the normal range. For values occurring outside the range, determine what they might indicate.*

Laboratory Test	TR's Values	Normal Values	Comparison
Hemoglobin	13 g/dL	14–18 g/dL	Depressed
Hematocrit	37%	39–49 %	Depressed
Serum B$_{12}$	800 pg/mL	200–1000 pg/mL	WNL
Total lymphocyte count	3000 cell/mm^3	200–3500 cells/mm^3	WNL
Albumin	4.4 g/dL	3.5–5.0 g/dL	WNL
Glucose	90 mg/dL	70–100 mg/dL	WNL
Cholesterol	220 mg/dL	<200 mg/dL	Elevated

The significance of the depressed hemoglobin and hematocrit may be related to the dark blood in the stool. The dark blood indicates that a bleed is occurring in the proximal portion of the GI tract. This could be an indication of a bleeding ulcer. Blood losses are associated with lowering of hemoglobin and hematocrit. This may also be used to estimate the duration of the bleeding. The elevated cholesterol can result from dietary intake of fat, as well as a number of other non-nutritional factors.

3.   *What are the significant factors related to TR's social and diet histories?*

The social history includes a description of TR's work situation, which is one of high stress. The fact that he has two teenagers may also be a factor related to stress. The family history is not significant. The diet history reveals questionable eating habits.

SUGGESTED TEST QUESTIONS

1. Height assessments on children less than 2–3 years of age should be performed
* a. with the child in the recumbent position.
   b. using the arm spa.
   c. using a statiometer.
   d. using the sitting height.

2. In performance of a nutritional assessment, the use of body mass index (BMI) has the advantage of
   a. not being dependent on frame size.
* b. being a reliable predictor for lean muscle mass.
   c. being easier to calculate.
   d. being most effective for children.

3. A waist-to-hip ratio (WHR) of 1.0 or greater in men and 0.8 or greater in women is associated with a
   a. lower incidence of cardiovascular disease.
   b. increased longevity.
* c. increased risk for obesity-related diseases.
   d. less than adequate fat stores and marginal nutritional status.

4. Combining the mid-upper arm circumference with the triceps skinfold thickness measurement provides the health care team with information on
   a. risk of obesity-related diseases.
   b. measure of adiposity.
   c. body mass index.
* d. arm muscle and arm fat area.

5. The most objective measure of nutritional status is the
   a. dietary history.
* b. evaluation of biochemical tests.
   c. observation of meal consumption.
   d. evaluation of height and weight based on reference standards.

6. Anthropometric data are most valuable when accurately measured and recorded
   a. daily.
   b. weekly.
* c. over a relatively long period of time.
   d. upon admission and discharge.

7. When using the Quetelet Index, obesity is defined as a BMI of
* a. less than 25.
   b. 25–29.5 or greater.
   c. 30 or greater.
   d. 40 or greater.

8. Skinfold sites identified as the most useful measurements of body fat are
   a. at the biceps and triceps.
   b. below the scapula and above the biceps.
* c. at the triceps and below the scapula.
   d. at the iliac crest and the upper thigh.

9. The arm muscle area, which is a good indicator of lean body mass and thus skeletal protein reserves, is determined using
   a. weight and height measurements.
   b. triceps skinfold and weight measurements.
* c. triceps skinfold and mid-upper arm circumference measurements.
   d. knee height and weight measurements.

10. Measurement of head circumference is useful for
   a. children less than 3 years of age as an indicator of malnutrition.
* b. children less than 3 years of age as an indicator of primarily non-nutritional abnormalities.
   c. children more than 3 years of age as an indicator of nutritional deficiencies.
   d. adults only as an indicator of non-nutritional abnormalities.

11. Nutritional deficiency and nutritional overloads
   a. can result after only a few days of a poor diet.
   b. are easily diagnosed.
* c. are progressive and result in adaptations in functional levels.
   d. are evident in a three-day diet record.

12. Nutritional screening is used to
   a. identify patients at nutritional risk.
   b. determine a patient's nutritional problem.
   c. categorize patients as high or moderate risk.
   d. assess the patient's nutritional status.

13. The nutritional history and the diet history differ in that
    a. the diet history includes detailed information about intake for a minimum of 7 days.
    * b. the nutrition history includes a diet history, clinical findings, and laboratory data.
    c. the nutrition history is done by the physician while the diet history is done by the dietitian.
    d. the diet history is usually not accurate.

14. The 24-hour recall and the food frequency are limited by
    a. the patient's level of literacy.
    b. the time required to collect data.
    c. the lack of tools for these purposes.
    * d. reliance on the patient's recollection.

15. In a hypercatabolic patient, the nitrogen balance is
    a. zero.
    b. positive.
    c. positive 2–4 g.
    * d. negative.

16. Skin testing for evaluating immuno-competency
    a. is highly accurate.
    * b. has not been proven to be well correlated with nutritional status.
    c. is most useful in patients with food allergies.
    d. is inaccurate because most patients have no response.

CHAPTER

INTERACTIONS BETWEEN DRUGS AND NUTRIENTS

OVERVIEW

The purpose of this chapter is to provide the student with an understanding of the effects that drugs and medications have on nutritional status. The chapter begins with a brief introduction to pharmacology. The remainder of the chapter is devoted to two major concerns: effects of drugs on nutrients and effect of nutrients on drugs. The chapter concludes with a review of the potential incompatibilities of medications and enteral nutrition. A large number of drug names appear throughout the chapter.

LEARNING OBJECTIVES

This chapter will prepare the learner to be able to

1. Identify the three stages of drug action.
2. Identify individuals at greatest risk for drug-induced malnutrition.
3. State the ways in which a drug can cause an increase or decrease in dietary intake.
4. Categorize the type of drugs most likely to affect dietary intake.
5. Explain how drugs affect absorption of nutrients.
6. Categorize the type of drugs most likely to cause malabsorption of nutrients.
7. Explain how drugs affect metabolism and excretion of nutrients.
8. Categorize the type of drugs most likely to interfere with metabolism and excretion of nutrients.
9. Summarize the nutrition-related action of some common drugs.
10. State nutritional concerns related to drugs of abuse, botanicals, and alcohol.
11. Describe the effects of nutrients on drug absorption, availability, and metabolism.
12. Summarize the effects of drugs used with enteral feeding formulas.

107

CHAPTER OUTLINE ─────────────

(Drug names appearing in the textbook are included here for the convenience of the instructor.)

I.   Basic Pharmacology

pharmaceutical stage, pharmacokinetic stage, pharmacodynamic stage

II. Phases of Drug Actions

mixed function oxidase system (MFOS)

III. Risk Factors for Interactions

IV. Effects of Drugs on Nutritional Status and Requirements
     A. Drugs that affect dietary intake

Table 18-1 (Transparency) lists drugs that can cause a loss of appetite.
Table 18-2 (Transparency) lists drugs that can alter or diminish taste perception.
Table 18-3 (Transparency) lists drugs used to increase appetite.
dysgeusia, hypogeusia
methylphenidate (Ritalin), cis-platin, dexfenfluramine, fluoxetin, ephedrine, phenylpropanolamine, megesterol acetate

     B. Drugs that affect nutrient absorption
         1. Luminal effects

Key concepts: The three concepts presented here are influence on transit time, affect on bile acid activity, and change in the gastrointestinal environment.
cholestryramine, neomycin, mineral oil, cimetidine

         2. Mucosal effects

Key concepts: The two concepts presented here are damage to the intestinal mucosa and affects on intestinal transport mechanisms.
aspirin, colchicine, para-aminosalicylic acid (PASA), sulfasalazine, trimethoprim, pryimethamine

     C. Drugs that affect nutrient metabolism and excretion
         1. Antivitamins

Key concepts: The two concepts presented here are inhibition of synthesis of specific enzymes and formation of a drug–nutrient complex.
methotrexate, pyrimethamine, isoniazid (INH), hydralazine, penicillamine

         2. Monoamine oxidase inhibitors

Table 18-4 (Transparency) provides a list of the drugs that inhibit the action of oxidases.
Table 18-5 is a list of foods containing tyramine and categorized by degree of concern for use.

              tyramine, serotonin, histamine, norepinephrine, dopamine, reversible inhibitors of monoamine oxidase (RIMA)

3. Excretion of nutrients — **D-penicillamine, ethylenediaminotetraacetate (EDTA), cefotetan, cephalexin**

4. Drug-induced electrolyte alterations — **Appendix 31** contains additional information on the effects of drugs on nutritional status. **furosemide, ethacrynic acid, triamterene, thiazide, cisplatin**

5. Drugs of abuse — **Note:** Drugs of abuse listed in the textbook include caffeine, tobacco, and alcohol. This may require clarification for students. **Table 18-6** lists the effects of some of the more common drugs of abuse on appetite. **barbiturates, amphetamines**

D. Summary of nutrition-related action of some common drugs
  1. Anticonvulsants — **anticonvulsant drugs (ACDs)** **phenytoin, phenobarbitol, primidone**

  2. Oral contraceptives — **low-estrogen oral contraceptives**

  3. Antiinflammatory drugs — **glucocorticoids**

  4. Antihypertensives — **glucothiazide, beta-adrenergic blocking drugs (beta blockers)**

  5. Medications used in HIV — **AZT (zidovudine, Retrovir), bactrim, pentamidine, pyrimethamine, amphoteracin-B**

E. Botanicals — **aloe, ligustrum, taraxacum, prunella, ginseng, Ma huang, guarana, Kola nut, white willow, senna**

V. Effect of Food and Nutrition on Drug Therapy
  A. Effect on drug absorption and availability — **Table 18-7** summarizes the effects of various foods and beverages on drug action. **nitofurantoin, hydralazine, L-dopa, penicillin G, tetracycline, penicillamine, methldopa, carbidopa, captopril, thyroxine, phenytoin, griseofulvin**

  B. Effect on drug metabolism — **phenytoin, warfarin, propanolol, theophylline, levodopa**

  C. Effect on drug excretion — **lithium carbonate, barbiturates, theophylline, phenyutoin, amphetamines**

D. Alcohol interactions	**phenytoin, disulfuram (Antibuse), metroiadazole, griseofulvin, procarbazine**
VI. Medication and Enteral Nutrition Incompatibilities	
A. Physical incompatibilities	**mellaril, thorazine, Feosol, Dimetapp Elizir, Robitussin, pseudoephedrine, Kaopectate**
B. Pharmaceutical incompatibilities	**theophylline, phenytoin**
C. Physiologic incompatibilities	
D. Pharmacokinetic incompatibilities	**phenytoin, warfarin**
VII. Nutrition Counseling	

CASE STUDY INSIGHTS

1. After reviewing Ms. S's medications and her intake at lunch, which foods may be responsible for her symptoms of headache and palpitations?

The symptoms of palpitations and headache are associated with the use of monoamine inhibitors (MAOI) following ingestion of foods containing tyramine. In the lunch meal, the sausage and beer would be contraindicated with the use of nardil (MAOI); the yeast bread and potato salad (salad dressing and boiled egg) may also be under suspicion.

2. Which physical exam findings may relate to a nutrient deficiency, and which nutrient may be involved? Which medications could have potentially caused this deficiency?

The glossitis, elevated MCH, pale conjunctiva, and depressed Hgb are all associated with folate deficiency, which can be induced by phenytoin. Folate deficiency produces a megaloblastic anemia. The MCV is not associated with folate deficiency but would be expected to be decreased in this patient due to a depressed Hgb.

3. Which medication could produce weight gain as a side effect?

The nardil.

4. What type of anemia is characterized by an elevated MCH and MCV? Which nutrient and which medications may be involved?

An increased MCV and a decreased MCH are associated with macrocytic anemias. The megaloblastic anemia associated with folate deficiency is a macrocytic (large cell) anemia. The folate deficiency suspected here could result from the phenytoin being used to treat the seizure disorder.

5. *How would you evaluate the adequacy of Ms. S's vitamin D intake? What factors influence her requirements for vitamin D?*

   Ms. S's poor intake of milk, fruits, and vegetables is suggestive of a poor intake of vitamin D. While phenytoin is thought to interfere with the conversion of cholecalciferol to 25-OHD in the liver, there does not appear to be a high risk for vitamin D deficiency. People at risk for vitamin D deficiency are those with highly pigmented skin or inadequate exposure to sunlight. The case study does not provide sufficient information to consider these factors.

6. *How may the chronic antacid ingestion influence the patient's absorption of phenytoin?*

   Absorption of most drugs is dependent on transport across the gastrointestinal epithelium. The process is pH dependent since ionization is required for absorption. The use of antacids can threaten absorption of drugs, including phenytoin, by altering the gastric pH.

7. *How does low serum albumin affect drug disposition?*

   Drugs are usually found bound to a protein, most often albumin. When albumin levels are depressed, the result is an increase in serum levels of the drug which, in turn, results in an increased pharmacological action. A drug such as phenytoin, which is highly protein bound, is most affected by a depressed albumin. In this case, Ms. S exhibits a depressed albumin and an increased serum level of phenytoin, as expected.

8. *What nutritional care would you recommend for the patient? Be sure to include educational needs.*

   Ms. S is in need of a more thorough nutritional assessment so that potential deficiencies of additional nutrients, particularly protein, can be identified. Dependent on the outcome of such an assessment, a nutrition care plan should be developed that will improve her overall nutritional status. Apparent at this time is education on the importance of avoiding foods high in tyramine (she will need to know what these are). She is also in need of education about healthy eating habits.

SUGGESTED TEST QUESTIONS

1. A child who is diagnosed as hyperactive may be treated with methylphenidate (Ritalin). Parents of the child should be cautioned to
   * a. have frequent anthropometric measurements of the child to ensure adequate growth.
   b. be sure that immunization status is current before the medication regimen is begun.
   c. monitor the child for weight gain secondary to the decrease in activity.
   d. ensure that the child's intake of fat is adequate.

2. A patient assigned to your care complains of decreased acuity of taste sensation (hypogeusia). Since she is also receiving penicillamine, you would suspect a deficiency of
   a. sodium.
   b. potassium.
   * c. zinc.
   d. iron.

3. As you are assessing your patient, she tells you that she has used cathartic agents for years. Recently she has noted free fat in her stools (steatorrhea); you would be concerned that the steatorrhea may also cause an increased loss of
   a. vitamin C.
   b. sodium.
   c. vitamin B$_6$.
 * d. calcium.

4. Patients who are diagnosed with peptic ulcer disease and treated with one of the H2 antagonists (Cimetidine) should have their red blood cell status monitored for
 * a. vitamin B$_{12}$ deficiency.
   b. vitamin C levels.
   c. iron deficiency.
   d. folate deficiency.

5. Patients who have been treated long-term with the anti-TB agent isoniazid (INH) may be at risk for
   a. vitamin K deficiency.
   b. vitamin E toxicity.
 * c. vitamin B$_6$ deficiency.
   d. folic acid deficiency.

6. A patient to be treated for depression with a monoamine oxidase inhibitor should be instructed to avoid
   a. milk, soy protein, and grapefruit.
 * b. cheese, smoked or pickled fish, and Chianti wine.
   c. tomatoes, onions, and poultry.
   d. cantaloupe, canned pineapple, and dried beans.

7. Hypertensive patients who are taking diuretics for reduction of blood pressure may experience low potassium (hypokalemia). A second nutrient deficiency that may be concurrent is
 * a. magnesium.
   b. sodium.
   c. phosphorus.
   d. chloride.

8. A diuretic that may be used to reduce an elevated serum calcium level is
   a. D-penicillamine.
   b. chlorpromazine.
   c. EDTA.
 * d. furosemide.

9. The proper technique for administering oral medications through a feeding tube is to
 * a. stop administration of the formula and irrigate the tube before and after administering the medication.
   b. add the medication to the feeding.
   c. crush the medications and mix them with water before administration.
   d. add Dimetapp Elixir, Sudafed Syrup, or Robitussin Expectorant to the feedings.

10. Patients who are taking tetracyclines should be taught to avoid taking their mediations with
    a. fruit juices.
    b. meat.
 * c. milk.
    d. sucrose-containing desserts.

11. The bioavailability of a drug indicates the proportion of the drug that is
 * a. available to the target tissue.
    b. transported bound to protein.
    c. metabolized by the liver.
    d. oxidized within body cells.

12. Certain tranquilizers, such as lithium carbonate and chlorpromazine,
    a. induce weight loss.
 * b. induce weight gain.
    c. decrease appetite.
    d. induce anorexia.

13. The cancer chemotherapeutic agent methotrexate acts as an antagonist of the vitamin
    a. pantothenic acid.
    b. biotin.
 * c. folate.
    d. pyridoxine.

14. Healthy women using low estrogen oral contraceptives have
    a. a need for two to three times the RDA for folate.
*   b. no significant increase above the RDA for folate.
    c. higher levels of serum folate.
    d. significant abnormalities in their folate metabolism.

15. Within 8–10 days of starting therapy with glucocorticoid drugs,
    a. bone mass increases.
    b. bone resorption is suppressed.
    c. calcium absorption is increased and calcium excretion decreased.
*   d. calcium absorption is reduced and calcium excretion increased.

16. Beta-adrenergic blocking drugs (beta-blockers) used to lower blood pressure may cause
    a. decreased serum triglycerides.
    b. increased concentrations of HDL cholesterol.
*   c. increased serum triglycerides.
    d. decreased concentration of LDL cholesterol.

17. Tetracycline derivatives should be taken without milk or diary products because
*   a. calcium chelates tetracycline and prevents its absorption.
    b. lactose interferes with the absorption of the drug.
    c. the protein content reduces the drug's bioavailability.
    d. the fat content interferes with the absorption of the drug.

18. Conditions such as malnutrition or liver disease in which serum albumin levels are decreased can lead to
    a. decreased serum levels of certain drugs.
*   b. increased serum levels of certain drugs.
    c. decreased mtabolism of the drug by the liver.
    d. decreased pharmacological effects.

19. Anticonvulsant drugs, such as phenytoin and phenobarbitol, have been shown to induce biochemical or clinical deficiencies of
    a. ascorbic acid and vitamin A.
    b. ascorbic acid and vitamin D.
*   c. folate, biotin, and vitamin D.
    d. pyridoxine, iron, and vitamin A.

THE NUTRITIONAL CARE PROCESS

OVERVIEW

The purpose of this chapter is to introduce the student to the process by which nutritional care is delivered in order to meet the nutritional needs of the patient. The process is presented in five steps: (1) assessing nutritional status, (2) identifying nutritional needs or problems, (3) planning and prioritizing objectives of nutritional care to meet these needs, (4) implementing nutritional activities necessary to meet the objectives, and (5) evaluating the nutritional care. (Assessment of nutritional status was presented in depth in Chapter 17.) The chapter also includes information related to charting and documentation, modification of diets for nutrition intervention, and nutritional care for hospitalized patients.

LEARNING OBJECTIVES

This chapter will prepare the learner to be able to

1. Define the nutritional care process and Standards of Care.
2. State the purpose of nutrition screening and identify who is responsible for nutrition screening.
3. Identify the characteristics of objectives for nutritional care.
4. Explain how nutritional care is implemented.
5. Relate the evaluation of nutritional care to the development of nutritional care objectives.
6. State the function of the nutritional care record.
7. Describe how nutritional care is documented in the medical record.
8. Describe how modified diets are related to the normal diet.
9. State the purpose of a diet prescription.
10. List the standard hospital diets and describe their characteristics.
11. State the purpose of each of the standard hospital diets.
12. State the goal of nutritional care for the terminally ill or hospice patient.

CHAPTER OUTLINE	NOTES, TERMS, & TRANSPARENCY MASTERS
I. Nutritional Care Process	**Figure 19-1** is an example of Standards of Care for the General Patient. This will provide a good beginning for students as they begin to grasp the scope of the nutritional care process. **nutritional care, nutritional care process, Standards of Care, nutrition support teams (NST)**
A. Identification of nutritional risk	**Table 19-1 (Transparency)** lists the basic information to be included in nutritional screening. This topic is also covered in **Chapter 17.** **nutritional screening, nutritional assessment**
B. Nutritional care plan	**patient focused care**
1. Assessment	**Table 19-2** summarizes nutritional screening and assessment, indicating the degree of risk. This is a useful tool for the student.
2. Objectives of nutritional care	**Key concept:** Objectives are intended to be written in behavioral terms, thus indicating what the patient can do when the objectives are met. **Note:** This section introduces a case study that illustrates the concepts presented. **patient-centered**
3. Implementation of nutritional care	**Key concept:** All the activities or interventions that are used to assist the patient in meeting the objectives are included in specific terms of when, what, where, and how.
4. Evaluation of nutritional care	**Key concept**: The evaluation of nutritional care is based on the behavioral objectives established in the plan. The evaluation should indicate whether the objectives have been met or not. **Table 19-3** summarizes the steps of the nutritional care process. Each step includes definitions, components, and factors to consider.
C. Nutritional care record	**Key concept:** The medical record is a legal document. The nutritional care process must be documented in the medical record. **Figure 19-2** is a photograph of a dietitian and a medical record. **Figure 19-3** is a sample nutritional care record. A record such as this is usually kept by the clinical dietitian and summarized periodically in the medical record.

II. Charting and Documentation

Key concept: There are a number of methods for documenting the nutritional care process in the medical record. The SOAP format is presented in depth here. The guidelines for documentation presented here can be considered as general guidelines. Students should be told that procedures for documentation may differ among institutions.

Figure 19-4 is an example of a form that can be used for assessment and documentation.

III. Nutrition Intervention—Diet Modification

Key concept: Modified diets, or therapeutic diets, are intended to be based on normal diets with only the minimal changes that are necessary to meet nutritional needs.

Clinical insight: This is a summary of dietary practices for various religions.

A. The diet perscription

Key concept: The diet prescription is intended to be a specific description of the diet to be provided to the patient. The information in the prescription will vary depending on individual patient needs.

1. Energy allowance

See **Chapters 2** and **30** for reviews of the determination of energy needs.

See **Appendix 16** for determination of desirable weight.

Table 19-4 is the table provided with the 1989 RDAs for energy needs for healthy people.

2. Protein allowance

Key concept: The energy to nitrogen ratio is introduced here with recommendations for hypermetabolic conditions. This calculation should be demonstrated to students.

3. Fat and carbohydrate allowances
4. Minerals and vitamins
5. Fluids

B. Modification of the normal diet

Key concept: Therapeutic diets are qualitative and/or quantitative modifications of the normal diet. Qualitative refers to food and nutrients present, while quantitative refers to amounts of nutrients.

C. Foods as nutrient sources

Key concept: Nutritional needs are met by foods, which are what people eat.

IV. Nutritional Care for the Hospitalized Patient
    A. Standard hospital diets   **general, soft, liquid**

        1. General or normal diet   See **Chapter 16** and **Table 16-8** for use in planning the nutritional adequate diet.

        2. Soft diet   **Table 19-5** provides a sample menu for a soft diet.
        3. Liquid diets
             a. full liquid diet   **Table 19-6** provides a sample menu for a full liquid diet.

             b. clear liquid diet   **Table 19-7** provides a sample menu for a clear liquid diet.
                                    Table 19-8 is a summary of the four standard hospital diets.

    B. Food intake
    C. Psychological factors
    D. Discharge planning and home care   **Key concept:** Nutritional care does not stop at the point of hospital discharge.

    E. Care of the terminally ill or hospice patient   **palliative care, hospice**

STUDENT ACTIVITIES

1. Obtain a sample medical record to show to students, indicating the organization, consistency, and preciseness of documentation. An alternative activity would be to have students meet at a local hospital and have clinical dietitians show them medical records of actual patients. This may need to be done in small groups to accommodate the hospital environment.

2. Obtain a diet manual from a local hospital or from the American Dietetic Association. Review the general, soft, full liquid, and clear liquid diets.

3. Obtain sample menus from a local hospital for the general, soft, full liquid, and clear liquid diets. Analyze the nutritional content of the diets. Have students make recommendations for improvement when the diets are not nutritionally adequate (complete nutritional adequacy is not always achieved with the liquid diets).

SUGGESTED TEST QUESTIONS

1. Which of these observations noted during a routine nutritional screening would warrant further assessment?
   a. weight gain of 2 lbs in seven days
   * b. unintentional weight loss of 10% or more in the past 6 months
   c. refusal to eat breakfast
   d. increased consumption of food served

2. In determining the nutritional requirements for the hospitalized patient, which of these should be included for wound healing?
   a. vitamin B_{12}, vitamin D, and potassium.
   b. vitamin E, vitamin A, and calcium.
   * c. vitamin A, vitamin C, and zinc.
   d. vitamin B_6, vitamin D, and magnesium.

3. Unless there is documented evidence of nutritional deficits at the time of admission, the patient should be screened for deficits every
   a. 24 hours.
   b. 48 hours.
   c. 3–5 days.
   * d. 7–14 days.

4. Which of these is a behavioral objective for the newly diagnosed diabetic who requires the administration of insulin on a twice daily basis?
   a. The caregiver will teach the patient to administer the insulin.
   b. The caregiver will demonstrate the correct administration technique for insulin.
   * c. The patient will demonstrate correct technique for insulin preparation and administration.
   d. The patient will understand how to administer insulin before leaving the hospital.

5. Patients who are experiencing moderate stress may have energy requirements that exceed their BEE by
   a. 20%.
   b. 30%.
   c. 40%.
   * d. 50%.

6. To provide adequate fluid for a patient who is not experiencing accelerated fluid loss, the total quantity ingested should be
   a. 500–800 mL/day.
   b. 1000–1500 mL/day.
   * c. 1800–2500 mL/day.
   d. 2500–3500 mL/day.

7. A newly admitted patient is observed to have poorly fitting dental plates. The most appropriate diet for this patient is a
   a. general diet.
   b. full liquid diet.
   c. clear liquid diet.
   * d. soft diet.

8. A full liquid diet provides all nutrients for maintenance except for
   * a. fiber.
   b. protein.
   c. B vitamin complex.
   d. fat.

9. If the patient cannot tolerate diets beyond clear liquid, which of these may be indicated for long-term use?
   a. addition of milk products
   * b. an elemental diet
   c. pureed proteins
   d. soft diet

10. Nutritional screening should be done on
   a. patients considered to be at nutritional risk upon admission.
   * b. all patients within 3–4 days of entering the hospital.
   c. patients who appear to be cachectic or malnourished.
   d. patients who are chronically ill.

11. Nutritional screening should be conducted by
   a. dietitians only.
   b. dietitians and diet technicians.
   * c. diet technicians and other hospital personnel trained in the procedure.
   d. physicians only.

12. The most important determination in nutritional screening is the
*   a. percentage change from usual weight.
    b. percent of ideal body weight.
    c. percent of desirable body weight.
    d. percent of ideal body weight based on
      NHANES II standards.

13. The first step in the nutritional care plan is to
    a. identify nutritional problems.
    b. set objectives for education and coun-
      seling.
    c. determine nutrient needs.
*   d. conduct a nutritional assessment.

14. Information on the nutrition care plan should
be documented
    a. only upon admission.
*   b. throughout the patient's stay.
    c. only if there is no progress.
    d. only upon a physician's order.

15. Patients with mild stress, such as those with
uncomplicated surgery, require how much
additional energy over their BEE?
*   a. 0–20%
    b. 20–40%
    c. 20–50%
    d. 50–60%

16. The average clear or restricted liquid diet
contains
    a. 20–30 g protein, 1000-1200 kcal.
*   b. 5–10 g protein, 400-500 kcal.
    c. 40–50 g protein, 800-1000 kcal.
    d. no protein, 500–700 kcal.

17. When providing nutritional care for the terminally ill patient, dietary restrictions
    a. must be maintained throughout the illness.
*   b. are rarely appropriate.
    c. should be followed whenever possible.
    d. should be followed without exception.

18. The daily intake of water needed by a normal
healthy adult is about
    a. 1000 mL.
    b. 1500 mL.
*   c. 2200 mL.
    d. 3000 mL.

CHAPTER

METHODS OF NUTRITIONAL SUPPORT

OVERVIEW

The purpose of this chapter is to introduce the student to methods of meeting nutritional needs without the use of actual foods. The chapter begins with identifying the alternatives available for nutritional support. Information presented on the use of enteral nutrition includes choice of products, routes of access, formula composition, administration, and monitoring. This is followed by parallel information on the use of parenteral nutrition. The procedures for transitioning patients from enteral and parenteral feedings to use of actual foods are covered. The chapter concludes with presentation of information related to long-term and home care use of nutritional support methods.

LEARNING OBJECTIVES

This chapter will prepare the learner to be able to

1. Identify criteria for choosing a method of nutritional support.
2. State the uses of oral supplements and enteral formulas.
3. List the nonsurgical placements for enteral feeding tubes.
4. List the surgical placements for enteral feeding tubes.
5. Identify nutritional components of enteral feedings and the criteria used for their selection.
6. Identify the methods of administration for enteral tube feedings.
7. Explain the method for evaluation and monitoring of enteral tube feedings.
8. List the common problems associated with enteral tube feedings and their probable causes.
9. List the routes of access for parenteral nutrition feedings.
10. Identify nutritional components of parenteral feedings and the criteria used for their selection.
11. Identify the methods of administration for parenteral feedings.
12. Explain the method for evaluation and monitoring of parenteral feedings.
13. List the common problems associated with parenteral feedings and their probable causes.
14. List the recommended methods for transitional feeding.
15. State the methods for nutritional support in long-term and home care.

CHAPTER OUTLINE	NOTES, TERMS, & TRANSPARENCY MASTERS
I. Choosing the Method of Nutrition Support	**Table 20-1** provides a listing of physiological problems and the recommended method of feeding.
	total parenteral nutrition (TPN), enteral nutrition, parenteral nutrition, borborygmus, bacterial translocation
II. Enteral Nutrition	**Key concept:** The term *enteral* refers here to commercially available formulas, both supplemental and nutritionally complete. Since the meaning of enteral is "within or by the way of the GI tract," the intake of food by oral route is also an enteral feeding.
A. Oral supplements	**Key concept:** Oral supplements are intended to be used in addition to solid foods. By themselves, the supplements are not nutritionally complete.
B. Tube feeding 1. Routes of access	**Figure 20-1 (Transparency)** is a diagram showing the various routes of access for tube feedings.
a. nasogastric route	**Table 20-2** lists ingredients that might be used to prepare a blenderized formula for a tube feeding. The issue of sanitation and safe food handling practices must be emphasized.
	nasogastric tube
b. nasoduodenal or nasojejunal route	**nasoduodenal, nasojejunal**
2. enterostomies a. surgical gastrostomies	**gastrostomy, Stamm technique, Witzel technique, Foley catheter, Malicot catheter, Janeway procedure**
b. surgical jejunostomies	**jejunostomy, needle catheter jejunostomy**
c. percutaneous endoscopic gastrostomy (PEG) or jejunostomy (PEJ)	**percutaneous endoscopic gastrostomy, percutaneous endoscopic jejunostomy**
d. multiple lumen tubes 3. Enteral formula composition	**Appendices 33–40** provide a listing of current commercially available enteral formulas.
	Table 20-3 is a list of the factors to be considered in selecting an enteral formula.
a. protein b. carbohydrate c. fat	

    d. vitamins and minerals
    e. fluids
    g. osmolality   **Chapter 8** provides an explanation of osmolality.

    h. renal solute load   **renal solute load**
  4. Administration
    a. continuous drip   **continuous drip**

    b. intermittent drip or bolus   **intermittent drip, bolus**

  5. Monitoring and problem solving   **Table 20-4 (Transparency)** provides recommended guidelines for monitoring the enterally tube-fed patient.
    Table 20-5 summarizes the complications associated with enteral tube feedings and provides indications, explanations, and solutions.
    Figure 20-2 is a sample enteral nutrition support order form, which is used to ensure that all aspects of the feeding have been determined.

III. Parenteral Nutrition   **Key concept:** Parenteral nutrition is an alternative for nutritional support only when the patient cannot be sustained by enteral means. A patient with impaired digestion or absorption may be unable to use an enteral feeding.
    Table 20-6 is a list of the indicators used to determine the route of access.

  A. Parenteral access
    1. Peripheral access   **peripheral vein**

    2. short-term central access   **Figure 20-3 (Transparency)** is a diagram showing the various routes of access for parenteral feedings.

    3. long-term central access   **Hickman catheter, Broviac catheter, PIC line**

  B. Parenteral nutrition solutions
    1. Protein   **crystalline amino acids**

    2. Carbohydrate   See **Clinical Insight:** "Calculation of the Osmolarity of a Parenteral Nutrition Solution."

    3. Fat
    4. Vitamins, trace elements, and electrolytes   **Table 20-7** provides guidelines for the addition of electrolytes to the parenteral solution.
    Table 20-8 provides guidelines for the addition of vitamins to the parenteral solution.
    Table 20-9 provides guidelines for the addition of trace elements to the parenteral solution.

Key concept: Recommended quantities of electrolytes, vitamins, and trace elements administered with the parenteral solution are lower than RDA since digestion and absorption are bypassed.

5. Fluid needs
6. Compounding methods

Figure 20-4 is a sample physician's order form used for prescribing the parenteral solution. This form is added to the medical record.

Figure 20-5 is also a sample physician's order for ordering TPN.

compounding, 3-in-1 solution

B. Administration
  1. Continuous infusion

continuous infusion

  2. Cyclic infusion

cyclic infusion

C. Monitoring and problem solving
  1. Monitoring

Table 20-10 lists the parameters that are used in monitoring parenteral nutrition therapy.

Table 20-11 lists the complications associated with the use of TPN.

  2. Catheter care
  3. Refeeding syndrome

Table 20-12 lists the manifestations of refeeding syndrome.

refeeding syndrome, hypercapnia

IV. Transitional Feeding
  A. Parenteral to enteral feeding
  B. Parenteral to oral feeding

Table 20-13 lists common beverages and their osmolalities. This is useful in considering reintroduction of enteral feeding.

  C. Enteral to oral feeding

Table 20-14 defines the categories of enteral formulas and provides indications and descriptions of the formulas.

V. Nutritional Support in Long-Term and Home Care
  A. Long-term care
  B. Home care
  C. Ethical issues
  D. Nutrition support services
  E. Standards and guidelines
  F. Future trends

Table 20-15 lists the criteria for selection of patients suitable for home nutrition therapy.

practice guidelines

CASE STUDY INSIGHTS

*1. What is a typical scenario for progression of ulcerative colitis, and what are the nutritional
    ramifications?*

Ulcerative colitis is presented in Chapter 28. It is a chronic inflammation and ulceration of the mucosa
of the large intestine. It is manifested by rectal bleeding, diarrhea with pain and spasm, fever, ulcerative
lesions, dehydration, electrolyte imbalance, and anorexia. Additional concerns are malabsorption, steatorrhea, and protein losses in the gut. Drug therapy may also result in negative nitrogen balance and inhibition
of folate absorption. The combined effect of these manifestations is malnutrition related to a number of
nutrients.

*2. Make recommendations for choosing between an enteral feeding formula and a TPN prescription using
    standard solutions based on CB's assessed nutritional needs. What might need to be modified on
    follow-up?*

The placement of the tunneled catheter for long-term administration of TPN is an indication that enteral
feeding formula is not indicated. The severity of CB's disease and abnormal chemistries are indications that
a parenteral feeding would be most effective in delivering adequate nutritional support. Nutritional needs
can be determined using the Harris-Benedict equation (Chapter 2) and a stress or injury factor of 1.5–1.7
(Chapter 30).

3. What particular factors need close monitoring in CB considering her history?

CB has had a significant loss of weight (she is currently 67% of usual weight). Continued weight loss
should be avoided. Close monitoring of the adequacy of the energy provided by the TPN solution is important. Her elevated blood sugar is probably secondary to the use of steroids as an antiinflammatory.

*4. Would you recommend oral intake for CB while on TPN, and if so, what would you recommend? What
    about fiber?*

The case study does not give enough information to fully assess the patient or identify the long-term
treatment plan. Initially, withholding oral intake is recommended, primarily to reduce discomfort and allow
the bowel to rest. However, given the severity of the disease, CB is a candidate for surgical intervention,
specifically a colectomy. This method of treatment would eliminate the disease. The TPN is necessary
presurgery to replete nutritional stores and prepare the patient for surgery. After surgery, TPN would not be
indicated. A gradual transition to oral feedings would be implemented. The use of fiber in the diet would be
determined by the outcome of the surgical procedure and the placement of the stoma, as well as the
patient's tolerance.

5. Suggest the possible etiology of CB's severe hypoalbuminemia.

CB's decreased albumin has resulted from both a poor dietary intake of protein and increased losses of
protein in the gut.

STUDENT ACTIVITIES

1. Invite a representative from a formula manufacturer to present their product line to students. Ask the representative to bring equipment used in administration and products to sample.

2. Contact the pharmacy in a local hospital and determine how parenteral solutions are calculated and prepared. Arrange for students to visit the pharmacy or have the pharmacist come to class for a presentation.

SUGGESTED TEST QUESTIONS

1. The functions of which of these body systems are maintained better with enteral feedings than with parenteral feedings?
   a. cardiovascular system
   b. immunologic system
   * c. gastrointestinal system
   d. pulmonary system

2. For the patient with delayed gastric emptying, nausea and vomiting, or other indications that there is a risk for aspiration, the tube should be placed through the.
   a. mouth into the stomach.
   b. nose into the stomach.
   c. mouth into the duodenum or jejunum.
   * d. nose into the duodenum or jejunum.

3. The smallest tube compatible with the formula used is preferred for nasoenteric feedings. The reasons for this are patient comfort and
   * a. decreased reduction of gastroesophageal sphincter competence.
   b. increased gastroesophageal sphincter competence.
   c. increased rate of gastric emptying.
   d. decreased rate of tube obstruction.

4. It is widely accepted that enteral feedings are beneficial in maintaining the health of the GI tract. A nutrient of particular benefit to the gut mucosa is
   a. essential fatty acids.
   * b. intact protein.
   c. zinc.
   d. vitamin C.

5. Patients who may be adversely affected by a low fat formula for enteral feeding are those
   a. with hypoperistalsis.
   b. with small bowel resection.
   * c. who are ventilator dependent.
   d. with multiple fractures.

6. Patients on enteral tube feedings who are experiencing diarrhea may benefit from
   * a. the addition of fiber to the formula.
   b. a change in the formula.
   c. reduction in the volume of the water flush.
   d. an increase in the carbohydrate concentration of the formula.

7. Bolus enteral feedings are advantageous to patients who
   a. are not conscious.
   * b. desire mobility.
   c. cannot afford a pump.
   d. need a large volume of formula each day.

8. As you administer hyperosmolar enteral feedings to patients, a sign and symptom that you may note at the beginning of the feeding regimen is
   a. constipation.
   b. steatorrhea.
   * c. diarrhea.
   d. flatulence.

9. A measure that should be included in the care plan of a patient receiving nasogastric enteral feedings is to
   * a. remove residual gastric content and measure every 4–8 hours.
   b. add 100 mL of water to each feeding.
   c. elevate the head of the bed 30° during feedings and for 1 hour afterward.
   d. provide a 12-hour supply of formula at a time.

10. Whenever the digestive and absorptive capacities of the GI tract are still functional, the preferred route of feeding is
    a. peripheral.
    b. parenteral.
    c. peripheral or parenteral.
    * d. enteral.

11. For a patient to be solely maintained by enteral feeding, there needs to be a functioning small bowel of
    * a. 2–3 feet.
    b. 4–6 feet.
    c. 7–9 feet.
    d. 10–12 feet.

12. Placement of an enteral tube feeding beyond the stomach is indicated when
    * a. there is risk of aspiration.
    b. the patient will only require the feeding for a few days.
    c. the small intestine is blocked.
    d. the tube must remain in for a month or more.

13. Enteral feeding is preferred over parenteral feeding in maintaining gastrointestinal integrity because of the presence of
    a. carbohydrate.
    b. tryptophan.
    * c. intact protein.
    d. fat.

14. Isotonic enteral formulas may be initially administered to the patient at
    a. quarter-strength.
    b. half-strength.
    c. three-quarters strength.
    * d. full strength.

15. When determining fluid needs for an adult patient receiving an enteral formula, use the guideline of
    * a. 1 mL water/kcal ingested.
    b. 0.5 mL water/kcal ingested.
    c. 2 mL water/kcal ingested.
    d. 3 mL water/kcal ingested.

16. The most common complication of enteral tube feeding is
    a. hyponatremia.
    b. dehydration.
    * c. diarrhea.
    d. hypoalbuminemia.

17. When nutritional needs are not high, parenteral nutrition can be provided by
    a. percutaneous endoscopic jejunostomy.
    * b. peripheral access.
    c. a central catheter.
    d. a right atrial catheter.

18. To meet the essential fatty acid requirements of a patient receiving parenteral nutrition, the percentage of the total energy requirement that should be provided as essential fatty acids is
    a. 10%.
    b. 6–8%.
    c. 4–6%.
    * d. 2–4%.

19. An amino acid solution with a concentration of 15% provides
    a. 15 g of amino acids per liter.
    b. 15 g of amino acids per day.
    * c. 150 g of amino acids per liter.
    d. 150 g of amino acids per day.

20. The maximum recommended dosage of fat in a parenteral solution should not exceed
    a. 25% of total calories.
    b. 50% of total calories.
    c. 1 g/kg of ideal body weight.
    * d. 2.5 g/kg of body weight per day.

21. In the overly aggressive refeeding of patients who have been without food for a period of time, a characteristic of the nutritional recovery syndrome is
    a. overhydration.
    * b. hyperglycemia.
    c. hypernatremia.
    d. folic acid deficiency.

WEIGHT MANAGEMENT
AND EATING DISORDERS

OVERVIEW

The purpose of this chapter is to provide students with an understanding of the etiology, morbidity, and management strategies for conditions related to both excessive and insufficient body weight. The variations in body composition and fat distribution are presented along with the physiological factors affecting weight maintenance. Several methods of treatment are introduced. Anorexia nervosa and bulimia nervosa are presented as eating disorders.

LEARNING OBJECTIVES

This chapter will prepare the learner to be able to

1. List the components of body weight and their approximate proportions.
2. Identify the various types of body fat.
3. Identify the common types of fat deposition and the implications of each.
4. Explain the theories of fat cell development.
5. Describe the factors related to short-term and long-term maintenance of body weight.
6. State the criteria used to diagnosis overweight and obesity using BMI.
7. Describe the theories of how obesity develops.
8. Explain how a plateau or weight cycling relate to physiological adaptation to weight loss.
9. State the goals of treatment for obesity.
10. State the recommended dietary modifications for weight reduction.
11. List four examples of behavior modification strategies useful in weight reduction.
12. Explain how exercise affects body weight.
13. List the surgical procedures that have been used for weight reduction.
14. Describe the factors related to maintenance of weight loss.
15. Define excessive leanness and identify the assessment parameters used to identify the condition.
16. Compare and contrast the characteristic signs, symptoms, and behaviors of anorexia nervosa and bulimia.

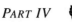

CHAPTER OUTLINE ———————————————— **NOTES, TERMS, & TRANSPARENCY MASTERS**

Key concept: *Obese* is defined as being 20% above desirable weight and *severely obese* is defined as being 40% or more above desirable weight.

Figure 21-1 is a graph showing the percentage of overweight (>85th percentile of weight for height) men and women from NHANES II.

I.   Components of Body Weight

lean body mass (LBM), fat-free mass (FFM)

II. Adipose Tissue: The Fat Depot

Figure 21-2 is Behnke's theoretical model for composition of a male and female body.

Key concept: There are significant differences in body composition for males and females. These are natural differences.

essential fat, sex-specific body fat, storage fat, adipocytes

   A. Structure

white adipose tissue, brown adipose tissue (BAT)

   B. Regional distribution

Key concept: Evidence suggests that the android type regional distribution of body fat may be a risk factor for hypertension, cardiovascular disease, and non–insulin dependent diabetes mellitus.

android, gynoid

   C. Adipocytes
       1. Hypertrophy and hyperplasia

hypertrophy, hyperplasia

       2. Fat cell development

adiposity rebound

   D. Fat storage
       1. Source of lipid in fat cells
       2. Role of lipoprotein lipase

lipoprotein lipase (LPL), very low density lipoprotein (VLDL), hormone-sensitive lipase (HSL), estrogens

III. Regulation of Body Weight

norepinephrine, dopamine, sympathetic nervous system (SNS)

   A. Short- and long-term regulation

Figure 21-3 illustrates the increasing body weight of Americans.

       1. Short-term regulation

satiety, hunger, hypophagia, hyperphagia

       2. Long-term regulation

adipose mass

3. Set-point theory
  A. Thermogenesis

    resting energy expenditure (REE), resting metabolic rate (RMR), diet-induced thermogenesis

  B. Thermogenic effect of food (TEF)
  c. Resting metabolic rate (RMR)
  d. Gut peptides

    gut peptides, cholecystokinin (CCK)

  e. Brain proteins

    galatin, enterostatin

  f. Thyroid hormones
  g. Insulin

IV. Weight Imbalance: Obesity

    overweight, obesity

  A. Assessment

    Table 21-1 provides the diagnostic criteria for classifications of overweight and obesity according to gender, percent IBW, and BMI.
    ideal body weight (IBW), body mass index (BMI), Quetelet's Index, waist to hip ratio (WHR)

  B. Risk

    Figure 21-4 is a graphic comparison of the mortality risk according to BMI.
    syndrome X

  C. Etiology
    1. Heredity

      genetic component, ob, oblob

    2. Factors affecting weight gain

      hyperphagia, externality theory, restraint theory, defect in thermogenesis

V. Tissue Adaption to Weight Loss
  A. Plateau effect
  B. Weight cycling

    yo-yo effect

VI. Management of Obesity

    Key concepts: The management of obesity is an expensive industry. The emphasis here should be twofold: (1) there are a variety of effective methods for weight loss that do not have medical risks and (2) loss of body weight should focus on loss of body fat with the least risk for overall nutritional status.

  A. Goals of treatment
  B. Rate and extent of weight loss
  C. Dietary modifications
    1. Recommendations
    2. Restricted-energy diets
      a. Energy-restricted diets

    high-carbohydrate, low-fat diet; calculating fat grams

b. Exchange system diets

Table 21-2 illustrates a 1200-kcal diet with 22% of total kilocalories from fat. Summary of the exchanges, a meal plan, and a menu are given.

Figure 21-5 is a photographic illustration comparing the meal planned in Table 21-2 with a typical American diet.

c. Formula diets

d. Commercial programs

Table 21-3 list the currently popular commercial diet programs. The general plan for administration of these programs is summarized.

e. Fad diets and practices

Table 21-4 is a list of recommended methods for evaluating fat diets.

Key concept: This is an opportunity to discuss the use of ketogenic diets in weight control. The ineffectiveness of these diets, along with the risk, should be pointed out.

low-carbohydrate, high-fat diet

f. Extreme energy restriction
   i.   Fasting
   ii. Very low calorie diet

very low calorie diet (VLCD), protein-sparing modified fast (PSMF), commercially formulated liquid diet

D. Behavior modification

Table 21-5 provides students with a list of techniques used in behavior modification programs for weight management.

self-monitoring, stimulus control, self-reward

E. Exercise

Figure 21-6 is a photograph of a person swimming, an example of an aerobic exercise.

aerobic exercise, resistance training

F. Pharmaceutical management

amphetamines, fenfluramine, mazindol, phenylpropanolamine, 5-hydroxytryptophan, dehydroepiandrosterone (DHEA)

G. Surgical procedures

intractable morbid obesity

1. Gastric restriction (gastric bypass and gastroplasty)

Figure 21-7 (Handout) is a set of drawings showing the types of surgeries used for treatment of obesity.

gastric restriction, gastroplasty, gastric bypass, dumping syndrome

2. Jaw wiring (maxillomandibular fixation)

maxillomandibular fixation

3. Liposuction

liposuction

H. Psychotherapy

cognitive structuring

I. Weight management in children

Key concept: Management of excessive weight in children must emphasize the adequacy of the diet for providing sufficient nutrients (including energy) for normal growth and development.

See **Clinical Insight:** "American Dietetic Association Criteria for Use of Very Low Calorie Diets."

J. Maintenance of reduced body weight

energy requirements, behavior modification, exercise, support groups

VII. Weight Imbalance: Excessive Leanness

Key concept: *Underweight* is defined as being 15–20% or more below accepted weight standards.

Key concept: The underweight individual is at risk for general malnutrition, a condition that can affect normal body functions, including the endocrine system.

A. Etiology
B. Assessment
C. Management
   1. High-energy diets for weight gain

VIII. Management of Eating Disorders

anorexia nervosa, bulimia nervosa

A. Occurrence

Figure 21-9 (Transparency) illustrates the spectrum of eating disorders that spans from anorexia nervosa (extreme leanness) to developmental obesity (severe obesity).

B. Characteristics

Table 21-7 lists the physical signs seen in anorexia nervosa.

Figure 21-10 is a series of photographs showing the emaciation associated with anorexia nervosa.

binge eating disorder (BED)

C. Etiology
D. Management
   1. Psychotherapy
   2. Nutritional care

Table 21-8 provides guidelines for nutritional management of both anorexia nervosa and bulimia nervosa.

   3. Energy requirements for weight gain
   4. Dietary intake
E. Prognosis

CASE STUDY INSIGHTS: WEIGHT MANAGEMENT

1. How would you address the concern about Mary L.'s medications?

It is likely that some of the medications she is taking have been prescribed for control of her hypertension. It is imperative that the exact drugs and dosages be known before making a final diet plan for Mary L. Her physician should be made aware of weight reduction strategies and progress in weight reduction.

2. What types of exercise would you be likely to discuss?

Exercise should be aerobic and weight bearing. She should be capable of walking as a routine exercise. Inclusion of resistance training would also be useful for increasing lean body mass and resting metabolic rate.

3. Which nutrients would you discuss with Mary (for example, total fat, saturated fat, sodium, potassium, and calcium)?

The use of low-fat diets are effective for weight loss, especially when used with calorie restrictions. Given the information about Mary's cardiac medications, you should find out more about her cardiac condition when considering the other nutrients. In general, the diet should be low in total fat, low in saturated fat, have a moderate intake of sodium, and include liberal intakes of potassium and calcium.

4. What would be the goals of her treatment?

Mary L. should use a combination of a calorie-restricted, nutritionally balanced diet along with exercise and behavior modification to achieve a weight loss of 0.5 to 1 pound per week (daily energy deficit of about 500 kcal).

CASE STUDY INSIGHTS: EATING DISORDERS

1. What suggestions would you offer to Jenny? Develop a care plan that could be followed in the outpatient setting.

The care plan would consist of the following goals:

  a. Assess current intake and adjust to provide a minimum of 800–1200 kcal per day with slow progression to meet total energy needs within 2 weeks.
  b. Use patient preferences to plan a nutritionally balanced diet.
  c. Supplement with multivitamin and mineral preparation.
  d. Suggest small, frequent feedings as tolerated.
  e. Limit daily activities and exercise routines.
  f. Plan incentives (rewards) for meeting recommended caloric intake.
  g. Maintain daily records for all foods, beverages, and exercise.
  h. Return to clinic once per week with daily records to be seen by dietitian.

2. *How does the starvation of anorexia nervosa compare with the starvation of AIDS? Discuss how you would care for Jenny if she had AIDS instead of anorexia nervosa.*

(Note: AIDS is presented in Chapter 37. Students may need to review this chapter before answering this question.) The major difference between the starvation of anorexia nervosa and that of AIDS is that the former is self-induced. The weight loss seen in AIDS is involuntary and usually part of the wasting syndrome seen in that condition. In AIDS, the malnutrition results from a combination of factors, including poor intake, malabsorption, increased metabolic demand, and increased losses. The starvation in anorexia nervosa exhibits many of the normal adaptations of long-term fasting.

In AIDS, aggressive medical nutritional therapy can be used to minimize the effects of the compromised nutritional status and prevent PEM. In anorexia nervosa, aggressive medical nutritional therapy such as parenteral or tube feedings are avoided unless the condition reaches a life-threatening level.

3. *What do you suggest for including Jenny in the treatment plan? At this point, she does want to be well and is willing to work with you.*

See answer to question #1. You should take the opportunity to work with Jenny to educate her about nutrition and planning a balanced diet. You can also work with her to find appropriate incentives for achieving treatment goals. Look for things that she likes to do and will be supportive of her need to increase intake and decrease or minimize excessive activity.

4. *How would you include Jenny's family in the nutritional care plan?*

Jenny's entire family should be included in the treatment plan, including psychotherapy. The family should be part of the goal-setting sessions for nutritional care. The family's role in being supportive but not forcing Jenny to eat should be emphasized. The family can plan meals together that are satisfactory to everyone, including Jenny. Meal preparation can also be a shared activity. There should be an emphasis on family meal times where everyone is involved.

SUGGESTED TEST QUESTIONS

1. For obese patients, the cycle of weight gain and weight loss often results in
   a. restructuring of fat deposits from the abdomen to the hips.
   b. increased accumulation of visceral fat.
   c. decreased resistance to infections.
   * d. increased time needed to lose and decreased time to gain the same amount of weight.

2. The rate of weight loss for men on energy-deficient diets is more rapid than for women because men
   a. generally have less fat to lose.
   b. are more successful at weight reduction programs.
   * c. have higher RMR and LBM than women.
   d. are more likely to exercise while trying to lose weight.

3. Supplementation of vitamins and minerals is recommended for individuals whose daily caloric intake is
   a. 2500 kcal for both men and women.
   b. 2000 kcal for women and 2500 kcal for men.
   c. 1500 kcal for both men and women.
   * d. 1200 kcal for women and 1800 kcal for men.

4. The use of fasting as a means of weight loss results in
   a. excessive weight gain after refeeding.
 * b. an initial rapid weight loss from diuresis.
   c. a decrease in ketone formation.
   d. carbohydrate craving.

5. Fasting and very low calorie (VLC) diets may result in development of gout, which is a result of elevated ketones impeding the elimination of
   a. creatinine.
   b. sodium.
 * c. uric acid.
   d. potassium.

6. Exercise training programs used for weight loss would not be expected to show reductions in adipose tissue until
   a. after the first two weeks.
 * b. after the first two months.
   c. a severe calorie-restricted diet is initiated.
   d. liver and muscle glycogen stores are depleted.

7. Patients diagnosed with intractable morbid obesity may benefit from
   a. pharmacological treatment with amphetamines for an extended period of time.
 * b. gastric restrictive surgery.
   c. intestinal bypass that decreases the absorptive surface.
   d. liposuction on select areas of the body.

8. The success of maintaining a weight loss in a formerly obese individual is
   a. good for a high percentage of clients.
   b. depends on whether the individual lost weight intentionally.
 * c. about 5% for 5 years after a reduction program.
   d. excellent due to the risk of chronic disease for obese adults.

9. The occurrence of obesity in the United States can best be described as
   a. on the decline and more prevalent in women than in men.
   b. on the decline and more prevalent in men than in women.
 * c. on the rise and more prevalent in women than in men.
   d. on the rise and more prevalent in men than in women.

10. The effectiveness of exercise as part of a weight management program is that the resting metabolic rate is
    a. increased as adipose tissue is increased with exercise.
    b. decreased as adipose tissue is decreased with exercise.
    c. decreased as lean body mass is decreased with exercise.
 * d. increased as lean body mass is increased with exercise.

11. The regional distribution of fat that promotes rapid mobilization of free fatty acids and is associated with significant risk for hypertension is
 * a. the android type.
    b. the gynoid type.
    c. brown adipose tissue.
    d. white adipose tissue.

12. Dietary triglyceride is transported to the liver as part of the chylomicrons and is removed from the blood by the enzyme
    a. hormone-sensitive lipase.
 * b. lipoprotein lipase.
    c. cholecystokinin.
    d. insulin.

13. Feeding behavior is affected by several factors, including hormonal controls from the
    a. pituitary gland.
    b. parotid gland.
 * c. hypothalamus gland.
    d. adrenal glands.

14. During starvation, the body's adaptive response is
* a. a drop in the RMR as much as 15% in two weeks.
b. a rise in the RMR as much as 15% in two weeks.
c. a drop in the RMR as much as 45% in one month.
d. a rise in the RMR as much as 45% in one month.

15. One of the gut peptides released when food comes into contact with the muscles of the stomach and small intestine that has an immediate effect on satiety is
* a. cholecystokinin.
b. gastrin.
c. secretin.
d. insulin.

16. If resting metabolic rate decreases during a period of weight reduction, then it can be concluded that
* a. lean body mass is lost.
b. lean body mass increases.
c. adipose tissue is lost.
d. the thermogenic effect of food increases.

17. Weight reduction programs having the highest rates of success include
a. diet and exercise.
b. behavior modification and diet.
* c. diet, exercise, and behavior modification.
d. behavior modification and exercise.

18. To achieve a weight reduction of 1 lb per week, the diet should have how many kilocalories less than maintenance requirements?
a. 1000 kcal/day
* b. 500 kcal/day
c. 1000 kcal/week
d. 500 kcal/week

19. Fasting can lead to serious hypotension because
* a. more than 50% of the rapid weight loss is fluid.
b. lack of caloric intake depletes energy reserves.
c. it results in rapid loss of lean body mass.
d. more than 50% of the rapid weight loss is carbohydrate.

20. Aerobic exercise is effective in weight management because it
* a. lowers glycogen stores and promotes the use of fat for fuel.
b. decreases lean body mass in proportion to fat.
c. increases resistance to insulin.
d. decreases sensitivity to insulin.

21. The recommended treatment goal for a child who is overweight but has not yet reached adult weight is
a. weight loss of 1 lb per week.
* b. weight maintenance or a slower rate of weight gain.
c. weight loss of 2 lb per week.
d. no treatment until adult weight has been reached.

CHAPTER **22**

NUTRITION FOR ATHLETIC TRAINING AND PERFORMANCE

OVERVIEW

The purpose of this chapter is to provide students with an overview of the metabolic demand associated with athletic performance. The focus is on the competitive athlete, not the casual exerciser. The chapter begins with a review of the physiology and biochemistry of muscle contraction, including choice of energy substrate. Specific nutritional requirements for exercise are given, followed by nutritional considerations for before, during, and after an athletic event. Some attention is given to the effect of exercise on weight loss and gain.

LEARNING OBJECTIVES

This chapter will prepare the learner to be able to

1. Explain the basic mechanism of muscle contraction.
2. Compare and contrast aerobic and anaerobic metabolism.
3. Explain how the energy substrates used for muscle contraction during exercise change with intensity and duration.
4. List the dangers of dehydration and the proper methods to rehydrate an athlete.
5. Describe how the body meets the demand for energy using carbohydrate substrate during prolonged exercise.
6. Explain the concept of glycogen loading and the proper method to do it.
7. Describe the protein needs for an athlete and how they differ from a nonathlete.
8. Explain the effects of iron deficiency in an athlete.
9. State the possible role of antioxidants in recovery from exercise.
10. List the characteristics of the preevent meal.
11. Explain when and how nutrition should be provided during an event.
12. Describe the role of exercise in weight gain or loss.

CHAPTER OUTLINE	NOTES, TERMS, & TRANSPARENCY MASTERS
I. Physiology and Biochemistry of Exercise Muscle Contraction	**fibrils, filaments, myosin, actin, sarcomeres, sliding filament theory, adenosine triphosphate (ATP), actomyosin, adenosine diphosphate (ADP)**
A. Muscle fiber types	**Table 22-1** provides a summary of types of muscle fibers and their characteristics. **Type I (slow twitch), Type IIA (fast twitch), Type IIB (pure fast twitch)**
B. Phosphagen energy sources	**Figure 22-1** is a graphic classification of activities based on duration of performance (minutes) and predominant energy pathways (aerobic versus nonaerobic). **glycolysis, pyruvic acid, lactic acid**
C. Oxygen requirements 1. Aerobic metabolism	**Figure 22-2 (Handout)** is a schematic presentation of the pathways of energy production (glycolysis, Krebs' cycle, and electron transport) **aerobic metabolism**
2. Anaerobic metabolism	**Figure 22-3** is a graphic presentation of the contribution of aerobic and anaerobic energy during exercise (total energy yield in percent versus maximal work time in minutes). **glycogenolysis, respiratory exchange ratio (RER), respiratory quotient (RQ)**
3. Excess postexercise oxygen consumption	**Figure 22-4** is a photograph of soccer players, demonstrating a strenuous form of exercise requiring anaerobic energy production. **excess postexercise oxygen consumption (EPOC)**
D. Fuel of muscle contraction 1. Sources of fuel 2. Choice of fuel	**Key concept**: Carbohydrate is the preferred fuel and is most efficient with oxygen consumption. Available carbohydrate is limited to blood sugar and glycogen. Intensity and duration are factors in the choice of fuel.
3. Effect of training	
II. Nutritional Requirements of Exercise A. Fluid and electrolytes 1. Fluid 2. Electrolytes	**sweat**

B. Energy

Table 22-2 presents classifications of physical work based on energy expenditure.
Figure 22-5 is a photograph of a runner, demonstrating an exercise that requires repetitive muscle contractions and requires more energy.
Figure 22-6 is a photograph of a gymnast, demonstrating an exercise that requires muscle contraction maintenance, requiring less energy.
Figure 22-7 is a graphic prediction of calories burned during exercise based on pulse rate.
See **Clinical Insight** on metabolic equivalents.
metabolic equivalents (MET)

C. Carbohydrate

Figure 22-8 is a graphic illustration of sources of energy used during 4 hours of exercise.

1. Glycogen loading

Key concept: Many students are familiar with the term glycogen loading. Careful explanation of its theory is important; this regimen is not without risks.

D. Fat
E. Protein

Table 22-3 provides estimates of protein requirements for athletes (adolescent males).

F. Minerals and vitamins
   1. Iron
      a. Sports anemia

sports anemia

   2. Calcium
   3. B vitamins
   4. Antioxidant vitamins and beta-carotene
   5. Vitamin C
   6. Vitamin E

III. Nutritional Considerations for an Event
  A. Preevent meal
  B. Nutrition during performance

Table 22-4 summarizes the guidelines for proper hydration during physical performance.
Key concept: The appropriate composition of replacement fluid depends on the duration and intensity of an event, as well as the temperature and humidity of the environment.

  C. Postevent meal
  D. Other considerations
    1. Alcohol
    2. Caffeine
    3. Ergogenic aids

Key concept: An ergogenic aid is that which contributes to athletic ability.
Table 22-5 is a listing of unproven ergogenic aids for athletes.
carnitine, sodium bicarbonate

IV. Weight Gain or Loss

CASE STUDY INSIGHTS

1. Is it reasonable to expect LH to meet her goal weight before the marathon? Explain.

With 2 months left before the marathon, it is possible to have a safe weight loss of 8 lbs before the event. It is important to preserve lean body mass during the period of weight loss. You should also consider that you do not know much about the weight gain that LH has experienced. It is important to determine if the gain has been body fat or lean body mass. This can be estimated by determining her total body fat. If she is at or below the normal body fat for her condition, it may not be appropriate to promote weight loss before the event.

2. What would you recommend for fat intake for LH and why?

LH is currently consuming only 10–15% of her total kilocalories from fat. She could be compromising her performance at this intake. Ensuring that she receives a minimum of 15% of total kilocalories from fat will enhance intramuscular triglyceride storage. The recommended fat intake for athletes is 25–30% of total kilocalories.

3. Is calcium a concern for LH? How can you find out, and if it is a concern, what would you advise?

You need more information about her to determine if calcium is of concern. You need to know if she has experienced any menstrual irregularities and, if so, what they have been. You also need to know what her normal calcium intake is and whether she takes a calcium supplement. Your recommendations would then be based on your findings.

4. What protein intake would you recommend and how would you find out if LH is getting enough?

The recommended protein intake is 12–15% of total kilocalories to be provided by protein. In most diets, this meets or exceeds the RDA for protein (0.8 g/kg). A 24-hour recall and a food frequency would be helpful in determining whether her protein intake is adequate.

5. What vitamins might be of concern, and how would you advise LH to optimize her intake?

The vitamins most likely to be of concern are C, E, and A (also beta-carotene). Both vitamin A and C can be optimized by consuming the minimum recommendations in the Food Guide Pyramid for fruit and vegetable intake. Vitamin E supplementation can be used but should be limited to the RDA in the absence of conclusive evidence of its benefits to athletic performance.

6. LH has asked you specifically about her premarathon diet, both a few days ahead and just before the event. What would you recommend?

Glycogen loading can be done prior to the marathon since it is an endurance event. Beginning four days before the event, a high-carbohydrate diet with light exercise is undertaken for three days, followed by a final day of a high-carbohydrate diet with no exercise.

The preevent meal should be consumed 3–4 hours prior to the onset of the event and should contain 200–350 g of carbohydrate. Then, 30 minutes to 1 hour before the onset of the event, an additional 50–100 g of carbohydrate should be eaten.

SUGGESTED TEST QUESTIONS

1. After exercise that results in lactic acid build up and an increase in body temperature, recovery from the oxygen debt may require
   a. medical intervention.
   b. a short rest period.
   * c. several hours to one day.
   d. extra fluids to eliminate the lactic acid.

2. The choice of fuel during exercise is influenced by the intensity and duration of the exercise. In general,
   a. carbohydrate is the larger fraction of the energy source as the intensity decreases.
   b. fatty acids are the larger fraction of the energy source as the intensity increases.
   * c. carbohydrate is the larger fraction of the energy source as the intensity increases.
   d. fatty acids are the larger fraction of the energy source as the intensity decreases.

3. Inappropriate fluid replacement following athletic competition can result in
   * a. hypotension due to decreased blood volume and elevated core temperature.
   b. decreased calcium that can eventually lead to tetany.
   c. cerebral edema and bradycardia.
   d. diuresis and osmotic diarrhea.

4. During sustained exercise, an individual's fluid replacement should be guided by
   a. thirst and need to urinate.
   * b. urine color and changes in body weight.
   c. performance.
   d. formulations based on body weight.

5. The rate of electrolyte losses from sweating during athletic competition is
   a. usually high enough to require special salt tablets.
   b. a primary problem for experienced athletes.
   * c. less dramatic than the rate of water loss.
   d. highest for magnesium.

6. For athletes participating in events lasting more than 1 hour, preevent glycogen loading regimens can
   a. cause hyperglycemia.
   * b. increase muscle glycogen storage capacity.
   c. cause hypotension.
   d. improve strength during an event.

7. The preevent meal should be
   * a. eaten 3–4 hours prior to competition.
   b. restricted in carbohydrate.
   c. high in calories and protein.
   d. eaten 1–2 hours prior to competition.

8. Ingestion of fructose during competition may cause the athlete to experience
   a. improved performance.
   b. transient hypoglycemia.
   * c. osmotic diarrhea.
   d. increased endurance.

9. During exercise of low to moderate intensity, the primary source of energy comes from
   * a. fatty acids.
   b. glycogen.
   c. amino acids.
   d. glycerol.

10. The amount of fluid lost during exercise depends on
    * a. the intensity and duration of the activity and the temperature and humidity of the environment.
    b. the percentage of body water at the onset of the event.
    c. the ambient temperature.
    d. how much body surface is exposed to the environment.

11. The recommendation for fluid replacement during long, strenuous exercise is to replace water
    a. only in warm temperatures.
    b. if perspiration has been excessive.
    * c. in amounts sufficient to maintain pre-exercise weight.
    d. if hypertension occurs.

12. Sports requiring repetitive muscle contractions use more energy than those involving more muscle contraction maintenance because
    a. the metabolic equivalents are less.
 * b. more energy is needed to initiate a muscle contraction than to maintain it.
    c. the intensity of effort is greater.
    d. the intensity of effort is less.

13. The first source of glucose for the exercising muscle is
    a. blood glucose.
    b. liver glycogen.
 * c. muscle glycogen.
    d. muscle protein.

14. *Staleness,* in which even the smallest amount of exercise causes fatigue, can result from
 * a. insufficient replacement of glycogen stores.
    b. a decrease in dietary carbohydrate intake the day of exercise.
    c. consuming a diet that has 20–30% of calories from carbohydrate.
    d. consuming only carbohydrate for 3 days.

15. Carbohydrate intake immediately after a training session is important because
    a. energy stores are depleted.
    b. carbohydrate is needed to reverse the feeling of fatigue.
    c. hypoglycemia is a common end result of prolonged exercise.
 * d. glycogen stores must be replaced and lean body mass preserved.

16. The preevent meal should contain
    a. 100–200 g of carbohydrate.
 * b. 200–350 g of carbohydrate.
    c. only carbohydrate and fat.
    d. only protein and fat.

17. ATP for energy is most rapidly obtained from
    a. gluconeogenesis.
    b. lipolysis.
 * c. glycolysis.
    d. glycogenolysis.

18. An increased level of lactic acid during exercise can lead to fatigue because the lactic acid
 * a. lowers the pH to a level that interferes with enzymatic action.
    b. raises the pH to a level that interferes with enzymatic action.
    c. exceeds the capacity for oxidation.
    d. prevents aerobic oxidation of glucose.

19. The appropriate rehydration drink for correcting excessive weight loss during heavy training in a hot climate should contain
    a. 2 teaspoons of salt per liter of water.
    b. sodium and potassium.
    c. 2–3 teaspoons of salt per liter of water.
 * d. no more than 1/2 teaspoon of salt per liter of water.

20. Which of the following best characterizes the role of iron in exercise?
 * a. Low serum ferritin levels can have a detrimental effect on exercise performance, even when anemia is not present.
    b. Exercise performance is affected only in cases of severe iron-deficiency anemia.
    c. Mild iron-deficiency anemia has no detrimental effects.
    d. Iron plays no significant role in muscle activity.

CHAPTER 23

NUTRITION IN CARDIOVASCULAR DISEASE

OVERVIEW

The purpose of this chapter is to provide students with a comprehensive understanding of the significance of cardiovascular disease in the population. The chapter provides an opportunity to gain knowledge in the pathophysiology, etiology, morbidity, mortality, treatment, and nutritional care principles related to cardiovascular disease. A important part of the chapter is devoted to the current findings on blood lipids and lipoproteins. The National Cholesterol Education Program's Step I and Step II diets are included.

LEARNING OBJECTIVES

This chapter will prepare the learner to be able to

1. State the significance of cardiovascular disease as it relates to morbidity and mortality.
2. Explain the pathophysiology of atherosclerosis and its diagnosis.
3. Define thrombosis and state its significance.
4. Identify the five classes of lipoproteins and their relative composition.
5. State the risk factors for cardiovascular disease.
6. State the criteria for assessing risk for cardiovascular disease according to serum lipid levels.
7. Explain the relationship of diet to development of cardiovascular disease.
8. Identify the significant dietary factors related to development of cardiovascular disease.
9. State the recommended treatment for cardiovascular disease based on NCEP criteria.
10. State the principles of the NCEP Step I and Step II diets.
11. List the medications used for treatment of cardiovascular disease and state their purpose.
12. Explain the surgical procedures used to treat cardiovascular disease.

CHAPTER OUTLINE ——————————— NOTES, TERMS, & TRANSPARENCY MASTERS

I. Prevalence and Incidence

Figure 23-1 illustrates worldwide male and female deaths from cardiovascular disease compared to all causes of death.
Figure 23-2 illustrates the morbidity and mortality related to coronary heart disease by age and sex (taken from the Framingham study follow-up).
See **Focus On:** "Framingham Heart Study."

142

II. Mortality	**Table 23-1** summarizes the deaths (per 100,000 people) from diseases of the heart by race and ethnicity.
III. Physiology and Etiology	**Figure 23-3 (Handout)** shows a drawing of three arteries ranging from normal to major blockage and a drawing of the heart indicating the location of the coronary arteries. **coronary heart disease (CHD)**
A. Atherosclerosis	**atherosclerosis, plaque, atheroma**
1. Pathology	**Figure 23-4** is a summary of the progression of atherosclerosis, from normal artery to fatty streak, fibrous plaque, and then calcification. The outcomes are myocardial infarction, stroke, gangrene, and aneurism. **fatty streaks, fibrous plaques**
2. Clinical determination	**invasive angiography (cardiac catheterization)**
3. End points	
B. Thrombosis	**thrombosis**
IV. Risk Factors for Coronary Heart Disease	
A. Blood lipids and lipoproteins	
1. Definitions	**Table 23-2** lists the five classes of lipoproteins and their compositions and atherogenicities. **lipoproteins, apolipoproteins**
2. Total cholesterol	**Figure 23-5** illustrates the relationship of serum cholesterol level to the rate of CHD death.
3. Total triglycerides	**familial dyslipidemias**
4. Lipoproteins and metabolism	See **Table 23-2.**
a. Chylomicrons	**chylomicron, lipoprotein lipase (LPL)**
b. Very low density lipoproteins	**very low density lipoproteins (VLDL)**
c. Intermediate-density lipoproteins	**intermediate density lipoproteins (IDL)**
d. Low-density lipoproteins	**low-density lipoproteins (LDL), phenotype A, phenotype B**
e. High-density lipoproteins	**high-density lipoproteins (HDL), protective effect, reverse cholesterol transport**

B. Assessing risk

Table 23-3 lists the adult reference percentiles for total cholesterol by age, gender, and ethnicity.

Table 23-4 lists the adult reference percentiles for LDL cholesterol by age, gender, and ethnicity.

Table 23-5 lists the adult reference percentiles for HDL cholesterol by age, gender, and ethnicity.

See **Clinical Insight** on the corresponding levels of lipids in mg/dL and mmol/L.

See **Clinical Insight** on the NCEP recommendations for detection and management of hypercholesterolemia in children and adolescents.

Table 23-6 lists the classifications for primary prevention of CHD based on serum total cholesterol and HDL cholesterol.

    1. Lipoprotein profile
C. Related blood analytes as risk factors
    1. Apolipoproteins
    2. Lp(a)
D. Nonlipid risk factors
    1. Nonmodifiable risk factors

age, gender, premature menopause, family history

    2. Modifiable risk factors
        a. Cigarette smoking
        b. Hypertension
        c. Diabetes

Key concept: Hypertension is defined as average blood pressure that is greater than or equal to 140/90 mmHg.

    3. Adiposity
    4. Inactivity

V. Genetic Hyperlipidemias
  A. Classification and diagnosis

Table 23-7 summarizes the phenotype classification of the hyperlipidemias by lipoprotein abnormality and blood lipids.

  B. Familial hypercholesterolemia

familial hypercholesterolemia (FH): type IIa or high LDL-C, normal TG

  C. Polygenic familial hypercholesterolemia

polygenic familial hypercholesterolemia

  D. Familial combined hyperlipidemia

familial combined hyperlipidemia (FCHL)

  E. Familial dyslipidemia

familial dyslipidemia, familial hypertriglyceridemia

  F. Familial dysbetalipoproteinemia

familial dysbetalipoproteinemia: type III hyperlipoproteinemia

VI. Relationship of Dietary Factors to Serum Lipids
  A. Type of fatty acids
    1. Saturated fatty acids (SFA)

stearic acid, palmitic acid, myristic acid, lauric acid

2. Polyunsaturated fatty acids
   a. Omega-6 polyunsaturated fatty acids — **linoleic acid**
   b. Omega-3 polyunsaturated acids — **eicosapentanoic acid (EPA), docosahexanoic acid (DHA), hypotriglyceridemic effect**

3. Monounsaturated fatty acids
   a. *Cis*-monounsaturated fatty acids — **oleic acid**
   b. Trans-fatty acids — **stereoisomers (trans-forms)**

B. Amount of dietary fat

Key concept: The effects of a low-fat diet vary depending on the type of fatty acids in the diet. A diet low in fat can lower LDL-C only when there is also a decrease in saturated fatty acids.

C. Dietary cholesterol
D. Other dietary factors
   1. Fiber

Table 23-8 summarizes the types and amounts of soluble fiber that show lipid-lowering effects.
soluble fibers, insoluble fibers

   2. Alcohol
   3. Coffee — **boiled coffee, filtered coffee**
   4. Antioxidants
   5. Calcium

VII. Prevention of Coronary Heart Disease
A. Primary prevention

clinical or patient-based strategy, primary prevention, secondary prevention

   1. National Cholesterol Education Program Adult Treatment Panel-II

National Cholesterol Education Program (NCEP)

   a. Rationale
   b. Assessment of risk

Figure 23-6 is an algorithm from NCEP that uses total cholesterol and HDL-C to assess risk for CHD.
Figure 23-7 is an algorithm from NCEP that uses LDL-C to assess risk for CHD.
Table 23-9 lists the criteria for dietary therapy and drug therapy based on LDL-C and presence of other risk factors.

   c. Step I and Step II diets

Table 23-10 summarizes the dietary recommendations for high blood cholesterol. Nutrients include total fat, saturated fatty acids, monounsaturated fatty acids, polyunsaturated fatty acids, carbohydrates, protein, cholesterol, and total calories.
Figure 23-8 is an example of a form used for quick dietary assessment in the NCEP.
Step I diet, Step II diet

B. Secondary prevention
C. Treatment
D. Diet and life-style changes
    1. Step I and II diets

        Table 23-11 presents the actual food choices for the Step I and Step II diets.

        Table 23-12 lists the total fat, saturated fat, cholesterol, and iron content of 3-oz portions of selected animal protein foods.

        Table 23-13 provides an eating plan for the Step I and Step II diets using the exchange system.

        Table 23-14 summarizes the recommended levels of total fat and saturated fat on the Step I and Step II diets based on total calories.

        Table 23-15 gives information on the nutrition label useful in assessing foods for the diet.

        Table 23-16 is a sample menu for both the Step I and Step II diets for a female consuming a traditional American diet.

        Table 23-17 is a sample menu for both the Step I and Step II diets for a male consuming a Mexican-American diet.

        Table 23-18 is a sample menu for both the Step I (male) and Step II (female) diets for a person consuming an Asian-American diet.

    2. Aggressive diets

        Table 23-19 is a food plan for a diet containing less than 10% of total calories from fat (aggressive low-fat diet).

        Table 23-20 provides quick tips for using the aggressive low-fat diet.

E. Pharmacological management

        Table 23-21 summarizes the effects of selected cholesterol-lowering medications on nutrition status.

        Key concept: The side effects of bile acid sequestrants should be viewed within the context of the role of bile in digestion, absorption, and excretion.

        bile acid sequestrants (cholestyramine), nicotinic acid, HMG CoA reductase inhibitors (lovastatin, pravastatin, fibric acid derivatives (clofibrate, gemfibrozil), probucol

F. Medical intervention
    1. Coronary angioplasty (PCTA)

        percutaneous transluminal coronary angioplasty (PCTA)

    2. Coronary bypass surgery (CABG)

        coronary artery bypass surgery (CABG)

CASE STUDY INSIGHTS

1. What are Mrs. W's risk factors for coronary heart disease?

Mrs. W has many risk factors for CHD: positive family history, obesity, diabetes, hypertension, age (over 55 years), and elevated serum lipids. One might also suspect that she has a sedentary lifestyle. No information is given on her diet, activity level, drinking, or smoking habits.

2. What type of diet would you recommend for Mrs. W? What additional information needs to be obtained before teaching about a new eating plan?

Mrs. W's lipid profile and medical history are most closely associated with a type IIb hyperlipoproteinemia (elevated LDL-C, elevated TG, obesity, hypertension, and diabetes). This would normally require a treatment plan that includes the Step II diet, weight reduction, management of the diabetes, increased activity, elimination of alcohol, and avoidance of estrogen therapy. The last two recommendations are specific for the elevated TG. Before beginning any therapy, more information is needed about Mrs. W's lifestyle and food preferences.

3. What suggestions for restaurant eating would help Mrs. W adhere to the eating plan?

Suggestions might include choosing restaurants that offer a variety of foods and preparation methods, avoiding fast food restaurants, selecting naturally low-fat foods prepared without added fat (such as fish and chicken), requesting larger serving sizes of vegetables and fruits to substitute for high-fat items normally served, and ordering from the á la carte menu to avoid unwanted foods. Students may have other suggestions.

4. What dietary factors could optimize Mrs. W's lipid profile?

Considering that you do not have a diet history for Mrs. W, it is difficult to assess the diet and identify the necessary changes. In general, the diet should be low in total fat, low in saturated fat, low in cholesterol, and include soluble fiber. All other factors related to a nutritionally balanced diet would apply.

SUGGESTED TEST QUESTIONS

1. The most reliable biochemical indicators for predicting cardiovascular disease are
 * a. serum concentrations of HDL and LDL cholesterol.
    b. serum potassium and blood glucose.
    c. serum levels of nicotinic acid and blood urea nitrogen.
    d. serum triglyceride and albumin levels.

2. In the NCEP Step I and Step II diets, the recommendations for intake of dietary saturated fatty acids is
    a. the same for each step.
    b. increased from 8–10% of total calories in Step I to 10–12% in Step II.
 * c. decreased from 8–10% of total calories in Step I to 7% in Step II.
    d. decreased from 30% of total calories in Step I to 20% in Step II.

3. In planning a diet for reduction of elevated serum lipids, the effect of increasing omega-3 fatty acids is
   a. decreased LDL cholesterol.
   b. increased HDL cholesterol.
   c. decreased bleeding time.
* d. decreased serum triglycerides.

4. Which oils should be used in food preparation by a patient who has been instructed to increase his intake of monounsaturated fatty acids?
* a. canola and olive oil
   b. cottonseed and palm oil
   c. coconut and palm oil
   d. safflower and palm oil

5. The use of bile acid sequestrants to lower serum cholesterol may cause
   a. decreased utilization of vitamin C.
   b. increased absorption of glucose.
* c. decreased absorption of calcium and fat soluble vitamins.
   d. increased absorption of fat.

6. When a patient presents with documented hypertriglyceridemia and hypercholesterolemia, the recommended treatment to lower both lipids is
   a. a bile acid sequestrant.
   b. nicotinic acid.
   c. a fibrate.
* d. a combination of medications.

7. Current research on the role of antioxidants in development of cardiovascular disease indicates that
   a. a decrease in intake is recommended.
* b. there is no conclusive evidence to support supplementation.
   c. supplementation is necessary but the exact level is not known.
   d. supplementation is very effective and should be aggressive.

8. The cause of the lipid abnormalities seen in familial combined hyperlipidemia (FCHL) is
* a. decreased clearance of LDL by the liver.
   b. overproduction of VLDL by the liver.
   c. excess intake of triglyceride and subsequent excess chylomicron synthesis.
   d. a decrease in LDL receptors on the cell.

9. The effectiveness of omega-3 polyunsaturated fatty acids (PUFA) in management of elevated plasma triglycerides appears to be
* a. inhibition of VLDL synthesis.
   b. acceleration of LDL clearance.
   c. acceleration of HDL catabolism.
   d. inhibition of LDL, VLDL, and HDL clearance.

10. The current research suggests that when substituted for SFA, monounsaturated fatty acids (MUFA) can
    a. increase LDL-C and triglyceride levels.
    b. increase total cholesterol levels.
*   c. decrease serum cholesterol, LDL-C, and triglyceride levels.
    d. decrease serum cholesterol and HDL-C levels.

11. Fibers shown to lower serum cholesterol levels include
    a. cellulose, pectin, psyllium, and gum.
    b. lignin, pectin, oat bran, and cellulose.
    c. guar gum, pectin, oat bran, and cellulose.
*   d. gum, pectin, mucilages, and algal polysaccharides.

12. The dietary modifications recommended by the NCEP Step 1 diet include
    a. <40% of kcal from fat and <200 mg of cholesterol.
    b. <40% of kcal from fat and <300 mg of cholesterol.
    c. <30% of kcal from fat and <200 mg of cholesterol.
*   d. <30% of kcal from fat and <300 mg of cholesterol.

13. The primary transport vehicle for cholesterol in the blood is the
* a. low-density lipoprotein.
  b. high-density lipoprotein.
  c. very low density lipoprotein.
  d. chylomicron.

14. The relationship of high HDL cholesterol to decreased risk of coronary heart disease suggests that these lipoproteins
  a. transport cholesterol into the arterial wall.
  b. remove some of the triglycerides for use by the cells.
* c. act as a reverse lipid transport system.
  d. are involved in the uptake of LDL into the intimal layer.

15. Saturated fats and cholesterol are thought to interfere with clearance of LDL cholesterol from plasma by
* a. down-regulating activity of LDL receptors in the liver.
  b. decreasing uptake of cholesterol into cells.
  c. interfering with the action of cholesterol esterase.
  d. suppressing the activity of lipoprotein lipase.

16. The effect of dietary cholesterol on serum cholesterol levels appears to be
* a. minor as compared to the intake of saturated fatty acids.
  b. major as compared to the intake of saturated fatty acids.
  c. nonexistent.
  d. minor in causing a decrease in serum levels.

17. The effect of coffee drinking on elevating serum cholesterol levels is
  a. very strong.
  b. strong.
  c. weak.
* d. nonexistent.

18. In the absence of other risk factors, the criteria for initiating diet therapy for treatment of high blood cholesterol is
  a. ≥100 mg/dL.
  b. ≥130 mg/dL.
* c. ≥160 mg/dL.
  d. ≥200 mg/dL.

NUTRITION IN HYPERTENSION

OVERVIEW

The purpose of this chapter is to teach the student the knowledge needed to provide medical nutritional therapy for hypertension. The prevalence, pathophysiology, etiology, and risk factors are included. The principle dietary factors associated with hypertension are presented. The recommended methods for dietary management of the condition are included, along with suggestions for patient education topics.

LEARNING OBJECTIVES

This chapter will prepare the learner to be able to

1. Define hypertension and state the criteria for its diagnosis.
2. State the significance of hypertension as it relates to morbidity and mortality.
3. Explain the mechanisms for control of blood pressure.
4. List the factors influencing the development of hypertension.
5. State the dietary factors related to hypertension.
6. Explain the role of sodium and sodium chloride in control of hypertension.
7. Identify the components of a plan for management of hypertension, including dietary management.
8. State the medications used to treat hypertension and state the potential nutritional side effects of the medications.

CHAPTER OUTLINE ———————————————— NOTES, TERMS, & TRANSPARENCY MASTERS

I. Definition and Classification

Table 24-1 is a classification of blood pressure for adults (over 18 years) using both systolic and diastolic pressure as criteria.
essential or primary hypertension, secondary hypertension, systolic blood pressure (SBP), diastolic blood pressure (DBP)

150

II. Prevalence

Table 24-2 is a tabulation of the prevalence of hypertension by age group.
Key concept: Differences in prevalence occur in males and females until about age 55, after which there is no gender difference.

III. Morbidity and Morality

Table 24-3 summarizes the manifestations seen in target organ systems resulting from hypertension.
Table 24-4 is a list of the factors associated with a poor prognosis in hypertension.

IV. Physiology

Figure 24-1 is an illustration of the renin-angiotensin mechanism for control of blood pressure.
peripheral resistance, left ventricular hypertrophy, congestive heart failure

V. Primary Prevention

Table 24-5 is a list of the factors influencing the development of hypertension.
Key concept: The genetic predisposition to hypertension interacts with obesity, life style, and dietary components, resulting in hypertension.

A. Diet-related factors influencing development of hypertension
   1. Overweight

Key concept: Increases in serum insulin result in increased sodium reabsorption in the kidney, thus increasing blood pressure.
Key concept: Body weight is a strong factor in the development of hypertension.
Figure 24-2 is a flow chart that can be used to identify children with high blood pressure.
Table 24-6 summarizes the strategies for prevention of obesity and hypertension in children.
National High Blood Pressure Education Program

   2. Excess consumption of sodium chloride

Key concept: Salt intake is not universally a factor in elevated blood pressure, nor does habitual use of salt increase risk of hypertension for all people.
INTERSALT, salt-sensitive

   3. Alcohol consumption

Key concept: The intake that is significant in causing an increase in blood pressure is 3 oz of alcohol (3 drinks) per day.

   4. Exercise

Key concept: Less active individuals are 30–50% more likely to develop hypertension.

5. Other dietary factors
   a. Potassium
   b. Calcium
   c. Magnesium
   d. Lipids
B. Combination of risk factors for cardiovascular disease

sodium to potassium ratio

Key concept: The three factors—hypertension, insulin resistance, and central body fat distribution—have been shown to increase the incidence of cardiovascular disease. This is referred to as syndrome X, or dyslipidemic hypertension.

syndrome X, dyslipidemic hypertension

C. Medications

VI. Management
   A. Life-style modifications

Table 24-7 summarizes the recommendations for life-style modification to control hypertension.

   1. Weight management

Table 24-8 summarizes two 10-session programs for patient education on hypertension: weight control intervention and low-sodium, high-potassium intervention.

   2. Salt restriction

Key concept: Restriction is addressed in terms of salt, not solely sodium. A 6-g/day salt diet contains about 40% sodium, or 2400 mg.

   3. Other dietary modifications
      a. Minerals

Table 24-9 summarizes recommendations for sodium and potassium intakes based on body weight.

      b. Lipids
      c. Alcohol
   4. Exercise

   B. Pharmacological treatment

Table 24-10 lists the potential nutritional side effects of drugs used to treat hypertension.
Table 24-11 is a summary of the effects that the five classes of antihypertensive drugs have on altering risk for cardiovascular disease.

   C. Treatment of blood pressure in the elderly
   D. Compliance

CASE STUDY INSIGHTS

1. *Write a week's set of menus that Bob can follow, including a meal at home for breakfast, lunch at a restaurant, and a late-night carry-out deli meal.*

The following guidelines should be applied to the students' answers: limit intake of sodium to 2400 mg/day, promote weight loss, decrease intake of processed foods, increase potassium intake by including fresh fruits and vegetables, select restaurants that offer a variety of foods and preparation methods, emphasis fresh foods that do not have added salt and fat, and breakfast should be low in fat or fat free.

2. *Bob generally consumes one or two beers before bedtime and is willing to give up that habit. What healthy snack habits might he incorporate into his evening?*

Examples include fresh fruits, fresh vegetables, low-fat or nonfat yogurt, bagels, no-salt pretzels, rice cakes, fruit juice, and artificially sweetened beverages. Although his intake of alcohol does not exceed recommendations related to hypertension, alcoholic beverages are high in calories and low in nutrient density and thus should not be used when weight reduction is desired.

3. *Since Bob is on the road so much, food safety might be a problem. What tips would you suggest for him to keep his meals and snacks in his truck?*

Bob could carry a small ice chest with him to keep snacks. There are also small refrigerated units available that use the electrical system of the vehicle. If he does not have a means of maintaining safe temperatures for foods susceptible to food pathogens, he should avoid all perishable foods for snacks while working.

SUGGESTED TEST QUESTIONS

1. The segments of the U.S. population that have the highest incidence of hypertension are
   a. African-Americans and native Americans.
   b. the elderly and Hispanics.
 * c. African-Americans and the elderly.
   d. Southeast Asians and Hispanics.

2. Electrolyte alterations that are associated with a lowering of blood pressure include
   a. decreased calcium and sodium.
 * b. a sodium to potassium ratio of 1.
   c. increased magnesium and potassium.
   d. decreased sodium with an increase in all other electrolytes.

3. In collecting data in the assessment process, one observation that may be significant in causing the patient's hypertension is
   a. intake of large amounts of ocean fish.
   b. a vegetarian diet.
 * c. excessive alcohol intake.
   d. ingestion of large amounts of citrus fruits.

4. The use of a diuretic to control blood pressure in a hypertensive patient could put them at risk for
   a. increased serum potassium.
 * b. decreased serum potassium.
   c. bradycardia.
   d. tachycardia.

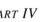

5. When developing the treatment plan following a hypertensive crisis, the primary emphasis is on
    a. increasing potassium intake.
    b. decreasing potassium intake.
*   c. reducing weight to within 15% of desired weight.
    d. initiating a strenuous exercise program three to five times per week.

6. Including fish in the diet of an individual attempting to reduce blood pressure may be of benefit because
*   a. most fish is naturally low in fat and is a good food choice for weight reduction.
    b. increased consumption of fish oil results in a significant lowering of diastolic blood pressure.
    c. the sodium found in ocean fish is very effective in lowering blood pressure.
    d. fish oils are more highly saturated than any other protein source.

7. One of the most predictable risk factors in hypertension is
    a. body weight.
    b. dietary sodium intake.
    c. age.
*   d. heredity.

8. When the diet is increased in energy, the subsequent elevation in plasma insulin can be a potential natriuretic factor causing
    a. decreased sodium resorption by the kidney.
*   b. increased sodium resorption by the kidney.
    c. increased sodium excretion through the kidney.
    d. increased potassium resorption by the kidney.

9. Habitual high salt intake may affect blood pressure in certain individuals, referred to as
    a. high-risk sodium users.
*   b. salt sensitive.
    c. salt wasters.
    d. sodium intolerant.

10. The current research on dietary intake of calcium in the development of hypertension strongly suggests that
*   a. higher calcium intake for the purpose of preventing hypertension is not justifiable.
    b. calcium supplementation is justifiable in women.
    c. calcium supplementation to levels higher than the RDA are most effective.
    d. calcium intake should be limited in some people.

11. One causal factor of hypertension that is reversible is
    a. a high-sodium intake.
    b. a low-potassium intake.
*   c. alcohol consumption.
    d. excess leanness.

12. Thiazide diuretics are most likely to cause
*   a. increased urinary potassium excretion, especially with high salt intake.
    b. decreased urinary potassium excretion, especially with high salt intake.
    c. increased urinary potassium excretion, especially with low salt intake.
    d. decreased urinary potassium excretion, especially with low salt intake.

13. When treating hypertension, the recommendation for sodium intake is
    a   no sodium restrictions needed for most hypertensives.
    b. 3–4 g of sodium per day.
*   c. based on salt and is 6 g of salt per day.
    d. 1 g or less of sodium per day.

14. In the regime of hypertension management, reducing intake of dietary salt can best be accomplished by
    a. purchasing salt-free foods at the health food store.
*   b. avoiding processed foods.
    c. using canned fruits and vegetables.
    d. avoiding salt altogether.

15. For the patient with hypertension, intake of potassium, calcium, and magnesium should be
    a. increased above the RDA.
 * b. maintained at the RDA for calcium and magnesium and generous from food sources for potassium.
    c. increased for calcium and potassium to twice the RDA.
    d. increased for magnesium only.

16. One of the most effective means of preventing the development of hypertension throughout the life cycle is to
    a. decrease dietary sodium intake.
    b. increase the intake of potassium and magnesium.
 * c. promote normal weight and prevent obesity.
    d. consume calcium at twice the RDA.

17. In treating hypertension, fish oil supplementation is
    a. considered beneficial for all ages.
 * b. not recommended because of its affect on bleeding time, weight control, glycemic control, and LDL-C.
    c. not recommended for patients with iodine sensitivity.
    d. recommended only along with other forms of treatment.

CHAPTER

NUTRITION IN BONE HEALTH

OVERVIEW

The purpose of this chapter is to provide students with background and information on the maintenance of skeletal health. The physiology of bone metabolism, including remodeling and calcium homeostasis, are reviewed. Osteoporosis is defined and the methods for prevention and treatment are presented. The chapter also includes recommendations for calcium intake and suggestions for foods and supplements.

LEARNING OBJECTIVES

This chapter will prepare the learner to be able to

1. State the relationship of nutrition to bone health.
2. Explain the mechanisms for calcium homeostasis.
3. Describe the accumulation of bone mass and the factors affecting peak bone mass.
4. Define osteoporosis and state its significance.
5. Identify the types of osteoporosis and their primary causes.
6. State the risk factors for development of osteoporosis.
7. Explain the role of estrogen replacement therapy (ERT) in treatment of osteoporosis.
8. Explain the role of calcium in treatment of osteoporosis.
9. List methods of treatment in addition to ERT and dietary calcium.

CHAPTER OUTLINE ———————————————————— NOTES, TERMS, & TRANSPARENCY MASTERS

I. Bone Physiology
    A. Composition of bone

        hydroxyapatite

    B. Kinds of bone

        cortical bone, trabecular or cancellous bone

    C. Calcium homeostasis
    D. Bone remodeling

        Key concept: The concept of bone remodeling is essential to understanding the metabolism of calcium.

        osteoclasts, osteoblasts, activation, resorb, rebuilding, osteoid tissue, parathyroid hormone (PTH), estrogen, calcitonin

156

E. Bone mass
  1. Accumulation
  2. Peak bone mass

  3. Loss of bone mass

III. Osteoporosis
  A. Definition and occurrence

  B. Classification

  C. Etiology
    1. Possible causes
    2. Risk factors

     a. Menstrual status

     b. Lactation
     c. Calcium intake

     d. Vitamin D intake
     e. Trace mineral intake
     f. Lack of exercise

     g. Medications
     h. Alcohol and cigarettes

     i. Other dietary factors

---

hereditary component

Figure 25-1 shows photographs of normal bone tissue and osteoporotic bone.
Key concept: Bone loss is a normal part of the aging process. This natural loss is related to deterioration of the collagen forming the matrix of bone and the uncoupling of the remodeling process.

osteoporosis

Figure 25-2 is an illustration of the normal female spine at age 40 years and the subsequent deterioration due to osteoporotic changes at ages 60 and 70 years.
Table 25-1 (Transparency) is a list of common drugs that promote calcium loss.
Type I (postmenopausal) osteoporosis, type II (age-associated) osteoporosis, kyphosis (dowager's hump), primary idiopathic osteoporosis, secondary osteoporosis

Table 25-2 is a list of the risk factors known to contribute to the development of osteoporosis.

Key concept: Interruption in menstruation due to any cause, not just menopause, can result in bone loss.

Key concept: The effects of calcium intake during adulthood are not well understood. In general, the recommendation is to supplement intake with 1000–1500 mg of calcium and 400–800 IU of vitamin D.

osteocalcin, uncarboxylated osteocalcin (ucOC)

Figure 25-3 is an x-ray of a hand before and after immobilization, illustrating the effects of disuse or lack of exercise on bone tissue.

Key concept: Alcohol and cigarettes are believed to exert a toxic effect on osteoblasts.
See **Focus On:** "The Impact of Cigarettes on the Skeleton."

D. Prevention and treatment
  1. Estrogen replacement therapy
  2. Exercise
  3. Calcium
      a. Recommended intake
      b. Calcium from supplements
      c. Other treatment modalities

estrogen replacement therapy (ERT),

Table 25-3 lists foods that contribute significant amounts of calcium to the diet when eaten.

Table 25-4 summarizes the risks associated with excessive calcium supplementation.
calcium citrate maleate

Key concept: The role of calcium in acid–base balance may have an effect on bone metabolism that can be reversed in cases of progressive decline in bone mass and osteoporosis.
calcitonin, sodium fluoride, calcitriol, etidronate, potassium bicarbonate

CASE STUDY INSIGHTS

1. How would you evaluate Janet's current calcium intake? What factors and foods would you assess?

Information on Janet's intake is sparse. Referring to Chapter 16, Table 16-10, the diets of Laotians include a wide variety of vegetables and tofu, all of which contain calcium. It can be assumed that her milk and dairy intake are not significant in providing adequate calcium. Fish paste made from small, whole fish (including bones) would be an additional calcium source if included in the diet.

2. What would you recommend about the use of dolomite? What is the concern?

Dolomite use should be discontinued; it is unnecessary because the physician has prescribed supplementation with calcium carbonate. The dolomite is a compound of minerals (calcium magnesium carbonate) found in limestone and marble and is popular with health food faddists as a mineral supplement. The problems with the compound are that it can contain toxic impurities, it is not well absorbed, and it can interfere with the absorption of other minerals.

3. Plan a set of menus for one week for Janet, considering her cultural background and beliefs (see Chapter 16).

Criteria for evaluation of the students' menus should include nutritional adequacy, calcium content, and consideration for client preferences (based on cultural background rather than individual preferences).

SUGGESTED TEST QUESTIONS

1. An inhibitory effect on parathyroid hormone (PTH) that increases osteoclast activity can be produced therapeutically with
   a. calcitriol.
   b. etidronate.
   c. sodium fluoride.
   * d. calcitonin.

2. Assessment of a female patient indicates that she is at risk for osteoporosis if she is
   a. African-American, was normal age at menopause, and has a large frame and poor intake of calcium.
   b. Caucasian and overweight, had multiple pregnancies and late menopause, and consumes alcohol.
   * c. Caucasian and underweight, had premature menopause, does not exercising, and smokes cigarettes.
   d. Asian and premenopausal and has a large frame, a high calcium intake, and a sedentary life style.

3. For women who are genetically predisposed to osteoporosis, a dietary recommendation might be to
   a. eat a high-fiber diet to reduce the absorption of calcium.
   * b. decrease sodium in the diet.
   c. consume caffeine to increase calcium absorption.
   d. increase protein intake to stimulate osteoblastic activity.

4. The most effective method of reducing bone resorption and possibly increasing bone mineral density is
   a. increasing intake of calcium.
   b. a formal exercise program.
   * c. estrogen replacement therapy.
   d. thyroid hormone replacement.

5. The most beneficial type of exercise to include in an exercise program for a patient at risk for osteoporosis is
   a. swimming.
   * b. weight bearing.
   c. non–weight bearing.
   d. isometric.

6. When considering calcium supplements, a patient should be aware that
   a. any of the preparations currently on the market are effective in increasing calcium absorption.
   b. for the older client, the calcium preparation should be taken on an empty stomach.
   * c. calcium carbonate may be constipating, but this can be decreased by dividing the dose.
   d. calcium supplements may increase non-heme iron absorption.

7. Etidronate may be added to the treatment regimen to reduce risk of fractures in high-risk osteoporotic women because it
   a. is effective in activating vitamin D.
   b. increases the absorption of calcium from the terminal ileum.
   c. stimulates the osteoblast resorption.
   * d. inhibits osteoclast-mediated bone resorption.

8. The patient with osteoporosis may experience painful fractures of the
   a. ribs.
   b. toes.
   c. long bones.
   * d. lumbar vertebrae.

9. The majority of the bone remodeling process occurs in the
   a. cortical bone.
   * b. trabecular bone located in areas subject to the greatest weight-bearing stresses.
   c. trabecular bone located in areas unlikely to be subjected to weight-bearing stresses.
   d. cortical bone found in shafts of the long bones.

10. The most important determinant of bone density at any given time is
    a. calcium intake.
    b. protein intake.
*   c. age.
    d. body weight.

11. The calcium loss from bone that occurs with aging amounts to
    a. 100 mg/day.
    b. 200 mg/day.
*   c. 300 mg/day.
    d. 400 mg/day.

12. Acceleration of the bone loss that occurs in women after menopause is directly related to
*   a. lack of estrogen.
    b. poor calcium intake.
    c. a diminished level of calcitonin.
    d. the low level of parathyroid hormone.

13. Bone mass in amenorrheic athletes has been measured at levels
    a. 10–15% below control levels.
*   b. 25–40% below control levels.
    c. 15–25% above control levels.
    d. 50% above control levels.

14. Normal protein intake is recommended in osteoporosis so that
*   a. serum albumins remain normal and do not affect serum calcium levels.
    b. phosphorus levels remain high.
    c. excess protein is not used for energy.
    d. calcium resorption is increased.

15. In postmenopausal women, estrogen replacement therapy is most effective when used during the first
    a. year after menopause.
    b. 5 years after menopause.
*   c. 5–15 years after menopause.
    d. 10 years after menopause.

16. In 1989, the RDA for calcium was *not* increased for
    a. anyone.
    b. adolescents.
*   c. adults.
    d. any of the above.

NUTRITION IN DENTAL HEALTH

OVERVIEW

The purpose of this chapter is to present students with information about the role of nutrition in the development of teeth, dental caries, periodontal disease, and the oral manifestations of systemic diseases. The role of fluoride in dental health is discussed. Guidelines for preventative dental care are included. Special attention is given to baby bottle tooth decay.

LEARNING OBJECTIVES

This chapter will prepare the learner to be able to

1. Identify the nutrients that are significant in the normal development of teeth.
2. Explain how dental caries develop.
3. Define cariogenic, cariostatic, and anticariogenic and give an example of each.
4. Describe how plaque forms and the result of its formation.
5. Explain how fluoride can improve dental health.
6. Identify sources of fluoride.
7. List the guidelines for preventing dental caries.
8. Define periodontal disease and explain how it develops.
9. State the nutritional care guidelines for periodontal disease.
10. Describe how baby bottle tooth decay occurs.
11. State the population groups that are most susceptible to baby bottle tooth decay.
12. Identify concerns about nutritional status for tooth loss and dentures.
13. Describe the oral manifestations of systemic diseases that can affect nutritional status.

CHAPTER OUTLINE

I. Nutritional Factors in Tooth Development

NOTES, TERMS, & TRANSPARENCY MASTERS

Table 26-1 is a summary of the effects that nutrient deficiencies have on tooth development.
Figure 26-1 (Handout) is a drawing illustrating the anatomy of a tooth.
edentulism, dentin, hydroxyapatite

II. Dental Caries

    A. Etiology

        1. Microorganisms

        2. Substrate

        3. Cariogenicity of individual foods

        4. Factors affecting cariogenicity of food

        5. Susceptible tooth

    B. The decay process

        1. Plaque formation
        2. Acid production
    C. Saliva function

    D. Caries patterns
    E. Fluoride
        1. Mechanism of action
        2. Water fluoridation
        3. Other sources of fluoride

    F. Preventive care

---

dental caries

Figure 26-2 (Transparency) is a drawing illustrating the formation of dental caries.

Streptococcus mutans, Lactobacillus casein, Streptococcus sanguis

Table 26-2 (Transparency) lists factors that affect food cariogenicity and an example of each.

cariogenic, cariostatic, anticariogenic

Key concept: Carciogenicity refers to the caries-promoting properties of a food or diet. Several factors affect the cariogenicity of foods.

Key concept: In the presence of bacteria and fermentable substrate, the tooth itself is vulnerable to decay.

See **Figure 26-2** for reference to the decay process.

plaque, calculus

Table 26-3 is a list of medications that promote xerostomia (dry mouth).
fluoroapatite, Sjögren's syndrome

root caries, lingual caries

Key concept: There has been increasing concern about excessive fluoride intake because of the use of bottled water containing fluoride, fluoridation of community water sources, and the use of fluoridated water in food processing.
Table 26-4 provides the 1994 recommendations for fluoride supplementation.
fluorosis

Table 26-5 (Transparency) summarizes the guidelines for preventing dental caries.
Key concept: The five-carbon sugar xylitol has been shown to be resistant to oral bacteria. Xylitol-sweetened gum after meals and snacks containing fermentable carbohydrate can reduce the incidence of caries.

III. Periodontal Disease
   A. Etiology
   B. Nutritional Care

periodontal disease, gingivitis, periodontitis

See **Table 26-5**.

IV. Baby Bottle Tooth Decay (BBTD)

Figure 26-3 is a photograph of the teeth of a child with baby bottle tooth decay.

Key concept: The incidence of BBTD appears to be more prevalent in certain population groups. The highest incidence has been reported in Native Americans and Native Alaskans.

baby bottle tooth decay (BBTD)

   A. Management of BBTD

V. Tooth Loss and Dentures
VI. Oral Manifestations of Systemic Diseases

Key concept: Several diseases, including cancer, AIDS, diabetes mellitus, rheumatoid arthritis, and end-stage renal disease, may result in oral manifestations that can affect nutritional status.

stomatitis, xerostomia

CASE STUDY INSIGHTS

1. What are the cultural, educational, and environmental influences on the dental and nutritional health of this child?

This child's history indicates several factors consistent with poor dental health, including continued use of a bottle with fermentable carbohydrate-containing beverages; lack of fluoride supplementation; poor dietary intake of protein, calories, vitamins, and minerals; and poor dental hygiene. A more in-depth assessment of socioeconomic status may indicate additional factors, such as income and educational level of the caregiver.

2. What dental condition does the child have? What are the diet counseling recommendations for this condition?

The description of this child's teeth and dietary habits is strongly suggestive of baby bottle tooth decay (BBTD). The dietary recommendations for this child include discontinuing the use of a bottle at night and changing the frequency and content of bottles taken during the day. Since this child is 3 years old, an assertive effort should be made to discontinue the bottle completely.

3. What are the nutritional and dietary risk factors?

The combination of factors given for this child is suggestive of general malnutrition, not just baby bottle tooth decay. The diet must be well-balanced and should provide adequate protein and energy to promote normal growth and development. In regards to the dental condition, the most serious risk factor is the use of the bottle with fermentable carbohydrate-containing beverages during nap time.

4. Design a nutrition care plan to improve this youngster's dental health and growth.

The plan should incorporate educating the caregiver on the importance of proper nutrition and good dental hygiene. The dietary component of the plan should ensure that all nutritional needs of this child are met, including an opportunity for catch-up growth as appropriate.

SUGGESTED TEST QUESTIONS

1. Of the following sugars, the most cariogenic is
   a. xylitol.
   b. lactose.
   * c. sucrose.
   d. fructose.

2. An important factor in dental hygiene is
   a. eating small, frequent meals.
   * b. adequate saliva.
   c. adequate use of dentifrices.
   d. high intake of milk and dairy products.

3. The cariogenicity of a meal can be reduced when the meal is followed by ingestion of
   * a. cheese.
   b. fruit.
   c. bakery items made with honey.
   d. milk.

4. Fluoride generally occurs in minute amounts in foods. An exception to this is
   * a. seafood.
   b. beef.
   c. coffee.
   d. spinach.

5. When educating a patient on the prevention of dental caries, foods listed as potentially cariogenic should include
   a. raw carrots and apples.
   b. aged cheese and cottage cheese.
   c. fats and oils.
   * d. crackers and pretzels.

6. Secondary to gingival recession, a patient is at high risk for
   * a. root caries.
   b. flat occlusal caries.
   c. increased salivation.
   d. increased enamel production.

7. The prevention of baby bottle tooth decay requires that the infant be put to bed
   a. with a bottle of milk.
   b. with a bottle of apple juice.
   c. with a bottle of dilute fruit juice.
   * d. without a bottle.

8. Current research indicates that the incidence of dental caries is reduced at a fluoridation level of
   a. 3–5 parts per million (ppm) during the first 5 years of life.
   * b. 0.7–1 ppm during the first 12 years of life.
   c. 3–5 ppm during the first year of life.
   d. 0.7–1 ppm during the first 15 years of life.

9. The development of dental caries requires that the tooth is susceptible, bacteria are present in the dental plaque, exposure is long enough to promote acid production, and
   a. the environment is oxygen-free.
   * b. an appropriate substrate for bacterial metabolism is available.
   c. adequate saliva is present.
   d. the pH is alkaline.

10. Bacterial activity that promotes dental caries is most likely to occur with ingestion of
    * a. sucrose, glucose, and fructose.
    b. xylitol, lactose, and maltose.
    c. sorbitol, galactose, and lactose.
    d. xylitol, glucose, and fructose.

11. Acid begins to initiate the caries process when the pH drops below
    a. 7.
    b. 6.5.
    * c. 5.5.
    d. 5.

12. Foods high in fat decrease the cariogenic potential of foods containing carbohydrates by
    * a. forming a protective film over the surface of the tooth.
    b. lowering the pH below the critical point.
    c. raising the pH above the critical point.
    d. decreasing fermentation of carbohydrate.

13. The characteristics of foods having low cariogenic potential are
    * a. a high content of protein, calcium, and phosphorus.
    b. a low content of protein and a high content of calcium.
    c. a low content of phosphorus and protein.
    d. a high content of magnesium and fat.

14. The group of foods having the lowest cariogenic potential is
    a. fruits and vegetables.
    * b. beverages.
    c. breads, cereals, and vegetables.
    d. milk products, fruits, and grains.

15. Foods that initiate the chewing process are effective in promoting good dental health because they
    a. cleanse the tooth surface.
    * b. provoke saliva flow.
    c. lower the acidity level of the oral cavity.
    d. decrease the fermentation of carbohydrate.

CHAPTER

NUTRITIONAL CARE IN DISEASES OF THE
ORAL CAVITY, THE ESOPHAGUS, AND THE STOMACH

OVERVIEW

The purpose of this chapter is to present the major concerns about nutritional management and maintenance of nutritional health in the presence of diseases of the mouth, esophagus, and stomach. For each of
these three major organs, the pathophysiology, etiology, and nutritional management of the most commonly
occurring diseases are discussed. Peptic ulcer disease is emphasized.

LEARNING OBJECTIVES

This chapter will prepare the learner to be able to

1. State the factors affecting the normal function of the lower esophageal sphincter.
2. Define esophagitis and state the objectives of nutritional care.
3. Define hiatal hernia and state the objectives of nutritional care.
4. State the effects of cancer and cancer treatment on the oral cavity and esophagus.
5. Compare and contrast acute and chronic gastritis.
6. State the nutritional care for acute and chronic gastritis.
7. List the types of surgical procedures involving the stomach and identify the implications of each.
8. Explain the pathophysiology of dumping syndrome.
9. State the nutritional care objectives for dumping syndrome.
10. Define peptic ulcer disease, gastric ulcer, and duodenal ulcer.
11. Explain the pathophysiology of gastric and duodenal ulcers.
12. Explain the medical, nutritional, and surgical management strategies for treatment of peptic ulcer
    disease.

CHAPTER OUTLINE ——————————————— **NOTES, TERMS, & TRANSPARENCY MASTERS**

I. Diseases of the Esophagus
    A. Physiology

Table 27-1 is a summary of symptoms of gastrointestinal diseases and the possible disorder
that may exist.
lower esophageal sphincter (LES), dysphagia

B. Esophagitis	**heartburn, acute esophagitis, chronic or reflux esophagitis, *Helicobacter pylori*, nonsteroidal antiinflammatory drugs (NSAIDs)**
1. Nutritional care	**Table 27-2** is a summary of the nutritional care guidelines for treatment of esophagitis.
2. Drugs and other treatments	See **New Directions:** "Smoking and Gastrointestinal Function." **bethanechol, metoclopramide, cimetidine, antacids, alginates, Gaviscon, theophyllin, fundoplication**
C. Hiatal hernia	**Figure 27-1** is a drawing of the anatomical anomaly that occurs with hiatal hernia. **hiatal hernia, paraesophageal hernia**
D. Surgery of the mouth or esophagus	**Key concept:** Following surgery of the mouth or esophagus, a liquid formula is usually necessary for nutritional support. The student is referred to the appendices for a listing of current adult formulas.
E. Tonsillectomy	
F. Cancer of the oral cavity, pharynx, and esophagus	**mucositis**
II. Diseases of the Stomach	
A. Indigestion	**dyspepsia**
1. Nutritional care	
B. Acute gastritis	**Key concept:** The presence of *Helicobacter pylori* is associated with several gastric diseases. **gastritis, *Helicobacter pylori***
1. Nutritional care	**nasogastric lavage**
C. Chronic gastritis	See **Focus On:** "Endoscopy." **endoscopy**
1. Nutritional care	**atrophic gastritis, achlorhydria**
D. Gastric surgery	**Figure 27-3 (Handout)** is a series of drawings showing a variety of surgical procedures for treating gastric disease.
1. Dumping syndrome	**Key concept:** The side effects of gastrectomy are significant and can cause serious impairment to nutritional status. **dumping syndrome**
a. Symptoms	

2. Alimentary hypoglycemia

hypoglycemia

3. Malabsorption

Billroth II, truncal, selective or parietal cell vagotomy, pyloroplasty, antrectomy, Roux-en-Y esophagojejunostomy, loop esophago-jejunostomy

4. Anemia

pernicious anemia

5. Nutritional care

Table 27-3 is a summary of the guidelines for nutritional management of dumping syndrome and alimentary hypoglycemia.
acarbose, lactose intolerance

E. Carcinoma of the stomach
   1. Nutritional care

achylia gastrica, achlorhydria

III. Gastric and Duodenal Ulcers

Figure 27-4 (Handout) is a series of drawings of the stomach and duodenum showing eroded lesions, a gastric ulcer, and a duodenal ulcer.
peptic ulcer, gastric ulcer, duodenal ulcer

A. Pathogenesis of ulcer disease

mucosal barrier, melena, peptic ulcer disease (PUD)

B. Etiology
   1. Gastric ulcer

Figure 27-5 is a model of the pathogenesis of peptic ulcer disease.

   2. Duodenal ulcer

Table 27-4 is a summary of the pathogenic factors in the development of both gastric ulcers and duodenal ulcers.

C. Management
   1. Medical therapy

Key concept: The eradication of *H. pylori* has been shown to prevent recurrence of peptic ulcers in nearly 90% of patients.

   a. Antibiotics

colloidal bismuth, tinidazole, tetracycline, metronidazole, omeprazole, Zantac, Tagamet, Axid, Pepcid
antacids, aluminum hydroxide, calcium carbonate

   b. Antacids

   c. Other drugs

Table 27-5 is a list of some drugs used in the treatment of peptic ulcer disease and their intended action.
cimetidine (Tagumet), ranitidine, synthetic prostaglandins, sucralfate, arachidonic and linoleic acids, gastrointestinal peptides, carbenoxolone, sulfhydryl drugs

2. Nutritional care
   a. Reduction and neutralization of stomach acid secretion
   b. Foods that damage gastrointestinal mucosa
   c. Diet and eating pattern recommendations

3. Surgery

Table 27-6 summarizes the factors that both increase and decrease gastric acidity.

Key concept: Past recommendations for small, frequent feedings are no longer valid. It appears that gastric acid secretion does not differ significantly with three or six meals per day.

Figure 27-6 is a photograph of a clinical dietitian working with a peptic ulcer disease patient.

Table 27-7 is a summary of the principles of nutritional management of peptic ulcer disease.

vagal denervation, parietal cell vagotomy, truncal vagotomy with pyloroplasty, parietal gastric resection

---

CASE STUDY INSIGHTS

1. Is a low-fat diet appropriate for Jim? Why or why not?

Fat inhibits gastric secretion. However, the level of fat intake for Jim is not indicated. Depending on the level of fat in his diet, a low-fat diet may be appropriate for Jim. The Dietary Guidelines can be used for determining appropriate fat intake.

2. What other suggestions can you offer Jim about late-night eating and pain in the middle of the night?

The hiatal hernia may be partially the cause of the pain experienced during the night. Jim should avoid eating 3 hours before going to sleep or reclining. It would also be helpful to take his antacids before going to bed and 1–3 hours after a meal.

3. Should Jim be encouraged to regain his recent weight loss of 20 lbs?

There is no justification for him to regain the weight. Both his current weight (166 lbs) and his former weight (186 lbs) are within the normal recommended range (±10% of 178 lbs) for his height. A 20-lb loss in 2 years is not unhealthy. It would be helpful to determine what effort, if any, is being made to maintain the weight loss. Another consideration is the effect of excess body weight on aggravating the hiatal hernia.

4. What suggestions can you offer Jim for his traveling, including restaurant options, snacks, and breakfast choices?

Jim should focus on eating regular meals and avoiding foods that cause gastric irritation, such as alcohol, caffeine, chili powder, and black pepper. Other foods that cause distress should also be avoided. All meals should be well-balanced. Snacks are necessary only as desired.

5. Jim's mother suggests using a Sippy (milk-based) diet. What is the rationale for avoiding this regimen?

There is no longer a basis for the milk-based Sippy diet. It is now contraindicated because milk actually stimulates gastric acid secretion.

SUGGESTED TEST QUESTIONS

1. Foods that can cause a decrease in the pressure of the lower esophageal sphincter include
   a. high-acid foods.
   b. low fat milk and yogurt.
   c. high-protein foods.
   * d. fats and alcohol.

2. To minimize discomfort and reduce the incidence of bleeding after a tonsillectomy, recommended foods include
   * a. cold milk, fruit ice, and eggnog.
   b. cream soups, gelatin, and broth.
   c. warm pureed foods and hot chocolate.
   d. spicy foods and citrus fruits.

3. Surgery and radiation to the oral cavity, pharynx, or esophagus may result in decreased saliva production, which can be improved with
   a. carbonated beverages.
   * b. artificial saliva.
   c. coffee and tea.
   d. topical gels.

4. Medications used to treat oral fungal infections may affect dietary intake by causing
   a. pain on administration.
   b. loss of movement of the tongue.
   * c. residual metallic taste.
   d. nausea and vomiting.

5. Symptoms of dumping syndrome following removal of two-thirds or more of the stomach include
   * a. nausea, abdominal cramping, and diarrhea.
   b. elevated blood pressure, headache, and substernal pain.
   c. "heartburn", vomiting blood, and hypoglycemia.
   d. decreased salivation, steatorrhea, and bloating.

6. Following a gastrectomy with a vagotomy, problems with eating can be minimized by
   a. increasing carbohydrate intake, particularly simple sugars, and decreasing fat and protein.
   * b. decreasing intake of liquids and simple carbohydrates with meals.
   c. reducing the intake of fiber from fruits and vegetables.
   d. increasing the intake of milk at mealtime and between meals.

7. Dietary management of peptic ulcer disease requires elimination of
   a. coffee.
   b. high-acid foods.
   c. fried foods.
   * d. alcohol.

8. Damage to gastric mucosa can occur when a patient with peptic ulcer disease ingests
   * a. black or red pepper.
   b. high-acid foods.
   c. carbonated bevarages.
   d. coffee.

9. When an H_2 blocker is included in the regimen for peptic ulcer disease, the patient may be at risk for a deficiency of
   a. vitamin B_6.
   b. vitamin A.
   * c. vitamin B_{12}.
   d. vitamin D.

10. Treating esophagitis with cimetidine, a histamine H_2 receptor blocking agent, is effective because it
    a. provides a viscous protective barrier.
    * b. decreases gastric acid production.
    c. increases LES pressure.
    d. promotes gastric emptying.

11. Total parenteral nutrition may be required following gastric surgery for
  * a. patients with poor preoperative nutritional status or postoperative complications that delay enteral feeding.
  b. all patients.
  c. patients who have lost more that 5% of preoperative weight and are expected to begin enteral feeding shortly.
  d. only those patients who have had a total gastrectomy.

12. Alimentary hypoglycemia that occurs after meals in patients who have had a gastrectomy is caused by
  a. poor dietary intake.
  * b. rapid digestion and absorption of sugars and elevation of insulin levels.
  c. pancreatic insufficiency.
  d. elevated levels of secretin and pancreozymin.

13. Iron-deficiency anemia has been observed after gastric surgery and is most likely caused by a combination of blood loss and
  * a. impaired iron absorption.
  b. poor dietary intake of heme iron and ascorbic acid.
  c. bacterial overgrowth in the proximal small bowel.
  d. lack of intrinsic factor.

14. Guidelines for reducing the severity of dumping syndrome instruct the patient to
  a. consume a large amount of liquids with each meal.
  * b. limit the amount of liquids taken with meals.
  c. consume liquids only with solid foods.
  d. consume liquids only with the first meal of the day.

15. A diet used for management of dumping syndrome is
  * a. moderate-fat, low-carbohydrate, high-protein.
  b. high-carbohydrate, high-protein, low-fat.
  c. high-fat, low-protein, high-carbohydrate.
  d. moderate-fat, high-carbohydrate, high-protein.

16. The use of nutritional treatment in peptic ulcer disease is
  a. necessary for all patients .
  b. required along with medications.
  * c. secondary to medical management with medications.
  d. usually not effective.

17. Current diet therapy for peptic ulcer diseases is based on
  a. a bland diet.
  b. the Sippy diet.
  c. a low-fiber, high-fat diet.
  * d. avoiding foods that are poorly tolerated.

18. A side effect of the aluminum hydroxide antacids that are highly effective in neutralizing acids is binding of
  a. calcium.
  b. magnesium.
  c. iron.
  * d. phosphorus.

19. Calcium carbonate antacids are more desirable than those made of aluminum hydroxide even though they
  * a. stimulate gastrin secretion.
  b. decrease protein absorption.
  c. interfere with vitamin B_{12} absorption.
  d. have limited ability to buffer acid.

20. Esophagitis usually occurs in the lower esophagus as a result of
  * a. the irritating effect of acidic gastric reflux on the esophageal mucosa.
  b. oversecretion of secretin.
  c. a decrease in gastric acidity that decreases the lower esophageal sphincter pressure.
  d. peptic ulcer disease.

NUTRITIONAL CARE IN INTESTINAL DISEASE

OVERVIEW

The purpose of this chapter is to present the major concerns about nutritional management and maintenance of nutritional health in the presence of diseases of the small and large intestine. The chapter begins with an explanation of fiber modified diets. Nutritional management of symptoms of intestinal dysfunction (flatulence, diarrhea, constipation, and steatorrhea) are included. Several diseases of the small and large intestines, including inflammatory bowel disease, are described along with their nutritional care. The physiological effects of intestinal surgery (resection) and the nutritional implications are presented.

LEARNING OBJECTIVES

This chapter will prepare the learner to be able to

1. Describe the characteristics of the high-fiber and fiber-restricted diets.
2. List the foods most likely to cause flatulence.
3. Define constipation and state the guidelines for nutritional intervention.
4. Define diarrhea and state the guidelines for nutritional intervention.
5. Define steatorrhea and state the guidelines for nutritional intervention.
6. Explain the pathophysiology of celiac disease.
7. Describe the gluten-free diet.
8. Explain the pathophysiology of lactose intolerance.
9. Describe the lactose-free diet.
10. Define inflammatory bowel disease (IBD) and explain the pathophysiology of Crohn's disease and ulcerative colitis.
11. Describe the strategies used for management of IBD.
12. Define irritable bowel syndrome and state the guidelines for nutritional intervention.
13. Define diverticular disease and state the guidelines for nutritional intervention.
14. Describe the effects on nutritional status of surgically removing part of the intestines.
15. State the objectives of nutritional management following intestinal resection.

CHAPTER OUTLINE ——————————

I. Principles of Nutritional Care
   A. Fiber, roughage, and residue
   B. Modified fiber diets
     1. Restricted fiber diet

     2. High-fiber diet

     3. Minimal-residue diet

II. Common Symptoms of Intestinal Dysfunction
   A. Flatulence

   B. Constipation

     1. Etiology

     2. Treatment
     3. Nutritional care
     4. Laxatives

   C. Diarrhea

     1. Classification and etiology

     2. Nutritional care

       a. Adults
       b. Infants and children

NOTES, TERMS, & TRANSPARENCY MASTERS

dietary fiber

Table 28-1 summarizes the guidelines for a restricted-fiber diet.
restricted-fiber diet

Table 28-2 (**Transparency**) summarizes the guidelines for a high-fiber diet.
high-fiber diet, flatulence, borborygmus

Table 28-3 summarizes the guidelines for a minimal-residue diet.
Key concept: The nutritional inadequacy of the minimal-residue diet and the availability of nutritionally complete minimal-residue adult formulas has made this diet nearly obsolete.
minimal-residue diet

Table 28-4 (**Transparency**) provides a list of possible gas-forming vegetables and fruits.
aerophagia, eructed

constipation

Table 28-5 summarizes the causes of constipation, both systemic and gastrointestinal.

dihydroxyphenyl isatin, distention, encopresis

diarrhea

osmotic diarrhea, secretory diarrhea, exudative diarrhea, limited mucosal contact diarrhea

Key concept: Diarrhea is a symptom of an underlying disease that must be identified and treated. It can become life-threatening if fluid and electrolyte losses are not replaced.

Table 28-6 provides the composition and ingredients in a standard oral rehydration solution, recommended by the World Health Organization and the American Academy of Pediatrics.

D. Steatorrhea

Table 28-7 is a list of the diseases and conditions associated with malabsorption.

steatorrhea

1. Nutritional care
   a. Medium-chain triglycerides

medium-chain triglycerides (MCT)

III. Diseases of the Small Intestine
   A. Celiac disease (gluten-sensitive enteropathy)

Figure 28-1 shows two photomicrographs of duodenal mucosa: (A) normal villi and (B) the loss of villi associated with gluten enteropathy.

Table 28-8 is a summary of the extraintestinal manifestations of celiac disease showing organ system, manifestation, and probable cause.

celiac disease, gluten-sensitive enteropathy, nontropical sprue, gluten, gliadin, refractory sprue

   1. Symptoms

Key concept: The term *gluten sensitivity* is now used to describe patients with regular, atypical, and latent disease, as well as those with dermatitis herpetiformis.

   2. Nutritional care

Table 28-9 is a description of the gluten-restricted, gliadin-free diet that omits wheat, rye, oats, and barley.

Table 28-10 provides suggestions for the substitution of wheat flour in recipes and improvement of the eating quality of final products.

Table 28-11 lists gliadin-containing derivatives and includes typical nebulous terms used on ingredient labels and their possible meanings.

Table 28-12 is a description of a lactose-free diet. (Lactose intolerance is often seen with gluten sensitivity.)

gliadin-free diet

   B. Tropical sprue

tropical sprue

   1. Nutritional care
   C. Intestinal brush border enzyme deficiencies

intestinal enzyme deficiency state

   1. Lactase deficiency

Figure 28-2 is a schematic drawing of the pathogenesis, manifestations, and clinical implications of lactose intolerance.

   A. Lactose tolerance test

lactose tolerance test, breath hydrogen test

   B. Nutritional care

See Table 28-12 for a description of a lactose-free diet.

D. Inflammatory bowel diseases

inflammatory bowel disease (IBD)

1. Crohn's disease

Crohn's disease

2. Ulcerative colitis

Table 28-13 compares and contrasts the characteristics of Crohn's dieases and ulcerative colitis.
Figure 28-3 is a drawing of the location of the lesions associated with Crohn's disease and ulcerative colitis.
ulcerative colitis, megacolon, uveitis

3. Treatment

salicylazosulfapyridine (sulfasalazine), methotrexate, ileostomy

4. Nutritional care

Key concept: The avoidance of fiber is not necessary in IBD except during cases of acute flare-ups. A lack of dietary fiber may be a contributing factor to the development of IBD.

IV. Diseases of the Large Intestine
A. Irritable bowel syndrome

Figure 28-4 (Transparency) illustrates the abnormal colonic activity seen in irritable bowel syndrome.
irritable bowel syndrome (IBS)

1. Nutritional care
B. Diverticular disease

Figure 28-5 (Transparency) illustrates the intracolonic pressure that can contribute to the development of diverticula.
diverticulosis, diverticulitis, diverticula

1. Nutritional care

Key concept: Past recommendations on nutritional care for diverticular disease included a low-roughage diet. This is now considered inappropriate. A high-fiber diet results in soft, bulky stools that pass more easily and result in lower intracolonic pressure.
methylcelluose, psyllium, cefoxitin sodium, cephalosporin

C. Colon cancer and adenomatous polyps

V. Intestinal Surgery
A. Small bowel resection: short bowel syndrome

Key concept: A resection of the small bowel is used to treat many conditions, including cancer, diverticulitis, fistula, local abscess, ulcerative colitis, Crohn's disease, perforation, sclerodoma, radiation enteritis, mesenteric vascular accidents, and obstruction.
Figure 28-6 is a drawing showing the general characteristics of the feces as it is pushed through the colon. Output depends on the location of the stoma.
short bowel syndrome

1. Effects of decreased intestinal length

    Key concept: Consideration must be given to the absorption of vitamin B_{12} and bile salts when the terminal ileum is removed.

2. Other effects

    Key concept: The secondary conditions associated with short bowel syndrome may increase the malabsorption problem and result in significant nutritional problems.

3. Adaptation of the remaining small bowel

    Key concept: When a minimum of 60–100 cm (23–39 in.) of the small bowel remain, it is possible to provide nutritional support by the oral route.

4. Nutritional care

B. Blind loop syndrome (bacterial overgrowth)   **blind loop syndrome**

C. Fistula repair   **fistula**

D. Ileostomy or colostomy   **ileostomy, colostomy**

E. Rectal surgery   **hemorrhoidectomy**

CASE STUDY INSIGHTS

1. What presurgical dietary guidelines should Ted follow?

The presurgical guidelines should be based on attaining and maintaining normal nutritional status and minimizing the catabolic effect of the surgery. No information is given on his symptoms or present intake. In general, the diet should be adequate in protein and energy and provide all essential nutrients.

2. What lab values should be reviewed before surgery?

The lab values that are the best indicators of nutritional status should be reviewed before surgery. Serum albumin, TLC, hematocrit, and hemoglobin are necessary to screen for protein and iron deficiencies. Other lab tests may be indicated by the patient's medical history. Given Ted's use of beer, liver function tests may be useful in developing his total care plan.

3. After surgery, what types of foods may cause him difficulty?

His colostomy is suppose to be temporary, indicating that reanastomosis is expected. Immediately following surgery, the diet will need to be low residue to allow for healing of the surgical wound. A clear liquid diet will stimulate normal gastrointestinal function more rapidly than NPO. The diet should be progressed as tolerated to full liquids, soft foods, and then a regular diet with high fiber, avoiding foods that cause distress, blockage, and odor.

4. What are the long-term dietary changes that Ted can anticipate, and what symptoms should he monitor to know if his diet is suitable?

The complications of a colostomy include flatulence, blockage, odor, and skin irritation. The latter is related with hygiene and is not a dietary issue. The former three complications are diet-related and can be controlled by observing the cause and effect of the symptoms and eliminating foods known to be a problem. Some of the foods that might cause difficulty include gas forming foods (dried beans, cabbage family vegetables, onions, apples, and melons) and highly fibrous foods such as nuts, seeds, and corn.

SUGGESTED TEST QUESTIONS

1. When the terminal ileum has been resected, the patient is at risk for poor absorption of.
   a. calcium.
   b. vitamin B_6.
   c. potassium.
   * d. vitamin B_{12}.

2. When advised to eat a high-fiber diet, the patient should also be instructed to consume
   a. increased polyunsaturated fats.
   b. more vitamin C.
   c. 32 oz of water per day.
   d. more iron.

3. The type of diarrhea characteristic of dumping syndrome is
   * a. osmotic diarrhea.
   b. secretory diarrhea.
   c. excretory diarrhea.
   d. limited mucosal contact diarrhea.

4. For the adult patient with diarrhea, replacement of fluids should be accompanied by
   a. decreased intake of sodium.
   b. decreased intake of sodium and potassium.
   c. increased intake of potassium.
   * d. increased intake of sodium and potassium.

5. A patient on a gliadin-free diet is allowed to have
   a. rye flour.
   b. oatmeal.
   c. pearl barley.
   * d. cornmeal.

6. Patients who have lactose intolerance may be able to tolerate
   * a. small amounts of milk.
   b. frozen yogurt.
   c. normal intake of skim milk.
   d. cottage cheese.

7. When a patient with Crohn's disease is experiencing steatorrhea, the nutrition care provider should monitor for
   a. increased calcium absorption and oxalate depletion.
   b. increased magnesium absorption and decreased fat excretion.
   * c. decreased calcium, zinc, and magnesium absorption.
   d. hyperlipidemia and elevated serum sodium.

8. When resection of major portions of the jejunum results in decreased production of cholecystokinin and secretin, the patient is most likely to experience symptoms of
   a. gastric atony.
   b. lowered gastric secretion of hydrochloric acid.
   c. decreased oxalate absorption.
   * d. increased peristalsis and diarrhea.

9. The recommended daily fiber intake of a restricted fiber diet is
   * a. 5–10 g.
   b. 10–15 g.
   c. 15–25 g.
   d. 20–30 g.

10. The effectiveness of a high-fiber diet to combat constipation is increased with
    a. a vitamin mineral supplement providing 100% of the RDA.
    * b. eight 8-oz glasses of water daily.
    c. three meals plus two or three snacks per day.
    d. a mineral supplement containing all the trace elements.

11. The nutritional adequacy of the minimal residue diet is compromised by excluding foods of moderate to high fiber and
    a. all sugars.
    b. fresh fruits and vegetables.
    * c. milk, milk products, and meat.
    d. whole grains.

12. The type of diarrhea that results from active secretion of electrolytes and water by the intestinal epithelium is classified as
    * a. secretory diarrhea.
    b. osmotic diarrhea.
    c. exudative diarrhea.
    d. limited mucosal contact diarrhea.

13. The initial treatment of diarrhea should be
    a. a low-fat, low-fiber diet.
    * b. replacing lost fluids and electrolytes.
    c. giving high-pectin foods.
    d. a high-fiber diet to increase stool bulk and restore normal bowel motility.

14. The tissue affected by gluten-sensitive enteropathy is primarily the
    a. mucosa of the stomach.
    * b. mucosa of the small intestine.
    c. mucosa of the large intestine.
    d. pancreas.

15. A gliadin-free diet used to treat celiac disease eliminates
    * a. wheat, rye, oats, and barley.
    b. corn, rice, soybeans, and tapioca.
    c. potatoes, hydrolyzed vegetable protein, and arrowroot starch.
    d. wheat, rice, barley, and corn.

16. Some milk products such as aged cheese may be tolerated by a lactose-intolerant individual because
    a. cheese has no lactose.
    * b. cheese has a low content of lactose.
    c. the lactose in cheese is unavailable for hydrolysis.
    d. the calcium in cheese prevents hydrolysis of lactose.

17. Guidelines for the nutritional care of Crohn's disease include
    a. a low-fat, low-calorie, high-protein diet.
    b. a high-calorie, high-fat, moderate-protein diet.
    * c. a high-calorie, high-protein diet.
    d. a low-calorie, low-fat, high-protein diet.

18. Recommendations for treatment of patients with constipation include
    * a. a normal diet high in soluble and insoluble fiber.
    b. a normal diet high in soluble fiber.
    c. a diet restricted in crude fiber and simple carbohydrates.
    d. a diet moderate to high in fat, low in wheat bran.

19. Fluid replacement for acute diarrhea in infants and small children should be done with a solution of
    a. vitamins, minerals, and electrolytes.
    * b. glucose and electrolytes in water.
    c. chemically defined nutrients.
    d. lactose-free formula.

20. The normal amount of fat that is excreted daily in the stool is
    a. 30–35 g.
    b. 20–25 g.
    c. 10–15 g.
    * d. 2–5 g.

21. Medium-chain triglycerides are useful in the treatment of pancreatic disease because they hydrolyze more rapidly, need only small amounts of intestinal lipase for digestion, and
    a. contain 16–18 carbon atoms.
*   b. do not require pancreatic lipase.
    c. do not require digestion.
    d. do not contain glycerol.

22. For a lactose-intolerant individual, a lactose tolerance test would show that the blood glucose level increases how much per 100 mL of serum above the fasting level?
*   a. less than 25 mg/100 mL.
    b. more than 25 mg/100 mL.
    c. more than 50 mg/100 mL.
    d. less than 50 mg/100 mL.

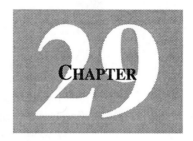

CHAPTER 29

NUTRITIONAL CARE IN DISEASES OF THE LIVER, BILIARY SYSTEM, AND EXOCRINE PANCREAS

OVERVIEW

The purpose of this chapter is to present the major concerns related to nutritional management and maintenance of nutritional health in the presence of diseases of the liver, gallbladder, and exocrine pancreas. Liver diseases included are hepatitis, alcoholic liver disease, cirrhosis, and hepatic failure. Nutritional management for liver disease focuses on the management of both the disease and the secondary conditions, such as malabsorption. The pathophysiology of gallbladder and exocrine pancreatic diseases are presented with guidelines for nutritional management.

LEARNING OBJECTIVES

This chapter will prepare the learner to be able to

1. Interrelate the functions of the liver and the possible metabolic outcomes of liver disease.
2. Define hepatitis and explain the pathophysiology of both acute and chronic hepatitis.
3. State the nutritional guidelines for management of hepatitis.
4. Describe the metabolic consequences of excess alcohol consumption.
5. Describe alcoholic liver disease and its progression.
6. State the characteristics, signs, and symptoms of end-stage liver disease.
7. State the nutritional guidelines for management of liver disease.
8. State the nutritional guidelines for management of liver resection and transplant.
9. State the functions of the gallbladder.
10. Describe the consequences of gallbladder disease related to digestion and absorption.
11. Define biliary dyskinesia, cholelithiasis, cholecystitis, and cholestasis.
12. State the nutritional guidelines for management of biliary disease.
13. State the exocrine functions of the pancreas.
14. Describe the pathophysiology of pancreatitis.
15. State the nutritional guidelines for management of pancreatic disease.

CHAPTER OUTLINE ———————	NOTES, TERMS, & TRANSPARENCY MASTERS
I. Functions of the Liver	**Key concept:** The liver is responsible for more functions than any other organ in the body. Its role in metabolism is extensive. See **Focus On:** "Metabolic Consequences of Alcohol Consumption." **glycogenesis, gluconeogenesis, transamination, oxidative deamination, Kupffer cells**
II. Disease of the Liver A. Hepatitis	**Figure 29-1 (Transparency)** is a drawing illustrating the normal liver, the liver with viral hepatitis, and the cirrhotic liver. **hepatitis A virus (HAV), hepatitis B virus (HBV), non-A, non-B hepatitis, chronic hepatitis, chronic active hepatitis (CAH), end-stage liver disease (ESLD), jaundice, hepatitis C**
B. Alcoholic liver disease	**Figure 29-2** is a flowchart showing the progression of metabolic consequences of alcohol consumption. **Figure 29-3** is a set of photographs showing the microscopic appearance of the normal liver and the fatty liver. **alcoholic liver disease (ALD), hepatic steatosis, alcoholic hepatitis, cirrhosis, acetaldehyde, fatty infiltration**
1. Cirrhosis	**Key concept:** Progression of alcoholic liver diseases to Laennec's cirrhosis occurs in only about 15% of heavy drinkers. There are other causes of cirrhosis besides alcohol. **cirrhosis, portal hypertension, balloon tamponade, endoscopic sclerotherapy, therapeutic shunts, ascites, jaundice, Laennec's cirrhosis**
C. Hepatic failure and end-stage liver disease (ESLD)	**Table 29-1 (Transparency)** lists the currently known amino acids that have altered metabolism as a result of liver disease. **hepatic failure, fulminant hepatic failure, portal systemic encephalopathy (PSE), hepatic encephalopathy (HE), asterixis, ammonia, lactulose, neomycin, altered neurotransmitter theory, branched-chain amino acids (BCAA), aromatic amino acids (AAA), mercaptans, phenols, gamma-aminobutyric acid (GABA)**

1. Liver function tests

Table 29-2 lists the tests used to determine liver function. The names of the tests and functions evaluated are given.

D. Nutritional management in liver disease
    1. Malnutrition

See **Focus On:** "Malnutrition in the Alcoholic."
Key concept: The metabolic alterations seen in liver disease that lead to malnutrition can result from drugs prescribed for management of the disease and from altered metabolism secondary to liver dysfunction.

    2. Assessment of nutritional status

Key concept: The assessment of nutritional status in the liver disease patient should be thorough and comprehensive. See Chapter 17 for additional assessment information.
subjective global assessment (SGA)

    3. Nutritional therapy in liver disease
       a. Energy
       b. Carbohydrate

See **Clinical Insight:** "Fasting Hypoglycemia."

       c. Lipid

Table 29-3 describes a fat-restricted diet used to control malabsorption in the liver patient.

       d. Protein

Key concept: The former practice of restricting protein intake in liver disease has been shown to be unnecessary in stable cirrhosis and hepatitis. In the absence of encephalopathy, a protein intake of 0.8–1.0 g/kg of dry body weight per day promotes nitrogen balance. If positive nitrogen balance is desired, the recommendation is 1.2 g/kg per day.

       e. Vitamins and minerals

Tables 29-4 is a summary of the vitamin and mineral deficits that can occur in severe hepatic failure. The predisposing factors and signs of deficiency are given.
Table 29-5 lists the copper content of commonly consumed foods.
cholestatic liver disease, primary biliary cirrhosis, primary sclerosing cholangitis, Wilson's disease

       f. Fluids and electrolytes

hyperaldosteronism, dilutional hyponatremia, Aldactone, Spironolactone

       g. Problems in feeding
E. Nutrition in portal systemic encephalopathy

portal system encephalopathy (PSE), ammonigenic amino acids

F. Nutritional management in liver
resection and transplantation

Key concept: In liver transplantation, a low-bacteria diet may be required if neutropenia is present. There are many nutrition-related side effects of medications used for post-transplant patients.

Table 29-6 is a list of the medications commonly used after liver transplants, the possible side effects, and the recommended nutritional therapy for control and correction.

liver resection, hepatocellular carcinoma, cholangiocarcinoma, liver transplantation, neutropenic

III. Physiology and Functions of the Gallbladder

Figure 29-4 (Transparency) is a schematic drawing of the organs in the upper abdomen and their relationships to one another.

bilirubin, bile salts, sphincter of Oddi, ampulla of Vater

IV. Diseases of the Gallbladder
  A. Biliary dyskinesia

biliary dyskinesia

  B. Cholelithiasis

cholelithiasis, choledocholithiasis, unpigmented cholesterol stones, pigmented stones, cholecystectomy, litholytic therapy, extracorporeal shock wave lithotripsy (ESWL), endoscopic retrograde cholangiopancreatography (ERCP), choledochotomy

  C. Cholecystitis

cholecystitis, jaundice

  D. Cholestasis

cholestasis

  E. Nutritional management of gallbladder disorders
    1. Acute cholecystitis
    2. Chronic cholecystitis
    3. Gallbladder surgery

V. Physiology and Function of the Pancreas

Key concept: The pancreas is involved in both exocrine and endocrine functions. This section is devoted to the abnormalities that can occur in exocrine functions, although some conditions can impair endocrine function as well.

VI. Diseases of the Exocrine Pancreas

Table 29-7 is a list of tests used to determine pancreatic function and the significance of each.

pancreatitis, edema, cellular exudate, fat necrosis

  A. Pancreatitis

B. Nutritional management in pancreatic
    disorders
    1. Acute pancreatitis
    2. Chronic pancreatitis

> **Key concept:** Cystic fibrosis (CF) is not discussed here (see Chapter 34), but reference to this section may be useful in discussions of CF.
> **pancreatic enzyme replacement, pancreatic protease, pancreatic bicarbonate secretion, glucose intolerance**

3. Pancreatic surgery

> **pancreaticoduodenectomy (Whipple procedure)**

CASE STUDY INSIGHTS

1. Based on the available data, what vitamin and mineral deficiencies may exist?

The data provided for the patient suggests the potential for several deficiencies. His stomatitis may be the result of riboflavin deficiency. The megaloblastic anemia profile suggests either folate or vitamin B_{12} deficiency. The characteristics of this disease also suggest potential deficiencies of fat-soluble vitamins, thiamin, and niacin. There is insufficient data to fully assess vitamin and mineral status.

2. What nutritional therapy would you prescribe?

The medical nutritional therapy should include elimination of alcohol from the diet, limited fat intake as appropriate to control malabsorption, replacement of long-chain triglycerides (LCT) with medium-chain triglycerides (MCT) adequate protein intake of 0.8–1.0 g/kg per day as long as encephalopathy is absent, and supplementation with vitamins and minerals. Fluid restriction may also be indicated.

3. What nutritional parameters are affected by the patient's liver dysfunction?

There are several indicators that this patient has protein malnutrition. This is most likely a result of the liver dysfunction and a decrease in protein synthesis in the liver. The parameters include muscle wasting, decreased serum albumin, decreased serum transferrin, depressed total lymphocytes, and delayed hypersensitivity in skin testing.

4. What is this patient's overall nutritional status?

Given the data presented, the nutritional status of the patient is poor.

5. What conditions may be leading to his frequent loose stools?

His frequent loose stools are most likely the result of malabsorption secondary to pancreatitis. His elevated bilirubin may be indicative of his liver dysfunction or biliary tract obstruction. This could also be a cause of the malabsorption.

6. What additional information would you need to complete your assessment?

Minimal information needed includes glucose tolerance, hemoglobin, hematocrit, serum ammonia, and hydration status.

SUGGESTED TEST QUESTIONS

1. When portal hypertension occurs secondary to cirrhosis, a common sign is
   * a. ascites.
   b. cardiac arrhythmias.
   c. increased gastrointestinal motility and peristalsis.
   d. pulmonary fibrosis.

2. Impending portal systemic hypertension is characterized by mild confusion and
   a. increased blood pressure.
   b. cyanosis.
   * c. asterixis.
   d. hypovolemia.

3. Excessive alcohol consumption results in an increased need for
   a. protein.
   b. fats and potassium.
   c. vitamin C and sodium.
   * d. B vitamins.

4. When portal systemic encephalopathy occurs, the diet may need to be
   * a. restricted in dietary protein.
   b. increased in dietary protein.
   c. restricted in branched-chain amino acids.
   d. increased in aromatic amino acids.

5. Patients who have cirrhosis with ascites should be monitored for fluid retention by measuring
   a. vital signs every 2 hours.
   b. the depth of edema.
   * c. weight.
   d. wrist circumference.

6. In the postliver transplant who exhibits neutropenia, the diet should be
   a. higher in protein.
   b. restricted in carbohydrate.
   c. high in water-soluble vitamins.
   * d. low in bacteria.

7. The patient with cholecystitis may experience pain when eating foods high in
   a. protein.
   * b. fat.
   c. complex carbohydrates.
   d. simple carbohydrates.

8. The patient with chronic pancreatitis may experience exacerbation of symptoms when consuming
   a. fried foods, foods with a high-sucrose content, and caffeine.
   b. carbohydrates, low-fat dairy products, and coffee.
   * c. large meals, fatty foods, and alcohol.
   d. red meat, sweets, and coffee.

9. When pancreatitis progresses to where the ability to secrete a sufficient quantity of enzymes is impaired, the most obvious symptom is
   a. constipation.
   b. hypervitaminosis A.
   * c. steatorrhea.
   d. elevated serum ammonia.

10. When blood glucose concentration cannot be maintained by glycogenolysis, liver cells convert protein to glucose by means of
    a. glycolysis.
    * b. gluconeogenesis.
    c. proteolysis.
    d. deamination.

11. The liver synthesizes cholesterol, and an appreciable amount occurs in
    * a. bile salts.
    b. bile acids.
    c. glycerol.
    d. chylomicrons.

12. Ascites is an accumulation of fluid, serum protein, and electrolytes in the
    a. intravascular system.
    * b. peritoneal cavity.
    c. portal vein.
    d. liver.

13. A diet that provides high levels of aromatic
    amino acids with low levels of branched-chain
    amino acids may result in
    a.   hepatitis.
    b.   cirrhosis.
    c.   a fatty liver.
*   d.   encephalopathy.

14. The energy requirements in alcoholic liver
    disease are about what percentage of the rest-
    ing energy expenditure?
    a.   100%
    b.   110%
*   c.   120–150%
    d.   150–170%

15. As a last resort in treatment of encephalopathy,
    daily protein intake may be restricted to
    a.   1.2–1.5 g/kg.
    b.   1.0-1.2 g/kg.
    c.   0.8-1.0 g/kg.
*   d.   0.6-0.8 g/kg.

16. Hepatic steatosis in alcoholic liver disease can
    be reduced by
    a.   decreasing fat to <30% of total calories.
    b.   decreasing fat to <20% of total calories.
*   c.   abstaining from alcohol.
    d.   limiting alcohol to 1 oz per day.

17. Patients with cirrhosis that receive only
    medium-chain triglycerides as their fat source
    are at risk for a deficiency of
*   a.   linoleic acid
    b.   linolenic acid
    c.   arachidonic acid.
    d.   oleic acid.

18. The accumulation of fluid in ascites can be
    reduced by restricting
    a.   fluid.
    b.   sodium.
    c.   potassium and sodium.
*   d.   sodium and fluid.

19. A low-fat diet (25–30% of total calories) is
    recommended for patients with chronic chole-
    cystitis because a more severe restriction may
    a.   lead to malnutrition.
    b.   lead to a mineral deficiency.
*   c.   not allow for drainage of the biliary tract.
    d.   not allow for adequate calories.

20. Along with pancreatic enzyme replacement for
    the steatorrhea associated with pancreatitis, the
    diet should be limited in daily fat intake to
*   a.   40–60 g and use MCT to replace LCT.
    b.   60–80 g.
    c.   20–30 g and use MCT to replace LCT.
    d.   10–20 g.

Nutritional Care in Metabolic Stress: Sepsis, Trauma, Burns, and Surgery

OVERVIEW

The purpose of this chapter is to present the major nutritional considerations associated with severe metabolic stress and methods for managing the condition. An explanation of the metabolic response to stress is given, including hormonal and endogenous mediators. The conditions of starvation and stress are contrasted, and multiple organ dysfunction syndrome is explained. Methods for determination of nutritional requirements during stress are presented. Specific information and recommendations are given for head injury, major burns, and surgery.

LEARNING OBJECTIVES

This chapter will prepare the learner to be able to

1. Explain the metabolic response to stress.
2. Compare and contrast the metabolic response to starvation and to stress.
3. Define multiple organ dysfunction syndrome and state its implications.
4. Explain how energy requirements are determined for hypermetabolic patients.
5. Explain how protein requirements are determined for hypermetabolic patients.
6. List the additional nutrients that may have increased requirements in hypermetabolic patients.
7. State the nutritional concerns for head injury and the recommended nutritional support.
8. State the nutritional concerns for thermal injury (major burn) and the recommended nutritional support.
9. Explain the metabolic effects of surgery.
10. List the guidelines for nutritional care for the preoperative and postoperative patient.

CHAPTER OUTLINE ——————————— NOTES, TERMS, & TRANSPARENCY MASTERS

I.   Metabolic Response to Stress

Figure 30-1 (Handout) is a flowchart showing the physiological and metabolic changes that occur immediately after an injury or burn.
Table 30-1 is a list of the characteristics of the ebb and flow phases of the metabolic response to severe injury.
ebb phase, flow phase

A. Hormonal and endogenous mediators

Figure 30-2 (Handout) illustrates the involvement of cytokines in response to injury.

adrenocorticotropic hormone (ACTH), catecholamines, epinephrine, norepinephrine, aldosterone, antidiuretic hormone (ADH), tumor necrosis factor (TNF), cytokines, interleukin-1

II. Starvation versus Stress

Table 30-2 is a comparison of the metabolic response to starvation and to stress (hypermetabolism).

Figure 30-3 illustrates the fate of the amino acids generated from muscle catabolism.

starvation, hypermetabolic state

III. Multiple Organ Dysfunction Syndrome

multiple organ dysfunction syndrome (MODS), gut hypothesis

A. Nutritional assessment

IV. Determination of Nutrient Requirements
A. Energy

corrective factors for stress, indirect calorimetry

B. Protein

Key concept: The optimal daily protein requirement for the critically ill patient is 1.5–2.0 g/kg of body weight. The suggested ratio of nonprotein kilocalories to grams of nitrogen (kcal:N) for critically ill patients is 100:1.

C. Vitamins, minerals, and trace elements

V. Nutritional Care Plan
A. Timing and route of feeding

bacterial translocation

B. Product selection

Key concept: Commercially available adult liquid formulas have been developed to specifically meet the nutrient recommendations of the critically ill patient.

C. Promoting anabolism

growth hormone

VI. Head Injury

traumatically brain injured (TBI), Glascow Coma Scale (GCS)

A. Energy requirements
B. Protein requirements
C. Vitamins, minerals, and fluid
D. Methods of nutritional support

VII.   Major Burns

Figure 30-4 illustrates the depth of thermal injuries diagnosed as first-, second-, or third-degree burns.

ileus

A. Fluid and electrolyte repletion
B. Wound management
C. Nutritional care

D. Energy

E. Energy sources
F. Protein
G. Assessment of energy and protein adequacy
H. Vitamins and minerals
I. Methods of nutritional support
J. Ancillary measures

VIII. Surgery
A. Preoperative nutritional care
B. Postoperative nutritional care

total body surface area (TBSA)

Table 30-3 summarizes the goals for nutritional care of the burn patient.

Figure 30-5 is a graphic illustration of the relationship between metabolic rate and burn size as it relates to ambient temperature.
Currier formula, Galveston formula, Polk formula

structured lipids

hyponatremia, hypokalemia, hypocalcemia, hypophosphatemia

Key concept: The nutritional status of the preoperative patient should be a factor in determining postoperative nutritional support. For the severely malnourished patient, support should be initiated within 1–3 days.

CASE STUDY INSIGHTS

1. What indications of hypermetabolism are evident in MP's history?

According to the Glascow Coma Scale, MP has a moderate head injury. This injury causes hypermetabolism and hypercatabolism due to catecholamine response. In addition, he has a fever, which will increase BMR by 7%/°F and 13%/°C. He is also ventilator dependent, which will increase metabolic needs.

2. Compare MP's measured energy expenditure to that calculated by the Harris-Benedict equation. What are the differences? Also compare it in kilocalories per kilogram.

The measured energy expenditure using indirect calorimetry is more accurate than the estimated energy needs calculated with the Harris-Benedict equation. The most likely explanation is that the injury or stress factor was underestimated when calculating energy needs from the equation. The calculated energy requirement would provide 36.4 kcal/kg/day, and the measured energy requirement would provide 40.6 kcal/kg/day based on admission weight (162 lbs, 73.6 kg).

3. What nutritional recommendations would you make for the remainder of his hospital stay?

Continue to monitor the patient's nitrogen status. The negative nitrogen balance should subside within 2–3 weeks if the diet is providing adequate protein. Monitor his weight status and increase enteral feeding to full volume and concentration to meet energy needs. If the patient regains consciousness, request feeding evaluation and adjust the nutritional care plan as appropriate.

SUGGESTED TEST QUESTIONS

1. The ebb phase of the metabolic response to severe injury is characterized by
* a. hypovolemic shock.
   b. fluid resuscitation.
   c. glycogenesis.
   d. lipolysis.

2. Shock stimulates the adrenal medulla to secrete catecholamines, which will
   a. increase insulin secretion.
   b. stimulate protein synthesis and glycogenesis.
* c. stimulate hepatic glycogenolysis, fat mobilization, and gluconeogenesis.
   d. inhibit fluid and electrolyte losses.

3. In contrast to stress, starvation is characterized by
   a. lethargy and fatigue.
* b. a decrease in both energy expenditure and protein wasting.
   c. an increase in fatty acid synthesis.
   d. an increase in use of protein for energy.

4. A urine urea nitrogen excretion in excess of 15 g/day in the injured patient is an indication of
   a. positive nitrogen balance .
* b. mild stress.
   c. multiple organ dysfunction syndrome.
   d. severe hypermetabolism.

5. The most accurate method of estimating energy needs in the hypermetabolic patient is
   a. total weight loss during a 24-hour period.
* b. indirect calorimetry.
   c. the Harris-Benedict equation.
   d. by using nitrogen balance.

6. The maximum rate of glucose oxidation in the hypermetabolic patient is
* a. 5–7 mg/kg/minute.
   b. 8–10 mg/kg/minute.
   c. 12–15 g/kg/day.
   d. 30–35 g/kg/day.

7. The optimal protein intake for the critically ill patient is
   a. 0.8–1.0 g/kg/day.
   b. 1.0–1.2 g/kg/day.
   c. 1.2–1.5 g/kg/day.
* d. 1.5–2.0 g/kg/day.

8. The recommended ratio of nonprotein kilocalories to grams of nitrogen (kcal:N) in the critically ill patient is
* a. 100:1.
   b. 150:1.
   c. 200:1.
   d. 300:1.

9. The integrity of the intestinal mucosa may be compromised during critical illness when
   a. the enteral route is used too soon for feeding.
   b. the diet does not provide sufficient carbohydrate.
* c. glutamine is not available as a fuel source for the enterocyte.
   d. the diet is not supplemented with zinc and selenium.

10. During the first 24–48 hours after a thermal injury, the primary objective is
   a. aggressive nutritional support.
   b. nutritional support to help the individual resist infection.
   c. nutritional support to offset the catabolism that follows trauma.
* d. maintaining blood volume and electrolyte balance.

11. Burn injury patients often develop an ileus following the injury, which is indicated by
    * a. decreased bowel sounds.
    b. increased bowel sounds.
    c. diarrhea.
    d. increased appetite.

12. Cortisol, released from the adrenal cortex in response to physiological stress, mobilizes
    a. fatty acids from adipose tissue.
    * b. amino acids from skeletal muscle.
    c. glycerol from adipose tissue.
    d. glycogen from the liver.

13. During the flow phase of the stress response, the rapid increase in hepatic glucose production is due to
    * a. an increase in glucagon secretion and a decrease in insulin release.
    b. a decrease in glucagon secretion.
    c. a decrease in secretion of epinephrine.
    d. an increase in insulin and glucagon secretion.

14. One advantage to enteral feeding is that patients develop fewer infections, probably because
    a. parenterally fed patients do not receive complete nutritional support.
    b. parenterally fed patients lack sufficient protein to maintain immune function.
    c. parenterally fed patients do not receive trace minerals.
    * d. translocation of gut bacteria is minimized.

15. The daily nitrogen losses from a 20% open wound can be estimated as
    a. 0.01 g N/kg.
    b. 0.02 g N/kg.
    * c. 0.05 g N/kg.
    d. 0.12 g N/kg.

16. The use of preoperative total parenteral nutrition is recommended for patients who
    a. are having bowel surgery.
    b. are over the age of 75.
    c. will have a long recovery period.
    * d. exhibit severe malnutrition prior to surgery.

CHAPTER

NUTRITIONAL CARE IN DIABETES MELLITUS AND REACTIVE HYPOGLYCEMIA

OVERVIEW

The purpose of this chapter is to provide an overview of the conditions of glucose intolerance and the resulting hyperglycemia and hypoglycemia. The chapter begins with an explanation of the range of glucose tolerance. Criteria for the diagnosis of specific types of diabetes mellitus are presented. The physiological activity of insulin, both endogenous and exogenous, are reviewed. The chapter covers in-depth descriptions of the management of diabetes (including nutrition, medications, exercise, and self-monitoring), the acute and long-term complications of diabetes, special considerations for pregnancy and childhood, and implementation of self-management of diabetes.

LEARNING OBJECTIVES

This chapter will prepare the learner to be able to

1. Identify the categories of glucose intolerance.
2. Explain the pathophysiology of insulin-dependent diabetes mellitus (IDDM) and non-insulin-dependent diabetes mellitus (NIDDM).
3. State the diagnostic criteria for diabetes mellitus.
4. Explain the effects of insulin on carbohydrate, protein, and fat metabolism.
5. List the goals for biochemical indices of glycemic control.
6. State the actions to be taken to correct abnormal blood glucose levels.
7. List the goals of medical nutrition therapy for diabetes.
8. Explain how insulin administration and food intake are coordinated.
9. State the recommended intake of carbohydrate, protein, and fat for medical nutritional management of diabetes.
10. State the action of endogenous insulin in terms of peak activity and duration.
11. Explain the mechanisms of the oral glucose-lowering medications and oral hypoglycemic agents.
12. State the methods for managing blood glucose when exercising.
13. Explain how self-blood glucose monitoring can be used to adjust insulin dosage.
14. State the cause of the acute complications of diabetes mellitus.
15. State the cause of the long-term complications of diabetes mellitus.
16. List the criteria for blood glucose control during pregnancy.
17. State the principles of medical nutrition therapy for children with diabetes mellitus.
18. List the steps for implementing a nutrition self-management plan for an individual.

192

CHAPTER OUTLINE ———————————

NOTES, TERMS, & TRANSPARENCY MASTERS

I. Categories of Glucose Intolerance

See **Focus on:** "Diabetes Does discriminate!"
Table 31-1 lists the classes of diabetes mellitus and other conditions of abnormal glucose tolerance. It also includes characteristics of each condition.

A. Diabetes mellitus
1. Insulin-dependent diabetes mellitus (IDDM)

Key concept: IDDM is seen less often than NIDDM. Of all people with diabetes, it is estimated that 10% or fewer have IDDM.
Key concept: The etiology of IDDM is complex and is still under investigation.
insulin-dependent diabetes mellitus, IDDM, type I diabetes mellitus, pancreatic beta cells, hyperglycemia, polyuria, polydipsia, ketoacidosis, histocompatibility locus antigens (HLA), autoimmune disease, islet cell antibodies (ICA), insulin autoantibodies (IAA), glutamic acid deoxycarboxylase (GAD), honeymoon period

2. Non-insulin-dependent diabetes mellitus (NIDDM)

non-insulin-dependent diabetes mellitus, NIDDM, type II diabetes mellitus, insulin resistance, polyphagia, euglycemia

3. Secondary and other types of diabetes
4. Malnutrition-related diabetes mellitus

endocrinopathies

B. Impaired glucose tolerance (IGT)

impaired glucose tolerance (IGT)

C. Gestational diabetes mellitus (GDM)

Key concept: If a woman has been diagnosed with diabetes mellitus prior to becoming pregnant, she is not considered to have gestational diabetes.
Key concept: In gestational diabetes, most women (90%) will have glucose tolerance return to normal after delivery of the baby.
gestational diabetes mellitus (GDM)

II Diagnosis of Diabetes Mellitus

Table 31-2 lists the diagnostic criteria for diabetes mellitus and impaired glucose tolerance.
Table 31-3 provides recommendations for screening and diagnostic criteria for gestational diabetes mellitus.
Key concept: Fasting plasma glucose levels are 10–15% higher than for whole blood.
fasting plasma glucose (FPG)

III. Insulin and the Counterregulatory Hormones

Table 31-4 (Transparency) summarizes the effects of insulin on carbohydrate, protein, and fat metabolism.
counterregulatory hormones

IV. Management of Diabetes Mellitus

Table 31-5 lists the goals for biochemical indices of glycemic control and indicates when action should be taken.
Diabetes Control and Complications Trial (DCCT), retinopathy, nephropathy, neuropathy, atherosclerosis, self-monitoring of blood glucose (SMBG), glycated hemoglobin (GHb), hemoglobin A1c (HbA1c)

  A. Nutrition

Table 31-6 is an overview of the historical changes in nutritional recommendations for diabetes management. Recommendations are shown in distribution of calories among carbohydrate, protein, and fat.
Key concept: The emphasis in nutritional management of diabetes is on individuality and flexibility.

    1. Goals

Table 31-7 lists the goals of medical nutritional therapy for diabetes mellitus.
Table 31-8 provides the identifying acceptable, borderline, and high lipid level for adults with diabetes.
exogenous, endogenous, macrovascular

    2. Strategies for nutrition therapy and IDDM

multiple injections, insulin infusion pump

    3. Strategies for nutrition therapy and NIDDM

    4. Protein

Key concept: The individual with diabetes who has no indication of renal dysfunction does not appear to need to reduce protein intake.

    5. Fat

    6. Carbohydrate

Key concept: It was once thought that sucrose in the diet increased blood glucose levels, but recent research has shown that this is not true. Carbohydrates vary in their effect on blood glucose (glycemic effect).
glycemic effect

    7. Fiber

alternative nutritive sweeteners, fructose, sorbitol, mannitol, xylitol, saccharin, aspartame, acesulfame K, sucralose, alitame, cyclamates

8. Sweeteners
9. Alcohol
10. Sodium
11. Vitamin and minerals

B. Medications
   1. Insulin

Syndrome X, sodium-sensitive individuals

Table 31-9 is a comparative listing of the actions of various types of human and animal insulin, including onset, peak, effective duration, and maximum duration.

Figure 31-1A illustrates the blood sugar changes that occur during a 24-hour period with two insulin injections, both containing regular and NPH insulin.

Figure 31-1B illustrates the blood sugar changes that occur during a 24-hour period with three insulin injections, the first containing regular and NPH insulin, the second with regular only, and the third with NPH only.

Figure 31-2A illustrates the blood sugar changes that occur during a 24-hour period with multiple insulin injections when regular insulin is taken before each meal and an intermediate-acting insulin is taken at bedtime.

Figure 31-2B illustrates the blood sugar changes that occur during a 24-hour period with multiple insulin injections when regular insulin is taken before each meal and long-acting insulin is taken in the morning.

Key concept: Insulin has four properties that are important in determining onset, peak, duration, and patient tolerance; they are action, concentration, purity, and source.

regular insulin, short-acting, intermediate-acting, long-acting, NPH, Lente, Ultralente, premixed insulin, U100, multiple daily injections (MDI), insulin infusion pump therapy, human insulin analogs

   2. Oral glucose-lowering medications and oral hypoglycemic agents (OHAs)

Table 31-10 is a comparative listing of the actions of oral hypoglycemic agents.

OHAs, sulfonylurea drugs, biguanide metformin, thiazolidinediones, troglitazone, alpha-glucoside inhibitors, acarbose

C. Exercise
   1. Benefits
   2. Potential problems with exercise

ketosis

3. Exercise guidelines

Table 31-11 provides guidelines for adjusting food intake for exercise. Criteria include blood glucose levels and type of exercise. Recommendations are made for amounts and types of nutrients, as well as specific food exchange lists.

self-blood glucose monitoring (SBGM)

4. Exercise prescription
D. Monitoring
    1. Self-blood glucose monitoring

Key concept: SBGM allows the patient to manage his diabetes more independently. The patient must be taught how to test, record results, identify patterns of glucose fluctuation, and make decisions about insulin doses based on the information.

ketonuria

E. Self-management education and behavior change

Table 31-12 lists the basic survival skills for medical nutrition therapy for all people with diabetes mellitus.

Table 31-13 lists the essential nutrition education topics for teaching patients how to self-manage their diabetes.

V. Acute Complications

diabetic ketoacidosis (DKA), hyperosmolar, hyperglycemic nonketotic syndrome (HHNK)

A. Hyperglycemia and diabetic ketoacidosis
    1. Diabetic ketoacidosis

Table 31-14 provides guidelines for managing diabetes on sick days.

hyperglycemia, diabetic ketoacidosis (DKA)

B. Hypoglycemia

Table 31-15 lists the common causes of hypoglycemia in diabetes.

Table 31-16 provides the recommended treatment for hypoglycemia resulting from diabetes medications.

hypoglycemia unawareness

1. Hyperglycemia after hypoglycemia

rebound, Somogyi effect

2. Dawn phenomenon

dawn phenomenon

VI. Long-Term Complications
A. Macrovascular diseases
    1. Dyslipidemia

fibric acid derivatives, Gemfibrozil, HMG-COA reductase inhibitors

2. Hypertension

B. Microvascular disease
  1. Retinopathy

retinopathy, laser photocoagulation, proliferative retinopathy, macular edema, nonproliferative diabetic retinopathy (NPDR), preproliferative diabetic retinopathy (PPDR), proliferative diabetic retinopathy (PDR)

  2. Nephropathy

end-stage renal disease (ESRD), microalbuminuria, macroalbuminuria

C. Neuropathy

Key concept: The term *brittle diabetes* has been used in the past to describe people with suboptimal glycemic control. The correct use of the term is to describe those who have severe episodes of ketosis or ketoacidosis and/or hypoglycemia that interfere with their ability to maintain a normal life-style.
peripheral neuropathy, autonomic neuropathy, gastroparesis, brittle diabetes

VII.   Surgery and Diabetes

VIII. Diabetes and Age-Related Issues
  A. Pregnancy

gestational diabetes

    1. Preexisting diabetes and pregnancy

Table 31-17 provides the criteria for blood glucose control during pregnancy for the woman who has preexisting diabetes or gestational diabetes.
starvation ketosis

    2. Gestational diabetes mellitus (GDM)

postprandial glucose levels

  B. Children and adolescence

Table 31-18 illustrates three methods for estimating caloric requirements for youth.
Key concept: Blood glucose levels should be controlled by adjusting insulin dosage, not by restricting food in children. Such restrictions can lead to poor growth and development.

  C. The elderly

Key concept: Malnutrition is seen more often in the elderly than obesity. It can be confused with normal physical changes during aging.

IX. Implementing Nutrition Self-Management

  A. Step 1: Assessment

Table 31-19 (Transparency) lists the data that should be included in the assessment of the diabetic patient.

B. Step 2: Medical and behavioral goals
C. Step 3: Implementation and education

D. Step 4: Evaluation
E. Step 5: Documentation

Figure 31-3 (Handout) is an example of a worksheet for assessing a patient's actual intake or planning a recommended intake. It is based on the exchange list method of diet calculation.

Table 31-20 provides three methods for determining adult caloric requirements.

Table 31-21 is a summary of four meal-planning approaches used in diabetes management and some examples of each.

Figure 31-4 illustrates a sample meal plan for a diet of 1800–1900 kcal/day.

Table 31-22 is a sample menu for the 1800–1900 kcal/day diet shown in Figure 31-4.

Table 31-23 shows the stages of change in the transtheoretical model of intentional behavior change.

Table 31-24 outlines the principles of adult learning.

Table 31-25 provides a list of types of nutritional intervention that require documentation.

CASE STUDY INSIGHTS: IDDM

1. What food and meal planning information needs to be shared with the health care team as insulin therapy is integrated into Ellen's normal eating and exercise habits?

Information on the diet prescription should include daily calories; grams of carbohydrate, protein, and fat; the distribution of the nutrients throughout the day; and the approximate timing of meals and snacks. This patient has a busy schedule, so all health care team members need to be aware of her daily activities and peak exercise times. There should be an emphasis on normal growth and development.

2. What guidance could you offer Ellen about her sports activities?

Ellen needs detailed instructions on the control of her blood sugar while exercising. If her schedule is predictable, she should be shown the most likely times for low blood sugar to occur. She should also be taught how to do SBGM and how to use the results of the tests to adjust her food intake.

3. Ellen is worried about keeping up with her peers. How can you help her adapt to the need for frequent snacks during a busy school day and during activities with her friends?

She needs to be aware that poor control of her blood sugar will limit her ability to keep up with her friends more than the recommended routine for maintaining her blood sugar. She can also elicit her friends support and assistance as needed.

4.   When Ellen travels on field trips or vacations, what types of snacks can she pack to take along?

The snacks need to provide all of the macronutrients—carbohydrates, protein, and fat. Food safety is also a concern. Good choices include peanut butter or cheese with crackers, rice cakes, bread, bagels or tortillas, fruits, and juices should be used with other foods or to treat low blood sugar.

5.   What signs and symptoms of lack of diabetes control must Ellen understand to manage her disease? Which problem is more likely for her—hyperglycemia or hypoglycemia?

Ellen is more likely to suffer from hypoglycemia due to her exercise and activity level and irregular eating habits. She must learn to be aware of the signs of hypoglycemia, especially those signs that are most likely to occur for her. Early intervention should be stressed to avoid disruptions in her routine. She may also have to deal with hyperglycemia related to her sexual maturation.

CASE STUDY INSIGHTS: NIDDM

1.   What advice would you offer for improving her metabolic parameters, particularly blood glucose control?

Student responses should include weight control, eating a well-balanced diet, and establishing a routine for eating meals and snacks.

2.   What suggestions would you have about fat intake?

Medical nutritional therapy for diabetes recommends that fat intake be controlled, particularly due to the long-term complication of atherosclerosis seen in this disease. The diet should be low in total fat with the least amount of fat coming from saturated fat. The dietary intake of cholesterol should also be limited.

3.   What should you discuss about exercise?

Mrs. Jones should increase her exercise. This will assist in weight reduction and may also result in lowering her serum lipid levels.

4.   What meal-planning method do you suggest for her?

Student responses should be evaluated on the rationale used to select the meal-planning method most appropriate for her.

5.   What would you recommend regarding her sugar intake?

While research has shown that intake of sugar may not result in an increase in blood glucose, there are still reasons for her to limit sugar intake. Foods containing sugar are often higher in calories and have lower nutrient density. These are not good foods for her to eat when weight reduction is a primary goal.

SUGGESTED TEST QUESTIONS

1. Among the symptoms of hyperglycemia, the patient may complain of
* a. blurred vision.
   b. loss of hair.
   c. elevated blood pressure.
   d. diarrhea.

2. An observation of body composition often associated with diabetes is
   a. a large frame.
   b. weight less than 90% of optimum.
* c. intra-abdominal obesity.
   d. increased fat in the hips and thighs.

3. The diagnosis of diabetes requires that an individual have a minimum of two fasting plasma glucose measurements greater than
   a. 75 mg/dL.
   b. 115 mg/dL.
* c. 140 mg/dL.
   d. 200 mg/dL.

4. When rebound hyperglycemia is seen following an episode of hypoglycemia, the condition is known as
* a. Somogyi phenomenon.
   b. Cushing's syndrome.
   c. acromegaly.
   d. Goodpasture's syndrome.

5. The patient who can be a candidate for oral hypoglycemic agents is one with
   a. functioning alpha cells in the pancreas.
* b. functioning beta cells in the pancreas.
   c. functioning chromaffin tissue in the liver.
   d. resistance to insulin in all tissue.

6. It is recommended that self-monitoring of blood glucose be done
   a. every morning and every night before bed.
   b. when there is a change in activity level or diet.
* c. before each meal, 1–2 hours after meals, and with exercise.
   d. 1 hour after each meal.

7. When regular insulin is administered before each meal to control blood glucose, the meal should be eaten within
   a. 3 hours of the time of administration.
   b. 2 hours of the time of administration.
   c. 1 hour of the time of administration.
* d. 30 minutes of the time of administration.

8. When planning to exercise, an insulin-dependent diabetic should
   a. strictly adhere to dietary restrictions.
* b. determine that her blood glucose level is <250–300 mg/dL.
   c. plan to exercise when the insulin is peaking.
   d. take an extra inject of insulin.

9. In the metabolism of lipids, insulin promotes
   a. lipolysis in the liver.
   b. an increase in serum free fatty acids.
* c. lipogenesis in the liver.
   d. the breakdown of fat stores in adipose tissue.

10. The effect of insufficient insulin on protein metabolism is that amino acids are
* a. deaminated in the liver.
   b. converted to glycogen.
   c. synthesized in the liver.
   d. stored in the liver.

11. The patient whose diabetes is uncontrolled may experience
   a. decreased appetite, weight gain, and urination.
   b. decreased thirst and weight loss and increased appetite.
* c. increased appetite, weight loss, and thirst.
   d. decreased thirst and urination and increased appetite.

12. One way that oral hypoglycemic agents help to lower blood glucose levels is by
* a. augmenting beta cell secretion of insulin.
   b. decreasing the insulin sensitivity of the receptor cell.
   c. increasing glucose formation from liver glycogen.
   d. decreasing deamination of protein.

13. The inclusion of alcohol in the diet has been shown to
* a. potentiate hypoglycemia in the fasting state when taking exogenous insulin.
   b. potentiate hyperglycemia in the fasting state when taking exogenous insulin.
   c. have no effect on the action of oral hypo-glycemic agents.
   d. stop the effect of oral hypoglycemic agents.

14. Determination of glycated hemoglobin is useful for
   a. assessing present blood glucose control.
   b. assessing blood glucose control for the past 3 days.
   c. adjusting daily insulin doses.
* d. assessing long-term blood glucose control.

15. Current recommendations for use of sucrose and other refined sugars are that they are
   a. never allowed.
   b. acceptable for all patients.
* c. acceptable if the patient is in metabolic control.
   d. acceptable only on rare occasions.

16. In the absence of gastrointestinal dysfunction, daily fiber intake for a person with diabetes should be
   a. about 5–10 g.
   b. about 10–20 g.
   c. about 15–50 g.
* d. about 20–35 g.

17. To reduce the risk of cardiovascular disease, the person with diabetes should follow the NCEP recommendation to restrict daily fat intake to less than
   a. 10% of total calories.
   b. 20% of total calories.
* c. 30% of total calories.
   d. 40% of total calories.

18. The diabetic patient should told that the use of alcohol is
   a. acceptable if body weight is normal.
   b. acceptable if consumed only once per day.
   c. acceptable if diabetes is well controlled.
* d. never acceptable.

NUTRITIONAL CARE IN ANEMIA

OVERVIEW

The purpose of this chapter is to provide students with a basic understanding of disorders related to blood cells and the nutritional management of such conditions. The chapter begins with a presentation of iron-related blood disorders, including both iron deficiencies and excess iron. Megaloblastic anemias are described with emphasis on the relationships of anemias caused by a deficiency of vitamin B_{12} and folate. Also presented are other nutritional anemias, including vitamin E, copper, and protein deficiencies, as well as sideroblastic anemia. The chapter concludes with information on non-nutritional anemias, particularly sickle cell anemia and the nutritional concerns for this condition.

LEARNING OBJECTIVES

This chapter will prepare the learner to be able to

1. Identify the classes of anemia using a morphological description of the condition.
2. Explain the changes in iron stores, circulating iron, and erythron iron as iron deficiency progresses.
3. State the criteria for diagnosis of iron-deficiency anemia.
4. List the method for treatment of iron-deficiency anemia.
5. Explain bioavailability of iron.
6. Define hemochromatosis and iron toxicity, and state the differences in the two conditions.
7. Explain the stages of deficiency of vitamin B_{12}.
8. List the method for treatment of anemia caused by a deficiency of vitamin B_{12}.
9. Explain the stages of deficiency of folate.
10. List the method for treatment of anemia caused by a deficiency of folate.
11. Name the nutritional anemias that occur in addition to iron, vitamin b_{12}, and folate.
12. State the nutritional care guidelines for treatment of sickle cell anemia.

CHAPTER OUTLINE ——————————

I. Iron-Related Blood Disorders

   A. Iron-deficiency anemia
      1. Etiology
      2. Stages of deficiency

      3. Clinical findings

      4. Diagnosis

      5. Treatment
        a. Medication

        b. Nutritional care

        c. Bioavailability of dietary iron
        d. Summary

   B. Hemochromatosis
      1. Etiology
      2. Clinical findings

      3. Diagnosis
      4. Treatment
      5. Nutritional care

   C. Iron toxicity

II. Megaloblastic Anemias

NOTES, TERMS, & TRANSPARENCY MASTERS

Table 32-1 lists the classifications of anemia based on morphology. The underlying abnormality, clinical syndromes, and treatment are indicated for four types of anemia.
anemia, erythrocytes, hemoglobin, macrocytic, normocytic, hypochromic, normochromic, nutritional anemias

iron-deficiency anemia

Figure 32-1 illustrates the sequential stages of iron status according to iron stores, circulating iron, and erythron iron. Accompanying biochemical indices are included.

Figure 32-2 is a photograph of the fingernails of an iron-deficient adult, illustrating koilonychia, and those of a normal adult.
koilonychia, glossitis, angular stomatitis, dysphagia

plasma ferritin, transferrin saturation (TS), TIBC, erythropoiesis, hemoglobin, hematocrit, ratio of zinc protoporphyrin (erythrocyte protoporphyrin) to heme (ZnPP/heme)

ferrous form, ferric form

Table 32-2 provides a list of the iron content of some common foods.

heme iron, MFP, nonheme iron, ethylenediaminetetraacetic acid (EDTA)

hemochromatosis

HLA-A gene, phlebotomy therapy

total iron-binding capacity (TIBC)

sideroblastic anemia, chronic hemolytic anemia, aplastic anemia, ineffective erythropoiesis, transfusional iron overload, porphyria cutanea tarda

megaloblastic anemias

A. Pernicious and other vitamin B_{12}
   deficiency anemias
   1. Etiology and metabolism

   Table 32-3 is a comprehensive list of the causes of vitamin B_{12} deficiency.
   pernicious anemia, macrocytic megaloblastic anemia, intrinsic factor (IF), holo-transcobalamin II (TCII), haptocorrin, transcobalamin I and III (TCI and TCIII)

   2. Stages of deficiency

   Figure 32-3 illustrates the sequential stages of vitamin B_{12} status according to liver B_{12}, holo TC II, and RBC + WBC B_{12}. Accompanying biochemical indices are included.

   3. Clinical findings

   paresthesia

   4. Diagnosis

   ***L. leichmannii, E. gracilis,* unsaturated B_{12} binding capacity (UBBC), intrinsic factor antibody (IFAB), serum homocysteine, serum methionine, Schilling test**

   5. Treatment
   6. Nutritional care

   Table 32-4 provides a list of the B_{12} content of some common foods.

B. Folic acid deficiency anemia
   1. Etiology and metabolism

   Table 32-5 is a comprehensive list of the causes of folate deficiency.
   folic acid deficiency anemia, pteroyl polyglutamate hydrolase, folate conjugase, 5-methyl-tetrahydrofolate (THFA)

   2. Methylfolate trap

   Figure 32-4 is a schematic drawing of how a vitamin B_{12} deficiency can cause folate to be trapped as 5-methyl THFA and result in folate deficiency.

   3. Stages of deficiency

   Figure 32-5 illustrates the sequential stages of folate status according to liver folate, plasma folate, and erythron folate. Accompanying biochemical indices are included.

   4. Clinical findings

   Key concept: Deficiencies of either vitamin B_{12} or folate result in the same clinical sign, a macrocytic megaloblastic blood cell.

   5. Diagnosis

   macrocytic megaloblastic anemia, formiminoglutamic acid (FIGLU)

   6. Treatment

   Table 32-6 provides a list of the folate content of some common foods.

III. Other Nutritional Anemias
    A. Copper-deficiency anemia   **ceruloplasmin**
    B. Anemia of protein-energy malnutrition
       (PEM)
    C. Sideroblastic anemia (pyridoxine-   **sideroblastic anemia, D-aminolevulinic acid synthetase, sideroblasts**
       responsive)

    D. Vitamin E responsive anemia   **hemolytic anemia**

IV. Non-Nutritional Anemias
    A. Sickle cell anemia (HB S disease)
       1. Clinical findings
       2. Treatment   "See **Clinical Insight:** "Nutritional Care for Sickle Cell Anemia."

    B. Thalassemia minor   **Thalassemia minor, red cell distribution width (RDW)**

    C. Sports anemia (hypochromic-microcytic   **Key concept:** It should be emphasized that iron
       transient anemia)   supplements for athletes are not warranted unless a iron deficiency is diagnosed.

CASE STUDY INSIGHTS

1. What are the dangers of taking a multiple vitamin and mineral supplement when one has sickle cell anemia?

In sickle cell anemia, supplemental intakes of iron and vitamin C can lead to increased problems related to iron metabolism. A multiple vitamin and mineral supplement is most likely to contain both of these nutrients. Folate needs may be increased for the patient. Folate supplementation may require a prescription due to the possibility of masking a deficiency of vitamin B_{12}.

2. What other lab data should you obtain before discussing Mary Jo's case with her doctor?

If would be helpful to have some indication of her liver function before discussing her case with the doctor. Liver function tests and tests that indicate iron status should be done.

3. What foods could she include in her diet that would be beneficial without giving her too much of any single vitamin or mineral?

Increasing her intake of milk, cheese, and eggs would increase her intake of vitamin B_{12} without contributing as much iron as meat products.

4. Are there any problems with her usual daily intake of one or two citrus fruits and juices?

Vitamin C improves the absorption of iron in the gastrointestinal tract. Citrus fruits and juices provide additional vitamin C in the diet. If iron intake is minimal, the use of these fruits can be encouraged.

5. What other suggestions would you offer Mary Jo?

The diet should include good sources of zinc and copper. She may also require increased fluid intake.

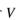

SUGGESTED TEST QUESTIONS

1. The absorption of dietary iron and iron supplements is enhanced by
   a. calcium containing foods.
   b. carbohydrates.
   * c. vitamin C .
   d. magnesium.

2. Among the side-effects of iron supplementation, a patient may complain of
   a. dry mouth.
   b. blurred vision.
   c. constipation.
   * d. headache.

3. The group of foods having the greatest proportion of absorbable iron is
   a. fresh citrus fruits, raisins, egg whites, and pork.
   b. cruciferous vegetables, tomatoes, and dried beans.
   * c. kidney, nuts, egg yolk,and liver.
   d. ocean fish, maple syrup, beef, and spinach.

4. Iron absorption may be reduced when consuming large amounts of
   * a. coffee or tea with meals.
   b. leavened bread.
   c. pork.
   d. fish.

5. Foods providing significant amounts of folate in the diet are
   a. fish and seafood.
   b. milk products.
   * c. fresh fruits and vegetables.
   d. eggs and poultry.

6. Pernicious anemia differs from folate deficiency in that it
   a. is easily treated by dietary alterations.
   * b. involves the central and peripheral nervous system.
   c. is reversible with treatment.
   d. results in microcytic and hypochromic red blood cells.

7. An individual with sickle cell anemia should avoid foods that are high in
   a. protein.
   b. folate.
   * c. iron.
   d. vitamin A.

8. If an anemia appears as microcytic and hypochromic, the most likely cause is a deficiency of
   a. folic acid.
   b. pyridoxine.
   * c. iron.
   d. vitamin B_{12}.

9. An adult male may be put at risk for iron-deficiency anemia if he has had
   * a. a recent blood loss.
   b. an inadequate intake of heme iron.
   c. malabsorption due to lack of ascorbic acid.
   d. an inadequate intake of nonheme iron.

10. The measurement of plasma ferritin when evaluating iron status provides a measure of
    a. the supply of iron delivered to developing red blood cells.
    * b. iron stores.
    c. total iron-binding capacity.
    d. iron supply to the tissues.

11. When symptoms of iron-deficiency anemia develop, the hemoglobin measurement is usually about
    a. 2–6 g/dL.
    b. 6–8 g/dL.
    * c. 8–11 g/dL.
    d. 12–15 g/dL.

12. Dietary components that may interfere with iron absorption include
    a. vitamin D and calcium.
    * b. phytates and carbonates.
    c. ascorbic acid.
    d. soluble fiber.

13. To maximize absorption of iron, a group of foods that should be limited is
    a. meat, fish, and poultry.
    b. ascorbic acid, tea, and vegetable fiber.
  * c. vegetable fiber, tea, and soybeans.
    d. fish, unrefined cereals, and egg yolks.

14. Pernicious anemia is a macrocytic, megaloblastic anemia that results from
  * a. a deficiency of vitamin B_{12}.
    b. a loss of blood through the gastrointestinal tract.
    c. a lack of iron from both heme and non-heme iron sources.
    d. interference with pyridoxine metabolism.

15. Normal mobilization of iron from storage sites to the plasma depends on the copper-containing protein
    a. hemoglobin.
    b. serum albumin.
    c. transferrin.
  * d. ceruloplasmin.

16. The patient with sickle cell anemia should be cautioned to consume
    a. iron-rich foods such as liver.
    b. iron-fortified cereals.
    c. ascorbic acid with meals.
  * d. a diet low in iron.

17. Vitamin B_6 is an effective therapy in sideroblastic anemia, which is a severe microcytic, hypochromic anemia in the presence of
  * a. iron overload.
    b. low serum iron levels.
    c. high serum iron and low tissue iron levels.
    d. low tissue iron levels.

CHAPTER 33

NUTRITIONAL CARE IN HEART FAILURE AND TRANSPLANT

OVERVIEW

The purpose of this chapter is to provide students with an understanding of heart failure, which can result from a number of conditions. The focus of the chapter is on congestive heart failure. The incidence, risk, progression, and treatment of the condition are presented. Specific information is given on the nutritional care of the individual with congestive heart disease. Definitions and explanations of various sodium-restricted diets are included. The nutritional care guidelines for cardiac transplantation are also discussed.

LEARNING OBJECTIVES

This chapter will prepare the learner to be able to

1. State the risk factors for congestive heart failure.
2. Define cardiac cachexia and explain its development.
3. List the types of medications used for treatment of congestive heart failure and their specific actions.
4. State the recommendations for energy intake for the individual with congestive heart failure.
5. Identify the various levels of sodium-restricted diets and state the amount of sodium allowed in each.
6. Explain how a nutrition label can be used to assess the sodium content of foods.
7. Define low-sodium or low-salt syndrome.
8. State the recommendations for potassium intake in congestive heart failure.
9. State the recommendations for fluid intake in congestive heart failure.
10. List the nutritional care guidelines for management of the cardiac transplant patient.

CHAPTER OUTLINE ——————————————— NOTES, TERMS, & TRANSPARENCY MASTERS

I. Congestive Heart Failure

    A. Prevalence and incidence
    B. Risk factors
    C. Disease progression

Figure 33-1 is a drawing of the blood flow into, through, and out of the heart.
congestive heart failure

Table 33-1 provides the classifications of heart failure based on patients' symptoms.
decompensation

D. Cardiac cachexia

Table 33-2 lists the factors that are involved in the development of cardiac cachexia.
cardiac cachexia, tumor necrosis factor

E. Symptoms

shortness of breath, dyspnea

F. Treatment

Table 33-3 lists the drugs commonly used in the treatment of CHF that can affect nutritional status.
diuretics, furosemide, vasodilators, enalapril, glycosides, digoxin, angiotensin-converting enzyme inhibitors

G. Nutritional care
    1. Assessment
    2. Energy

Key concept: Dietary intake of patients with CHF is affected by several factors secondary to the disease: anorexia, early satiety, ascites, altered taste, and labored efforts to eat. The patient should be monitored for oral intake and, when sufficient, started on an enteral nutrition support formula by duodenostomy.

    3. Sodium
        a. Sodium-restricted diets

See **Clinical Insight:** "Sodium and Salt Measurement Equivalents."

        b. Designing a sodium-restricted diet

Table 33-4 lists the serving sizes for high-sodium foods that can be used carefully in a sodium-restricted diet.
Table 33-5 lists additional foods high in sodium.
Table 33-6 (Transparency) lists sodium-containing additives to assist in label reading. Foods likely to contain the additive are listed.
Table 33-7 lists food groups and serving sizes with sodium content and suggested number of servings for each level of a sodium-restricted diet.
Table 33-8 provides the foods recommended and the foods to exclude on the 2-g sodium diet.
Key concept: The goal is to limit the total sodium intake, not to eliminate specific foods from the diet. Foods that are high in sodium can be used on sodium-restricted diets, provided that the total sodium intake does not exceed the prescribed intake.
Key concept: When salt is omitted during cooking and low-sodium foods are used but salt is allowed to be added at the table, studies have shown that the total salt intake is lower than when regular foods are served and salt is not allowed at the table.

c. Dietary sources of sodium
d. Sodium labeling

Table 33-9 (Transparency) gives the legal definitions of terms used in food labeling claims for sodium content.

Table 33-10 shows the equivalent amounts of sodium in milliequivalents (mEq) and milligrams (mg) and the approximate amount (in grams) of sodium chloride (salt) that would contain that amount of sodium.

Nutrition Labeling and Education Act of 1990, low sodium, moderately low sodium, reduced sodium

e. Non-nutrient sources of sodium
f. Nondietary sources of added sodium
g. Low-sodium or low-salt syndrome

salt substitutes

3. Potassium
4. Fluids
5. Other nutrients
6. Meal plan

hyponatremia, hypochloremia, azotemia, low-salt syndrome

II. Cardiac Transplantation

Table 33-11 summarizes the nutritional care guidelines for the cardiac transplant patient. It includes pretransplant care and immediate and long-term posttransplant care.

CASE STUDY INSIGHTS

1. What are the effects of Mrs. E's medications on nutritional status?

Zaroxlyn may increase urinary losses of sodium and potassium, thus a high-potassium diet may be recommended. Other nutrition-related effects include hypochloremic alkalosis, dry mouth, constipation, anorexia, nausea, and bloating. Lasix (furosemide) decreases glucose tolerance and increases loss of electrolytes, requiring foods high in potassium and magnesium. Additional effects include dizziness, anorexia, vomiting, nausea, dry mouth, increased thirst, and taste changes. Inderal (propranolol HCl) decreases glucose tolerance. Mrs. E should avoid natural licorice and should eat a low-sodium diet. Other possible effects on nutritional status include dizziness, fatigue, constipation, GI distress, dry mouth, and nausea.

2. She is currently on a 2-g sodium diet but will be following a "no added salt" diet at home. Her favorite foods are ethnic German foods, including sauerkraut, cabbage dishes, pork, and sausage. What dietary adaptation do you suggest?

Student responses should consider the sodium in sauerkraut and sausage. Other cabbage or pork dishes should be evaluated for the method of preparation, which may add sodium. The goal for therapy is to minimize her sodium intake so that total intake is 4 g or less. She could include a reasonable portion of sauerkraut and sausage in her diet without exceeding the restriction.

3. *Since shopping is a problem for Mrs. E, what types of agency referrals should you seek? What advice will you offer to her daughters who have called to talk about dietary changes?*

Available agencies will depend on your local area. Some suggestions include Area Agency on Aging, Meals on Wheels, and County Social Services or Health Department. Her daughters should be told to plan well-balanced meals, avoid purchasing high-sodium foods, and plan for small, frequent meals.

4. *If Mrs. E was discharged to a nursing home, write a draft discharge nutritional summary that you would send to the dietitian there. What key pieces of information are relevant?*

The discharge nutrition summary should include a review of her dietary course in the hospital, her response to the diet, her understanding of the diet, an assessment of her ability to comply with the diet, her weight status, and any other nutritional concerns identified.

SUGGESTED TEST QUESTIONS

1. For many patients, the edema associated with a failing heart can be reduced by administering a combination of
    a. vasopressors and restricted protein diet.
    b. anticholinergics and fluid restriction.
    * c. diuretics and sodium restriction.
    d. adrenergics and decreased potassium intake.

2. A patient placed on a moderate sodium restriction will need to limit
    a. foods high in potassium.
    b. fresh fruits and vegetables.
    c. regular bread and baked goods.
    * d. salt added at the table.

3. When the diuretics used for congestive heart failure are furosemide or hydrochlorothiazide, the patient should avoid
    * a. natural licorice.
    b. bran fiber.
    c. salt substitutes.
    d. magnesium supplements.

4. The condition in which severe congestive heart failure is characterized by a state of severe malnutrition is
    a. anorexia nervosa.
    * b. cardiac cachexia.
    c. hypoalbuminemia.
    d. tissue hypoxia.

5. The primary goals of medical nutritional therapy for the patient with congestive heart failure are to
    * a. provide adequate nourishment with as little work for the heart as possible while decreasing or preventing edema.
    b. restore protein stores and regain lost weight.
    c. return weight to desirable range and correct fluid and electrolyte imbalances.
    d. provide liquid foods that are easy to swallow and provide extra fluids.

6. In assessing the nutritional status of a patient with congestive heart failure, the greatest importance should be on
    a. serum transferrin and serum sodium.
    b. serum albumin and total iron-binding capacity.
    * c. dietary history and anthropometric measurements.
    d. retinol-binding protein and prealbumin levels.

7. The most reliable anthropometric measurements for a patient with edema and congestive heart failure are
    a. triceps and biceps skinfold.
    b. height to weight ratio and usual body weight.
    * c. calf, thigh, and mid-arm muscle circumference.
    d. weight and abdominal girth.

8. The patient with congestive heart failure should limit daily sodium intake to
   a. 4 g.
   b. 2–3 g.
   * c. 1 g.
   d. 500 mg.

9. Which of these rules is part of the no added salt (NAS) diet?
   * a. Up to 1/2 teaspoon of salt is allowed per day without high-sodium foods .
   b. No salt may be used in the preparation of food.
   c. Vegetables such as beets, carrots, and spinach should be omitted.
   d. All frozen vegetables should be omitted.

10. Among the vegetables that are recommended to be omitted on a 500-mg sodium diet are
    a. lettuce, green beans, and squash.
    * b. beets, carrots, and kale.
    c. peas, mushrooms, and tomatoes.
    d. scallions, peppers, and yellow beans.

11. A food group that is relatively high in naturally occurring sodium is
    * a. milk, cheese, and eggs.
    b. fruits and vegetables .
    c. grains and cereals.
    d. cereals and fruits.

12. The recommendation for fluid restriction in congestive heart failure is that fluids
    a. are always required.
    * b. may not be necessary if the patient complies with the low-sodium diet.
    c. need no restrictions if the patient is receiving diuretics.
    d. are restricted only in acute phases of the illness.

13. The patient undergoing cardiac surgery is at greatest risk for
    * a. cardiac cachexia.
    b. pulmonary thrombosis.
    c. abdominal aortic aneurism.
    d. hypotension.

14. A food labeled sodium-free must contain
    a. no sodium or sodium chloride at all.
    b. <1 mg of sodium per serving and no sodium chloride.
    * c. <5 mg of sodium per serving and no sodium chloride.
    d. <10 mg of sodium per serving and no sodium chloride.

15. A diet with 1000 mg of sodium contains how many milliequivalents of sodium?
    a. 23 mEq
    * b. 43 mEq
    c. 100 mEq
    d. 1000 mEq

CHAPTER 34

NUTRITIONAL CARE IN PULMONARY DISEASE

OVERVIEW

The purpose of this chapter is to provide the student with an understanding of the role of nutrition in pulmonary function and the effect of pulmonary function on nutritional status. Specific diseases covered in the chapter are cystic fibrosis (CF), bronchopulmonary dysplasia (BPD), chronic obstructive pulmonary disease (COPD), and respiratory failure (RF). Lung cancer is given minimal consideration here.

LEARNING OBJECTIVES

This chapter will prepare the learner to be able to

1. Explain the relationship of nutritional status to pulmonary function.
2. State the impact of pulmonary dysfunction on nutritional status.
3. Explain the pathophysiology of cystic fibrosis.
4. List the appropriate indices for nutritional assessment of a person with cystic fibrosis.
5. State the energy requirements for a person with cystic fibrosis.
6. State the recommendations and rationale for sodium intake with cystic fibrosis.
7. List the appropriate nutritional assessment parameters for a person with bronchopulmonary dysplasia.
8. State the energy requirements for an infant with bronchopulmonary dysplasia.
9. Describe the pathophysiology of chronic obstructive pulmonary disease.
10. List the appropriate nutritional assessment parameters for a person with chronic obstructive pulmonary disease.
11. State the principles of nutritional management of respiratory failure.

CHAPTER OUTLINE ———————————— NOTES, TERMS, & TRANSPARENCY MASTERS

I. Nutrition and the Pulmonary System

Figure 34-1 shows several illustrations of the anatomy of the pulmonary system. The series includes a chest roentgenogram, a schematic drawing of the lung, a diagram of the interstitial connective tissue compartments in the lungs, and a diagram of airway segmentation.
upper respiratory tract, lower respiratory tract

213

A. Impact of nutrition on pulmonary system status

B. Impact of malnutrition

vital lung capacity (lung volume), minute ventilation (volume exhaled per minute), efficiency of ventilation, compliance (distensibility), elasticity, surfactant, hypoxic ventilatory drive, pulmonary epithelium, cilia, alveolar macrophages

C. Impact of pulmonary system disease on nutritional status

Table 34-1 (Transparency) lists the adverse effect of lung disease on nutritional status.
albuterol, bronchodilator

II. Nutritional Care in Selected Pulmonary Diseases

tuberculosis (TB), bronchial asthma, aspiration, airway obstruction, anaphylaxis, cystic fibrosis (CF), chronic obstructive pulmonary disease (COPD), sputum, dyspnea, tachypnea, hemoptysis, nasal polyps

A. Cystic Fibrosis
  1. Description

cystic fibrosis (CF), cystic fibrosis transmembrane regulator (CFTR), bronchitis, bronchiectasis, pneumonia, atelectasis, peribronchial, parenchymal scarring, pneumothorax, sweat test, pilocarpine iontophoresis

  2. Nutritional status and assessment

Table 34-2 provides guidelines for nutritional assessment in cystic fibrosis using several indices.
Table 34-3 summarizes the categories of nutritional management of patients with cystic fibrosis.
pancreatic enzyme replacement, enteric-coated enzyme microspheres, meconium ileus equivalent

  3. Nutritional requirements and care
    a. Energy

See **Clinical Insight:** "Determination of Energy Requirements of Patients with Cystic Fibrosis."
Figure 34-2 is a set of three photographs of a child with CF showing the results of medical intervention. The child is shown at the ages of 4 months (time of diagnosis), 9 months, and 2 years.

    b. Macronutrients
    c. Micronutrients

Key concept: The patient with CF may be at risk for vitamin K deficiency due to chronic use of antibiotics, liver disease, and malabsorption. The patient should be monitored for abnormalities of prothrombin time.

Key concept: Sodium requirements increase in the CF patient due to increased losses in sweat. Infants require supplementation due to the low-sodium content of breast milk, formula, and baby foods.

Table 34-4 gives suggestions for vitamin and mineral supplementation for the patient with CF.

Table 34-5 lists suggestions for increasing energy intake in CF.

d. Diet modification

B. Bronchopulmonary dysplasia
1. Description

Table 34-6 provides a list of the nutritional assessment parameters for the infant with bronchopulmonary dysplasia.
bronchopulmonary dysplasia (BPD), respiratory distress syndrome (RDS), endotracheal intubation, patent ductus arteriosus

2. Nutritional status and assessment
3. Nutritional requirements and care
a. Energy
b. Macronutrients

Table 34-7 shows a variety of combinations of infant formulas that increase the energy concentration of the formula.
carnitine

c. Micronutrients
d. Diet modifications

gastroesophageal reflux

C. Asthma, bronchitis, and emphysema

asthma, bronchitis, emphysema, nonspecific lung disease, theophylline

D. Chronic obstructive pulmonary disease
1. Description

chronic obstructive pulmonary disease (COPD), chronic bronchitis, emphysema, cor pulmonale

2. Nutritional status and assessment

Table 34-8 provides a list of the nutritional assessment parameters for the adult with COPD.
pink puffer, blue bloater

3. Nutritional requirements and care
a. Energy
b. Macronutrients
c. Micronutrients
d. Diet modifications
E. Respiratory failure (RF)
1. Description
2. Nutritional status and assessment
3. Nutritional requirements and care
a. Energy
b. Macronutrients
c. Micronutrients
d. Diet modifications
F. Lung cancer

respiratory failure (RF)

lung cancer, oat cell carcinoma

CASE STUDY INSIGHTS

1. What nutritional screening and assessment information do you need before they arrive for your visit?

Since the three-day food record and dietary pattern for Sam is already available, additional information needed includes anthropometrics (height, weight, and TSF) and biochemical measurements (CBC, serum retinol, serum α-tocopherol, albumin, electrolytes, and acid–base balance).

2. What foods or nutrients would you highlight in Sam's diet?

Sam's diet should focus on providing adequate energy, protein, and moderate fat. The sodium chloride intake should also be sufficient. Foods included in the diet should have higher nutrient density to promote sufficient energy and nutrients for growth and development. Fluids should be increased.

3. What are the goals for weight gain? How long should it take if Sam's medicines are effective?

The goals are for Sam to have normal growth and development and to achieve his pre-CF growth potential. His growth channel prior to diagnosis may serve as a good indicator of the goal. It would be best to regain his lost weight. If his medications and medical management are effective and his diet adequate, he can return to his growth channel within one year.

4. Sam's family has recently heard about gene therapy. They ask you to discuss this issue with them. How would you respond?

This gives the instructor a good opportunity to discuss recent developments in treatment of cystic fibrosis and how these treatments can be used.

5. Sam is at a day care center. What types of lunches could his mother pack for the center staff to provide for him? What instructions should be shared with them?

Suggestions for lunch foods include low-fat or nonfat cheese and low-fat turkey and ham in sandwiches or as finger foods. Pretzels can be a good snack item. Emphasis should be on signs of the diet being poorly tolerated. It may be necessary to allow Sam to eat more often than the other children in order to meet his energy and nutrient needs.

SUGGESTED TEST QUESTIONS

1. Assessment of fluid needs in an infant with bronchopulmonary dysplasia (BPD) should be guided by
    a. respiratory rate.
    b. activity level.
    * c. urinary output.
    d. weight.

2. Potassium deficiency related to diuretic therapy in an infant with BPD may be indicated by
    a. metabolic alkalosis.
    * b. muscle weakness.
    c. hyperventilation.
    d. hypercalcemia.

3. An infant with BPD may suffer from gastroe-sophageal reflux, which can be minimized by
* a. using thickened feedings.
 b. supporting the infant in a supine position.
 c. diluting the feedings to reduce viscosity.
 d. keeping the head of the bed in a horizontal position.

4. Enzyme-replacement capsules that cannot be swallowed by a young child can be given by
 a. mixing the beads in milk.
 b. placing the beads directly on the child's tongue.
* c. mixing the beads in applesauce.
 d. mixing the beads in ice cream.

5. The vitamins most likely to be deficient in a child with cystic fibrosis are
 a. vitamins A, E, and C .
 b. the water-soluble vitamins and vitamin K.
 c. vitamins A, D, E, and K.
* d. the fat-soluble vitamins and vitamin B_{12}.

6. Symptoms indicating that the CF patient has an inadequate intake of sodium include
 a. increased activity and elevated blood pressure.
 b. increased peristalsis and good skin turgor.
* c. vomiting and lethargy.
 d. increased urinary output and elevated blood pressure.

7. Infants with CF require enzyme replacement supplements
 a. only if they are formula fed.
* b. at every feeding, whether breastfed or formula fed.
 c. only if they are breast fed.
 d. after they are 6 months old.

8. A significant finding in the nutritional assess-ment process for a patient with COPD is
 a. no changes in body weight for the past year.
 b. weight gain of about 5% of ideal body weight over the past year.
* c. a current body weight less than 90% of optimal body weight.
 d. frequent changes in body weight.

9. Discomfort from abdominal bloating in a patient with COPD can be reduced by
 a. decreasing activity and decreasing dietary fiber.
 b. increasing cruciferous vegetables and decreasing fluid intake.
* c. increasing activity and increasing dietary fiber.
 d. increasing rest periods after meals.

10. Patients being weaned from a mechanical ven-tilator benefit from a diet lower in carbohy-drate because it
 a. increases CO_2 production.
* b. decreases CO_2 production.
 c. increases O_2 consumption.
 d. decreases ventilatory compliance.

11. Manifestations of CF include malabsorption, frequent respiratory infections, and sweat characterized by
* a. elevated levels of sodium and chloride.
 b. decreased levels of sodium and chloride.
 c. elevated levels of sodium and potassium.
 d. decreased levels of potassium and chloride.

12. Nutrient absorption impaired by pancreatic enzyme insufficiency associated with CF include
 a. protein.
 b. fat and protein.
* c. fat, protein, and starch.
 d. protein and starch.

13. Malabsorption associated with CF is treated with
 a. a low-fat, high-salt diet.
* b. enzyme replacement therapy.
 c. IV enzyme therapy.
 d. a high-protein, low-fat, high-carbohydrate diet.

14. The medical nutritional therapy recommended for the patient with CF is a
    * a. high-calorie diet with 15–20% of calories as protein and 35–40% as fat.
    b. low-calorie diet with 10–15% of calories as protein and 35–40% as fat.
    c. high-calorie diet with 5–10% of calories as protein and 20–30% as fat.
    d. low-calorie diet with 25–30% of calories as protein and 10–15% as fat.

15. Most water-soluble vitamins are well absorbed in CF, with the exception of
    a. ascorbic acid.
    b. vitamin B_6.
    c. niacin.
    * d. vitamin B_{12}.

16. The basis for determining sodium requirements in CF is
    a. decreased losses in sweat.
    * b. increased losses in sweat.
    c. decreased losses from overhydration.
    d. increased losses from dehydration.

17. The nutritional wasting commonly seen in patients with COPD is a result of
    * a. increased energy expenditure, decreased energy intake, and impaired oxygenation.
    b. decreased oxygen consumption and increased energy expenditure.
    c. decreased energy expenditure and decreased oxygen consumption.
    d. increased oxygen consumption and increased energy intake.

18. In patients with fluid retention, biochemical indicators of nutritional status such as serum proteins and electrolytes are
    a. increased due to increased urinary output.
    b. depressed due to poor nutritional status.
    c. increased due to hemoconcentration.
    * d. depressed duet to hemodilution.

19. The most reliable nutritional screening parameter in patients with acute respiratory failure is
    a. serum albumin.
    b. serum transferrin.
    * c. weight.
    d. triceps skinfold.

20. The energy needs of the COPD patient may be as high as
    a. 100% of the calculated REE.
    b. 125% of the calculated REE.
    * c. 150% of the calculated REE.
    d. 200% of the calculated REE.

CHAPTER

NUTRITIONAL CARE IN RENAL DISEASE

OVERVIEW

The purpose of this chapter is to provide students with an understanding of the nutritional management of diseases of the kidney. The chapter begins with a review of the physiology and functions of the kidney. Diseases of the kidney are presented in three general groups: glomerular disease, including nephrotic syndrome and nephritic syndrome; diseases of the tubules and interstitium; and end-stage renal disease. Principles of nutritional management are presented for various types of therapy, such as hemodialysis, intermittent peritoneal dialysis, continuous ambulatory peritoneal dialysis, and transplantation. Renal disease with concurrent factors, such as childhood, diabetes, and AIDS, are also described.

LEARNING OBJECTIVES

This chapter will prepare the learner to be able to

1. Describe the functions of the kidney and how pathophysiological changes can affect renal function.
2. Explain the renin-angiotensin mechanism for control of blood pressure.
3. Define nephrotic syndrome and nephritic syndrome.
4. State the principles of nutritional management of diseases of the glomerulus.
5. Describe the clinical manifestations of acute renal failure.
6. State the principles of nutritional management of acute renal failure.
7. Explain the role of diet in nephrolithiasis, both as a cause and as a treatment.
8. List the options for medical treatment of end-stage renal disease.
9. State the principles of nutritional management for each of the medical treatment options for end-stage renal disease.
10. Describe how parenteral nutrition is used to manage the nutritional needs of the renal patient.
11. State additional concerns for nutritional management of the renal patient with diabetes.
12. State additional concerns for nutritional management of the child with renal disease.
13. State additional concerns for nutritional management of the patient with renal disease and AIDS.

CHAPTER OUTLINE ————————————

NOTES, TERMS, & TRANSPARENCY MASTERS

I. Physiology and Function of the Kidney

Figure 35-1 (Transparency) is a drawing of a nephron.

Figure 35-2 (Transparency) is a schematic drawing of the renin-angiotensin mechanism that controls blood pressure.

nephron, glomerulus, tubules, proximal convoluted tubule, loop of Henle, distal tubule, collecting duct, Bowman's capsule, ultrafiltrate, collecting tubules, renal pelvis, ureter, antidiuretic hormone (ADH), oliguria, urea, uric acid, creatinine, ammonia, azotemia, renal function, renal failure, renin-angiotensin mechanism, juxtaglomerular apparatus, angiotensin I, angiotensin II, aldosterone, erythropoietin, calcium–phosphorus homeostasis

II. Diseases of the Kidney
  A. Glomerular diseases
    1. Nephrotic syndrome

nephrotic syndrome, hypoalbuminemia, hypercholesterolemia, hypercoagulability, systemic lupus erythematosus, amyloidosis, membranous nephropathy, focal glomerulosclerosis, membrano-proliferative glomerulonephritis

      a. Nutritional care

edema, diuretics

    2. Nephritic syndrome

nephritic syndrome, acute glomerulonephritides, hematuria, IgA nephropathy, hereditary nephritis

      a. Nutritional care
  B. Diseases of the tubules and interstitium

medullary interstitium, extraosseous calcification

    1. Acute renal failure

Table 35-1 (Transparency) lists some of the causes of acute renal failure.
acute renal failure (ARF), glomerular filtration rate (GFR), ischemic acute tubular necrosis

      a. Nutritional care

hemodialysis, peritoneal dialysis, continuous arteriovenous hemofiltration (CAVH)

      b. Protein

Nephramine, Aminosyn-RF, Aminess

      c. Energy

Controlyte, Polycose, Cal-Power

d. Fluid and sodium balance

Table 35-2 provides a sample calculation for determining fluid requirements in acute renal failure.
water intoxication

e. Potassium balance

Table 35-3 (Transparency) lists the recommended dietary allowances for acute renal failure.
exchange resins, Kayexalate

2. Other tubular or interstitial diseases

chronic interstitial nephritis, vesicouretero reflux, medullary cystic disease, Fanconi syndrome, renal tubular acidosis (RTA), isolate proximal RTA

3. Pyelonephritis

pyelonephritis, *Escherichia coli*

C. Nephrolithiasis (kidney stones)

struvite

1. Calcium oxalate and calcium phosphate stones

Table 35-4 lists foods that raise the urinary oxalate excretion level.
calcium oxalate, hydroxyapatite, hyperparathyroidism, hyperuricosuria, idiopathic hypercalciuria, hyperoxaluria, primary hyperoxaluria, enteric hyperoxaluria, oxalobacter formigenes, hypercalciuria, renal leaker, idiopathic hypercalciuria

2. Uric acid stones

See **Clinical Insight:** "Acid Ash" and "Alkaline Ash" Diets.
uric acid stones, potential renal acid load (PRAL), renal net acid excretion (NAE)

3. Cystinine stones

cystinine stones

4. Struvite stones

Figure 35-3 is a diagram of a kidney showing a staghorn calculus.
struvite stones, Proteus, Klebsiella, staghorn calculi

III. Progressive Nature of Renal Disease

Modification of diet in renal disease (MDRD)

IV. End-Stage Renal Disease
A. Medical treatment
1. Transplantation

end-stage renal disease, uremia

transplantation

a. Nutritional care

immunosuppressive therapy, cyclosporine

2. Dialysis
a. Hemodialysis

Figure 35-4 is a drawing of a arteriovenous fistula with the temporary cannulas in place for hemodialysis.

Table 35-5 is a guide for nutrient requirements for adults with renal disease based on the type of therapy.
fistula

   b. Peritoneal dialysis

Figure 35-5 is a drawing of the peritoneal cavity and the placement of the catheter in peritoneal dialysis.
continuous ambulatory peritoneal dialysis (CAPD), peritonitis

B. Psychological support
C. Nutritional care

Figure 35-6 (Handout) is a simple menu plan for a patient on dialysis.

   1. Fluid and sodium balance

polycystic kidney disease, chronic obstructive uropathy

   2. Potassium
   3. Protein

See **Clinical Insight:** "Protein Calculation for a Dialysis Patient."

   4. Kinetic modeling

Table 35-7 presents the exchange lists for intake of protein, kilocalories, sodium, and phosphorus.
Figure 35-6 shows a simple menu plan for a dialysis patient.
KT/V, protein catabolic rate (PCR)

     a. Tube feeding
   5. Energy
   6. Calcium, phosphorus, and vitamin D

renal osteodystrophy, osteomalacia, osteitis fibrosa cystica, metastatic calcification, Basajel, Amphojel, calcitriol, Rocaltrol, Calcijex

   7. Fluoride
   8. Iron

erythropoietin (EPO), recombinant human erythropoietin (rHuEPO)

   9. Vitamins
  10. Carbohydrate
  11. Lipid

carnitine

C. Parenteral nutrition

Nephramine, Freeamine, Travasol 8.5, Aminosyn

   1. Vitamins and minerals

Table 35-8 provides the guidelines for daily parenteral vitamin supplementation in total parenteral nutrition for patients with renal failure.

   2. Intradialytic parenteral nutrition

Table 35-9 summarizes the regimen for parenteral nutrition via the peripheral vein for dialysis patients.

Table 35-10 summarizes the regimen for intermittent parenteral nutrition administered during hemodialysis therapy.

Table 35-11 summarizes the regimen for total parenteral nutrition via the subclavian vein for dialysis patients.

intradialytic parenteral nutrition

a. Complications

postdialysis hypoglycemia

D. End-stage renal disease in patients with diabetes

E. End-stage renal disease in children

Table 35-12 is a guide for nutrient requirements for children with renal disease based on the type of therapy.

rHeEPO, rDNA-produced growth hormone (rHGH)

V. Human Immunodeficiency Virus and Renal Disease

A. Nutritional care

See Chapter 37 for more on HIV and AIDS

AIDS-associated renal disease

CASE STUDY INSIGHTS: HEMODIALYSIS

1. What suggestions do you have for the dialysis nutrition prescription?

The nutritional prescription should be based on the prescribed method of treatment, in this case, hemodialysis. In the initial diet, energy requirements are 35 kcal/kg of body weight, protein requirements are 1.0–1.2 g/kg, fluid requirements are 800 cc plus the equivalent measure of urinary output, sodium and potassium requirements are each 2–3 g per day, and phosphorus requirements are 1.0–1.2 g per day. After initiation of diet, blood values are used to adjust nutrients for appropriate control.

2. His doctor suggests daily use of a multivitamin supplement containing B-complex vitamins but not fat-soluble vitamins. Why?

Generally, fat-soluble vitamins are not dialyzable. Water-soluble vitamins will be lost in the dialysate and should be replaced.

3. What level of protein would you suggest during dialysis? With this factor, how much should he be receiving in the way of protein foods?

The recommendation for protein intake while on hemodialysis is 1.0–1.2 g/kg per day. This patient requires 86–103 g per day. About 75% of the protein should be of high biological value (65–77 g). Student responses should be evaluated within the context of the entire diet prescription.

4. If he goes home without dialysis but has chronic renal failure, what might his doctor suggest for a protein level?

The predialysis patient with progressive renal failure demonstrated by decreasing GFR and elevated BUN and creatinine should be maintained on a diet providing 0.6–0.8 g/kg of body weight per day.

5. What foods would be monitored using the National Renal Diet?

The key nutrients are protein, energy, sodium, and potassium. Examples include milk, nondairy milk substitutes, meats, starches, vegetables, fruits, and fats. The food exchange lists in Table 35-7 in the textbook are from the National Renal Diet. The focus of student responses should be on meeting the diet prescription and rationale for selection of foods.

CASE STUDY INSIGHTS: PERITONEAL DIALYSIS

1. Explain why you would expect to see each of the lab value discrepancies and what could be done nutritionally to affect each value. Also assess the patient's weight and anthropometric values to determine appropriate nutritional therapy.

Laboratory values for some biochemical indices are altered as a result of dialysis. The serum sodium for this patient is slightly depressed. This may be a result of drinking too much fluid and excess weight gain between dialyses. Serum potassium is elevated, which may be due to excess potassium intake in the diet. The serum ferritin is depressed, which may result from the disease or be a side effect of the phosphate binders. Iron supplementation may be helpful.

The ideal body weight for this patient is 139 lbs. Her current weight is 126 lbs. She has been averaging 6.4-lb to 8.1-lb gains between dialyses. It is not known whether the recorded weight is pre- or postdialysis. Her arm muscle area suggests some protein depletion as well. Therapy should be based on these findings.

2. The patient takes the following medications: erythropoietin, Benadryl, folic acid, prednisone, Nephrocaps, Basagel, and Tums. The patient dialyzes against the following dialysate fluid: 3 mEq K, 3.5 mg calcium, bicarbonate, and 200 g dextrose. Comment on the appropriateness of each. What are they used for? Would you suggest any changes or additional medication?

The erythropoietin is used to improve the anemia that occurs with renal disease. Nephrocaps is a vitamin supplement that is designed to meet the needs of the renal patient and, along with folic acid, is being used to supplement water-soluble vitamins. The Basajel is a phosphate binder, and it along with the Tums and dialysate calcium are used to offset the osteodystrophy seen in renal disease. All are appropriate and no changes are needed.

3. The patient is currently awaiting a cadaveric transplant. She asks you how her diet will change with the transplant. If the transplant doesn't happen soon, she is considering peritoneal dialysis to give her more freedom from the machine. What would be the nutritional concerns if this were to happen?

When the patient receives a transplant, her dietary needs will change. Her initial needs will be higher protein and energy intakes. Her fluid, sodium, and potassium needs with be variable, and her calcium and phosphorus needs will remain about the same.

If we assume that the patient is already on intermittent peritoneal dialysis (IPD), then she must be considering a change to continuous ambulatory peritoneal dialysis (CAPD). If so, her energy needs will decrease, protein will stay the same, and fluid, sodium, potassium, and phosphorus needs will increase.

SUGGESTED TEST QUESTIONS

1. The accumulation of nitrogenous waste products in the blood of a patient with acute renal failure is directly affected by
   a. fat in the diet.
   b. carbohydrate in the diet.
   * c. protein in the diet.
   d. all the above.

2. To maintain appropriate fluid balance in acute renal failure with retention of sodium, it is important to
   a. administer all parenteral medications in electrolyte-free water.
   * b. administer parenteral medications in a balanced salt solution.
   c. reduce the amount of fluid added to medications by one-half.
   d. use potassium chloride in the diluent.

3. In acute renal failure, the serum potassium level can be reduced by administering
   a. chelating agents.
   * b. glucose, insulin, and bicarbonate.
   c. acidifying agents.
   d. sodium chloride solutions.

4. Guidelines for the patient who has a history of kidney stones include
   a. decreasing fluid intake to keep urine output to less than 1000 mL/day.
   b. decreasing intake of magnesium-containing antacids.
   * c. increasing intake of fluid to maintain urinary output at or above 2000 mL/day.
   d. using sodium bicarbonate to alkalinize urine.

5. Excretion of urinary calcium and uric acid is increased by
   * a. animal protein in the diet.
   b. carbohydrate in the diet.
   c. fat in the diet.
   d. increased intake of water.

6. A dietary modification that is beneficial in deteriorating renal function is to reduce the intake of
   * a. protein.
   b. carbohydrate.
   c. fat.
   d. sodium.

7. Following renal transplant, the patient taking cyclosporine will need to restrict dietary
   a. sodium.
   b. protein.
   * c. potassium.
   d. calcium.

8. Patients with ESRD who present with elevated blood pressure and edema may need to restrict dietary
   a. protein.
   b. potassium.
   * c. sodium.
   d. fat.

9. The demineralization that results from increased parathyroid action on bone calcium in renal disease can be minimized by
   a. eliminating carbonated beverages to decrease phosphates.
   b. using thiazide diuretics to eliminate calcium.
   * c. supplementing calcium early in the disease.
   d. decreasing protein products high in phosphate.

10. Regulation of water excretion through the kidney is mediated by
   * a. antidiuretic hormone secreted by the pituitary gland.
   b. antidiuretic hormone secreted by the adrenal glands.
   c. aldosterone secreted by the adrenal glands.
   d. angiotensin secreted by the pituitary gland.

11. The anemia present in chronic renal disease results primarily from a
   a. lack of heme and nonheme iron intake.
   b. loss of iron through the diseased kidney.
   * c. deficiency of the hormone erythropoietin.
   d. lack of the parathyroid hormone.

12. In nephrotic syndrome, a reduction of protein intake down to 0.6 mg/kg of body weight per day may result in
    * a. decreased proteinuria without adversely affecting serum albumin.
    b. increased proteinuria.
    c. protein malnutrition.
    d. disruption of calcium and phosphorus balance.

13. Guidelines for the management of edema in nephrotic syndrome include
    a. a no added salt diet.
    * b. mild sodium restriction.
    c. strict sodium restriction.
    d. severe sodium restriction.

14. Nephritic syndrome is most often manifested by
    a. hyperalbuminemia.
    b. hypotension.
    * c. hematuria.
    d. hypocholesterolemia.

15. The guidelines for nutritional care of the patient with acute glomerulonephritis include which of these?
    * a. Protein and potassium intakes do not need to be restricted unless significant uremia or hyperkalemia develops.
    b. Protein intake must be restricted in all patients.
    c. Potassium restriction is necessary for most patients.
    d. Protein and potassium intakes must be increased.

16. The recommended initial method for feeding the patient with acute renal failure is
    a. oral feedings as tolerated.
    b. enteral feedings as tolerated.
    c. parenteral administration of carbohydrate alone.
    * d. parenteral administration of glucose and essential amino acids.

17. Calcium restriction in the nutritional management of nephrolithiasis is indicated only when the condition is the
    a. resorptive form.
    b. resorptive form in which excess calcium is resorbed from the bone.
    c. absorptive form.
    * d. absorptive form in which hypercalciuria occurs only with a very high calcium intake.

18. Nutritional management of progressive renal insufficiency includes a protein requirement of
    a. 0.2–0.5 g/kg of IBW with 100% HBV.
    b. 0.4–0.6 g/kg of IBW with 50% HBV.
    * c. 0.6–0.8 g/kg of IBW with 75% HBV.
    d. 1–1.5 g/kg of IBW with 66% HBV.

19. The recommended protein intake for the patient on peritoneal dialysis is
    a. 0.2–0.5 g/kg of IBW.
    b. 0.4–0.6 g/kg of IBW.
    c. 0.8–1.0 g/kg of IBW.
    * d. 1.2–1.5 g/kg of IBW.

20. The goal for managing the calcium-phosphorus product in end-stage renal disease is
    a. >30.
    b. >40.
    c. <60.
    * d. <70.

Chapter 36

NUTRITIONAL CARE IN NEOPLASTIC DISEASE

OVERVIEW

The purpose of this chapter is to teach students the role of diet in the etiology of cancer and in the treatment of cancer. The dietary factors most often associated with the occurrence of cancer are examined, along with the nutritional effects of cancer. The nutritional effects of cancer treatment are presented, including chemotherapy, radiation therapy, surgery, immunotherapy, and marrow transplantation. General medical nutritional management of cancer is described with specific information provided for special situations.

LEARNING OBJECTIVES

This chapter will prepare the learner to be able to

1. Identify the role of diet in the etiology of cancer.
2. Discriminate between dietary factors that show strong evidence of an etiological relationship to cancer and those factors that do not show strong evidence.
3. Describe how nutrients functioning as antioxidants may play a role in cancer prevention.
4. Explain how fruit and vegetable intake may prevent cancer.
5. Describe cancer cachexia and how it develops.
6. List the major metabolic abnormalities that occur with cancer.
7. Identify the major nutritional concerns associated with various treatment methods for cancer.
8. State the goals of nutritional care of the cancer patient.
9. State the recommended nutritional care for the patient following marrow transplantation.
10. Characterize the patient who is most likely to seek unproven dietary treatments for cancer and the likely outcomes.

CHAPTER OUTLINE ――――――――――― NOTES, TERMS, & TRANSPARENCY MASTERS

tumorigenesis, carcinogenesis, initiation, promotion, progression

I. Nutrition in the Etiology of Cancer

Key concept: It has been estimated that at least 35% of cancer cases are related to diet and may be potentially preventable.

See **New Directions:** "Nutrients in Chemoprevention."

A. Energy

B. Lipids
C. Protein
D. Fiber
E. Nutrients with antioxidant functions
F. Fruits and vegetables

G. Calcium and vitamin D
H. Alcohol
I. Coffee
J. Artificial sweeteners

K. Preservatives

L. Nitrates, nitrites, and nitrosamines

M. Method of food preparation

II. Nutritional Effects of Cancer
  A. Cachexia

  B. Energy metabolism
  C. Substrate metabolism
  D. Other metabolic abnormalities
  E. Sensory changes

III. Nutritional Effects of Cancer Therapy

  A. Chemotherapy

estrogen-sensitive tissues

See **Clinical Insight: "Nutrition and Skin Cancer."**

Table 36-1 lists the results of studies on the intake of fruits and vegetables and cancer prevention. Data are organized by cancer site.
Table 36-2 is a summary of the case control evidence of the relationship between vegetable and fruit consumption and cancer.
phytochemicals, dithiolthiones, glucosinolate, indoles, isothiocyanates, flavonoids, phenols, protease inhibitors, plant sterols, allium compounds, and limonene

cyclamate, saccharin, aspartame

butylated hydroxytoulene (BHT), butylated hydroxyanisol (BHA)

nitrate, nitrite, *N*-nitroso compounds, nitrosamines, nitrosamides

polycyclic aromatic hydrocarbons, benzopyrene, heterocyclic aromatic amines

Figure 36-1 is a schematic illustration of the mechanism of cachexia in the cancer patient.
cancer cachexia, cytokines

carcinoid syndrome, Zollinger-Ellison syndrome

Table 36-3 lists the side effects of cancer therapy that may affect nutritional status.
autologous marrow transplantation, antineoplastic agents

Figure 36-2 is a photograph of the severe oral manifestations of marrow transplantation, chemotherapy, and radiation therapy.
Table 36-4 lists the common problems associated with drug therapy in cancer.
chemotherapeutic agents, mucositis, cheilosis, glossitis, stomatitis, esophagitis, oligophagy, adynamic ileus

B. Radiation therapy

xerostomia, radiation enteritis, short bowel syndrome

C. Surgery

steatorrhea, vagotomy, chylous fistula, dumping syndrome, colectomy

D. Immunotherapy

cytotoxic agents, monoclonal antibodies, alpha-interferon, melanoma

E. Marrow transplantation

leukemia, lymphoma, graft-versus-host disease (GVHD), venoocclusive disease (VOD), autologous marrow transplantation

IV. Nutritional Care of the Patient with Cancer
    A. Goals of nutritional care

Key concept: The overall goals of medical nutritional therapy in the cancer patient are to prevent or correct nutritional deficiencies and to minimize weight loss.
Table 36-5 presents guidelines for oral feeding during antitumor therapy. Specific problems with recommended diets, supplements or aids, and poorly tolerated foods are listed.
altered taste acuity, meat aversion, dysphagia, diminished salvation, intestinal damage, diarrhea, steatorrhea, ondansetron, granisetron, 5-hydroxytryptamine receptor antagonists

B. Timing of food presentation
C. Enteral tube feeding
D. Parenteral nutrition

bacterial translocation

E. Home enteral and parenteral nutrition
F. Pediatric patient
G. Terminal cancer patient

Key concept: While aggressive nutritional therapy in advanced cancer can prolong life, other factors must be considered. The foods provided should be well tolerated and be provided in an emotionally supportive environment.

H. Marrow transplant patient

allogenic marrow transplantation, mucositis, xerostomia, dysgeusia

I. Patient rehabilitation
J. Unproven dietary treatments

Key concept: Treatment of cancer is plagued with fraudulent claims that attract patients with false hope while often being expensive and unsuccessful.
metabolic therapy, amygdalin, Laetrile, oxymedicine, macrobiotic diet, mega–vitamin therapy

CASE STUDY INSIGHTS

1. What recommendations do you have to prepare Janice for surgery?

A primary goal in nutritional management of cancer is the prevention of protein-energy malnutrition. Although the patient is overweight, research shows that a weight loss as small as 5% can negatively affect the prognosis. Her protein stores should be assessed at this time. Depending on the outcome, her nutritional status should be maintained or improved before surgery.

2. What side effects might Janice experience from radiation therapy? List some dietary alterations that Janice can follow if she experiences weight loss, nausea, vomiting, and difficulty swallowing.

For nausea and vomiting, taking antiemetic drugs prior to meals, avoiding favorite foods when feeling bad, eating small frequent meals, and avoiding liquids with meals may help. For weight loss, it will help to eat high-calorie, protein-dense foods. For difficulty swallowing, use thick liquids and semisoft foods, use a straw for liquids, and add sauces and gravy. Additional side effects may include decreased appetite, taste and smell changes, dental problems, mucositis, xerostomia, esophageal stricture, and decreased immune function.

3. Is Janice at her ideal body weight (IBW)? If not, what suggestions would you recommend? Consider her hypertension, planned surgery, and radiation therapy.

The IBW for Janice is 140 lbs ± 10%, or 126–154 lbs. At her current weight, she is at 120% of IBW. While weight reduction would benefit her hypertension, it is mild and diet-controlled at this time. It would not be advisable for her to attempt weight loss prior to the planned surgery and radiation therapy.

4. What dietary recommendations, if any, should be provided for use with tamoxifen?

Tamoxifen is known to cause nausea and vomiting and may alter taste. Foods should be provided as tolerated, emphasizing high-nutrient density when nausea and vomiting are less. If taste alterations occur, work with patient to determine tolerances and increase or decrease flavorings as needed.

SUGGESTED TEST QUESTIONS

1. A middle-aged woman consuming a high-fat diet is at increased risk for
    a. lung cancer.
*   b. colon cancer.
    c. uterus cancer.
    d. pancreas cancer.

2. A factor not associated with an increased risk of cancer is
    a. cyclamates.
    b. alcohol.
*   c. coffee.
    d. nitrates.

3. When a cancer patient presents with anorexia, weight loss, anemia, and asthenia, it is likely that she has developed
   a. borborygmus.
   b. amyloidosis.
   c. Cushing's disease.
   * d. cachexia.

4. A common change in taste sensation in cancer therapy is decreased tolerance of bitter taste, resulting in the avoidance of
   a. starches.
   b. salty foods.
   * c. meats.
   d. dairy products.

5. When secretory diarrhea is severe for the patient with graft-versus-host disease (GVHD), implementing enteral feeding is contraindicated until the diarrhea is
   a. <3000 mL/day.
   * b. <1000 mL/day.
   c. <500 mL/day.
   d. absent for at least 48 hours.

6. The patient demonstrating or complaining of dysphagia may benefit from eating
   a. frozen dairy and fruit products.
   * b. foods that are soft or liquid at room temperature.
   c. cold liquid milk and cream soups.
   d. solid foods at warmer temperatures to stimulate swallowing.

7. Of the vitamins studied as chemopreventors of cancer, the one showing the greatest success is
   a. pyridoxine.
   b. pantothenic acid.
   * c. retinol.
   d. biotin.

8. Most evidence from current research on the relationship between drinking a large amount coffee and pancreatic cancer supports
   a. a strong causal role.
   b. a slight causal role.
   * c. no causal role.
   d. a strong causal role for decaffeinated coffee.

9. The results of studies on factors affecting the development of cancer of the gastric mucosa suggest that it may be inhibited by consumption of
   a. fresh vegetables high in dietary fiber.
   * b. fresh vegetables, especially those high in vitamin C.
   c. whole grain breads and cereals.
   d. milk and milk products.

10. The dysgnosia and dysgeusia experienced by cancer patients may include
   a. decreased threshold for sweet foods.
   b. increased threshold for bitter foods.
   c. decreased threshold for sour and salty foods.
   * d. increased threshold for sweet foods.

11. The temperature of foods best tolerated by the patient with dysphagia due to lesions in the oral and esophageal tissues is
   a. cold.
   b. hot.
   c. bland.
   * d. room temperature.

12. Use of macrobiotic diets for cancer treatment are generally not successful and are usually
   * a. low in energy and low in some vitamins and minerals.
   b. high in energy, fat, and protein and low in vitamin B_{12}.
   c. low in protein and high in energy and fat.
   d. high in protein and low in energy and fat.

13. Current epidemiological studies suggest an increased risk of stomach and esophageal cancers with frequent consumption of
   a. fruits and vegetables.
   * b. smoked and fried foods.
   c. refined sugars.
   d. microwaved foods.

14. The nutritional requirements of a child with cancer are
*   a.   similar to those of normal growing children.
    b.   much greater than those of normal growing children.
    c.   much less than those of normal growing children.
    d.   slightly less than those of normal growing children.

15. In the nutrition assessment process of the patient receiving radiation therapy, the use of immune function tests is limited because radiation
    a.   promotes immune function.
*   b.   depresses immune function.
    c.   induces malabsorption.
    d.   increases the total lymphocyte count.

CHAPTER 37

NUTRITIONAL CARE IN HIV INFECTION AND AIDS

OVERVIEW

The purpose of this chapter is to provide students with a general understanding of the pathophysiology of HIV and AIDS and associated nutritional factors. The chapter begins with a description of the etiology and classifications of HIV infection and AIDS. The manifestations of HIV are presented. The condition of malnutrition associated with AIDS is described with specific guidelines provided for nutritional assessment, management, and complications. The chapter ends with a description of some of the unproven nutritional therapies used to treat AIDS.

LEARNING OBJECTIVES

This chapter will prepare the learner to be able to

1. Describe the pathophysiology of AIDS.
2. Identify the classifications of HIV infection and AIDS.
3. State the manifestations of HIV infection, including opportunistic infections, malignancies, neurological disease, and other affected organ systems.
4. Explain the condition of cancer cachexia.
5. State the important nutritional assessment parameters for the HIV-infected or AIDS patient.
6. List the goals of nutritional therapy for the patient with AIDS.
7. State the guidelines of nutritional therapy for the patient with AIDS.
8. Describe the nutritional complications associated with AIDS and how they can be managed.
9. List the unproven methods for nutrition management of AIDS.

CHAPTER OUTLINE ─────────────── NOTES, TERMS, & TRANSPARENCY MASTERS

See **New Directions: "The Changing Face of
    AIDS."**
**acquired immunodeficiency syndrome (AIDS),
    Kaposi's sarcoma, human immuno-
    deficiency virus (HIV)**

I. Etiology and Classification

Table 37-1A provides a list of the recommended management for CD4+ and T-cell categories.

Table 37-1B is the 1993 revised classification system for HIV infection and AIDS for adolescents and adults.

Key concept: Current evidence indicates that HIV is present in the breast milk of women who are HIV-infected. The risk of transmission of the virus by this route is unknown. Present recommendations are that HIV-infected mothers should not breastfeed their infants.

CD4+, T-helper lymphocytes

II. Manifestations of HIV Infection

initial HIV infection, arthralgias, lymphadenopathy, constitutional disease, AIDS wasting syndrome

A. Opportunistic infections

Table 37-2 lists the AIDS-related infections seen in the syndrome and the associated physical problems and symptoms.

opportunistic infections

B. Malignancies

Figure 37-1 is a photograph of the forearm of an individual with the nodular lesions of Kaposi's sarcoma.

Kaposi's sarcoma, lymphomas, non-Hodgkin's lymphoma, Burkitt's lymphoma, squamous cell carcinoma, cloacogenic carcinoma

C. Neurological disease

HIV encephalopathy, AIDS dementia, myelopathy, peripheral neuropathy

D. Other affected organ systems

mycobacterium avium complex (MAC), cytomegalovirus (CMV), cryptosporidia, hepatitis B, HIV-associated nephropathy, AIDS enteropathy

III. Relationship Between Malnutrition and AIDS

protein-energy malnutrition (PEM), cachectin hypothesis, tumor necrosis factor

IV. Nutritional Assessment

Table 37-3 is a summary of the medications used for HIV therapy, their use, possible gastrointestinal interaction, and recommendations for minimizing effects.

V. Nutritional Management
    A. Nutritional screening
    B. Nutrition intervention
        1. Energy
        2. Protein

3. Fat
4. Fluids and electrolytes
5. Vitamins and minerals
C. Nutritional complications

doxorubin hydrochloride

1. Diarrhea and malabsorption

Table 37-4 is a summary of the nutrition intervention for diarrhea. Diarrhea that is treatable, nontreatable, and resulting from AIDS enteropathy is included.
Entamoeba histolytica, Salmonella, Campylobacter jejuni, Shigella, Cytomegalovirus, Mycobacterium aviumintracellular, Cryptosporidium parvum, microsporidioses, opitate, Lomotil, loperamide, Imodium, Octreotide

2. Disorders of the oral cavity and esophagus

Figure 37-2 is a photograph of the mouth of an HIV-infected person with oral pseudomembranous candidiasis.
Figure 37-3 is a photograph of the mouth of an individual with Kaposi's sarcoma.
Table 37-5 provides practical eating suggestions for managing various oral and gastrointestinal symptoms.
oral candidiasis, dysgeusia, Advera

3. Neurological disorders
D. Food handling and infection control

Key concept: The Centers for Disease Control (CDC) have recommended that all blood and body fluids be treated as potentially infective. Hospital employees may be at risk if infection control precautions are not applied.

VI. Unproven Nutritional Therapies

Table 37-6 lists nutritional therapy used by some individuals for the management of HIV infection and AIDS.

CASE STUDY INSIGHTS

1. Calculate Jon's reported daily intake of protein and calories. How does this compare with the recommended amount for his age, sex, and size?

Jon's intake for the past two days has been zero. No additional information is available that allows you to determine his intake prior to that time. His energy needs at this time are increased by an injury factor of about 1.3 when using the Harris-Benedict calculation. His protein needs are 1.0–1.4 g/kg of IBW.

2. *What recommendations would you make as this point about use of an oral diet?*

There is a suggestion here of intractable diarrhea or AIDS enteropathy. If he is able to tolerate oral feedings, the foods should provide adequate fluids to replace losses (also by IV), be low in fat and fiber, have no lactose or caffeine, and be at room temperature.

3. *What dietary suggestions would you offer to Jon ,who takes acyclovir, AZT, and Amphotericin-B? What side effects is Jon likely to experience with this therapy?*

Acyclovir may cause nausea and headache. Fluid intake should be monitored when using this drug. AZT may cause nausea, vomiting, and suppression of bone marrow. The patient needs to be monitored for anemia. Side effects associated with Amphotericin-B are anorexia, vomiting, hypokalemia, hypomagnesemia, and a metallic taste in the mouth.

4. *Would you recommend parenteral nutrition? Why or why not?*

Jon appears to be a good risk for TPN. When diarrhea is untreatable, it is not possible to provide adequate nutrients via the enteral route. It is assumed that he is malabsorbing. The TPN would reduce his risk for PEM.

SUGGESTED TEST QUESTIONS

1. Opportunistic infections seen in the AIDS patient may increase in the presence of malnutrition due to
    * a. further compromise of the immune system.
    b. reduction in available iron for the WBC.
    c. reduction in the RBC, causing the tissues to be inadequately oxygenated.
    d. decreased oncotic pressure in the intravascular space.

2. The least reliable parameters for determining the nutritional status of the AIDS patient are
    a. serum albumin, prealbumin, and transferrin.
    b. triceps skinfold fat measurement and mid-arm circumference.
    c. serial weight monitoring and protein status.
    * d. skin testing and TLC.

3. The AIDS patient who does not require repletion of protein stores should have a total protein intake of
    a. 0.5–0.75 g/kg of body weight.
    b. 0.75–1.0 g/kg of body weight.
    * c. 1.0–1.4 g/kg of body weight.
    d. 1.5–2.0 g/kg of body weight.

4. When fat malabsorption is manifested with diarrhea, it may be helpful to use
    a. polyunsaturated fats in the diet.
    b. a fat-free diet.
    * c. a low-fat diet and MCT oil.
    d. a larger dose of vitamin supplements.

5. The AIDS patient with oral candidiasis may complain of
    a. loss of appetite.
    b. dryness of the mouth.
    c. decreased saliva.
    * d. a burning sensation in the mouth.

6. Assessment of weight changes in the AIDS patient is most reliable when determined as
    a. percentage of ideal body weight.
    b. percentage of standard body weight.
    * c. percentage of usual body weight.
    d. percentiles based on NHANES II data.

7. Increased energy requirements for AIDS patients can be estimated as
   a. 0.8–1.0 times the BEE.
   b. 1.0–1.3 times the BEE.
 * c. 1.3–1.5 times the BEE.
   d. 2.0 times the BEE.

8. The recommendation for vitamin and mineral supplementation for the AIDS patient is to
 * a. provide 100% of the RDA.
   b. provide 200% of the RDA.
   c. use megadoses of all vitamins.
   d. not supplement.

9. For most patients who are HIV-infected or have developed AIDS, the common nutritional problems are
   a. dysgeusia and candidiasis.
 * b. diarrhea and malabsorption.
   c. psychomotor impairment and decreased liver function.
   d. weight gain and fatigue.

10. Diarrhea caused by the cytomegalovirus requires nutritional support using
   a. a liquid diet.
   b. a chemically defined diet.
   c. an enteral formula with MCT oil.
 * d. a parenterally administered diet.

11. A side effect of pentamidine, a drug used in the treatment of *Pneumocystis carnii* pneumonia, may include pancreatic dysfunction, resulting in
   a. hypercholesterolemia.
 * b. hypoglycemia or hyperglycemia.
   c. hypoalbuminemia.
   d. hyperkalemia or hyponatremia.

12. The human immunodeficiency virus that causes AIDS infects the genetic core of
   a. all lymphocytes.
   b. the T4 lymphocytes.
 * c. the CD4+ or T-helper lymphocytes.
   d. the CD4+ and T8 lymphocytes.

13. When counseling a pregnant woman who is HIV-positive, you should encourage her to
   a. breastfeed her baby.
 * b. not breastfeed her baby.
   c. breastfeed her baby only when she is asymptomatic.
   d. breastfeed her baby only if her disease is in its early stages.

14. The person with AIDS is more susceptible to foodborne pathogens because
   a. of drug effects.
 * b. of decreased immune function.
   c. the AIDS patient prefers room temperature foods.
   d. the production of HCl in the stomach is reduced.

15. In patients with diarrhea resulting from AIDS enteropathy, absorption may be satisfactory with the use of a
   a. standard enteral formula.
 * b. chemically defined enteral formula.
   c. blenderized diet.
   d. diet with whole protein and complex carbohydrates.

CHAPTER 38

NUTRITIONAL CARE IN FOOD ALLERGY AND FOOD INTOLERANCE

OVERVIEW

The purpose of this chapter is to provide students with an understanding of food allergy and food intolerance. The chapter begins with a definition of food hypersensitivity and an explanation of the immunological activities associated with food allergy. The common food allergies are identified and individuals at risk are identified. The nonimmunological reactions to food are presented along with those components of food most often involved in food intolerances. The diagnosis and treatment of food allergy are described. Recommendations for managing the infant with food allergy are included.

LEARNING OBJECTIVES

This chapter will prepare the learner to be able to

1. Discriminate between a food allergy and a food intolerance.
2. Explain the various immunological responses seen in food allergy.
3. Describe the phenomenon of an allergic reaction.
4. List the common food allergens.
5. State the factors that put an individual at risk for food allergy.
6. Explain the negative nonimmunological responses to foods.
7. List the common items causing food intolerance.
8. Explain the diagnostic procedures used to identify food allergy.
9. State the principles of nutritional management of food allergy.
10. State the concerns for infants having food allergy.

CHAPTER OUTLINE ———————————— NOTES, TERMS, & TRANSPARENCY MASTERS

I. Definition

Key concept: The term *food hypersensitivity* can also be used to describe immunologically mediated adverse reactions to foods.
food hypersensitivity

II. Immunological Basis
   A. Antigen exclusion

antigens, allergens

B. Immune system

Figure 38-1 is a schematic drawing of the immune response to an antigen.

B lymphocytes, T lymphocytes, macrophages, humoral pathway, antibodies, immunoglobulins, IgG, IgM, IgD, IgA, IgE, cellular immunity, lymphokines, cytokines, tissue macrophages, thymus, tonsils

C. Allergic reactions

Table 38-1 is a summary of the classification of allergic reactions. The mechanism of each type of reaction is described and examples are given for each.

Table 38-2 lists the symptoms associated with food allergy.

Figure 38-2 is a schematic drawing of what happens during an allergic reaction.

allergens, immediate hypersensitivity (type I), antigen-antibody complexes (type III reaction), cell-mediated hypersensitivity (type IV reaction)

III. Symptoms

Figure 38-3 is a set of photographs of a 3-year-old child's face showing contact urticaria from egg white.

IV. Common Food Allergens

Table 38-3 (Transparency) lists the most common food allergens. The list is divided into two parts: infants/children and adults.

cross-reactivity

V. Risk Factors for the Development of Food Allergy

atopy, antigen exposure, gastrointestinal permeability

VI. Food Intolerances

Table 38-4 lists the nonimmunological reactions to food. The causes, associated foods, and symptoms are presented.

A. Food additives

tartrazine, benzoic acid, sodium nitrates, butylated hydroxyanisol (BHA), butylated hydroxytoluene (BHT), sulfites, monosodium glutamate (MSG)

1. Sulfites

See **Focus On:** "Sulfite."
sulfite sensitivity

2. Carbohydrate intolerance

lactase

VII. Diagnosis

Figure 38-4 is an example of a food and symptom diary that is used to record any indications of food intolerance or allergy.

Table 38-5 lists the diagnostic tests used to diagnose food allergy. A description of the method of testing is given along with an indication of the test's reliability.

Table 38-6 illustrate two types of elimination diets. The first is for identifying allergy to milk, egg, or wheat. The second is a minimal elimination diet, eliminating all foods known to be allergenic.

Key concept: Elimination of the suspect food or foods is often used for diagnosing or confirming food allergy.

Key concept: Once symptoms clear using an elimination diet, a food challenge is done. The foods are reintroduced one at a time. One possible result of the food challenge is an anaphylactic reaction.

immunological testing, radioallergosorbent extract test (RAST), enzyme-linked immunosorbent assay (ELISA), weal, Nutramigen, Tolerex, double-blind placebo-controlled food challenge (DBPCFC), single-blind food challenge

VIII. Treatment

Table 38-7 is a reference for identifying foods likely to contain milk, eggs, wheat, soy, or corn. The list provides substitute foods and alternative names for the offending food items as stated on the ingredient panel.

Table 38-8 lists guidelines for use in managing food allergy diets.

rotation diet, desensitization treatments

IX. Natural History

X. Food Allergy in Infancy

Figure 38-5 is a photograph of an infant exhibiting abdominal distention and muscular wasting due to an allergy to cow's milk.

urticaria, angioedema

    A. Recommendations for infant feeding

Key concept: The use of goat's milk is not recommended when an infant demonstrates allergy to cow's milk. There is a potential for cross-reactivity with β-lactoglobulin in cow's milk.

protein hydrolysate, Pregestimil, Good Start, Alimentum

    B. Colic

XI. Diet and Prevention of Allergic Disease

CASE STUDY INSIGHTS

1. What is the best method of diet intervention for Sally?

Sally must eliminate peanuts and eggs from her diet.

2. What are some measures Mrs. J will have to take regarding Sally's food allergies in school?

Mrs. J should alert the school personnel, including Sally's teacher, to her daughter's allergies. Mrs. J should prepare lunch and snacks that are appropriate for Sally and send those to school with her.

3. What other circumstances may arise that warrant special instructions to caregivers?

The possibility of manifesting additional food allergies should be considered.

4. As Sally gets older, what can Mrs. J begin to teach her that will help Sally manage her food allergies independently?

Sally will need to be taught about the foods she must avoid and where they are likely to be found. She should also be taught to let her special needs be known to teachers or other adults who may have responsibility for her.

SUGGESTED TEST QUESTIONS

1. The age group most likely to develop food hypersensitivity is
    * a. 0–2 years of age.
    b. 3–12 years of age.
    c. adolescents.
    d. adults.

2. The most common antibodies in the humoral pathway that are involved in food allergy are
    a. IgG.
    b. IgM.
    c. T-cells.
    * d. IgE.

3. Symptoms of food allergies are most commonly seen
    a. in the respiratory system.
    b. on the skin.
    c. in the gastrointestinal tract.
    * d. in all of the above.

4. The onset of symptoms related to a food allergy is most likely to occur within
    * a. 2 hours.
    b. 2–24 hours.
    c. more than 24 hours.
    d. more than 48 hours.

5. The person intolerant of MSG is most likely to complain of
    a. decreased heart rate, constipation, and hives.
    * b. headache, flushing, abdominal pain, and nausea.
    c. steatorrhea, edema, proteinuria, and nausea.
    d. anaphylaxis, toxic shock syndrome, and headache.

6. When an adverse reaction to food is caused by a nonimmunological mechanism, it is called
    a. a food allergy.
    b. an allergenic reaction.
    * c. a food intolerance.
    d. a food sensitivity.

7. Limiting or avoiding exposure to allergenic foods during infancy
   a. may reduce the incidence of allergy during the first year of life.
   b. is likely to lead to malnutrition in the infant.
   c. includes eliminating all commercial infant formulas.
   * d. can prevent allergy after the first year of life.

8. When an infant is allergic to cow's milk, the use of goat's milk is
   a. recommended for the first 6 months.
   b. recommended for the first year of life.
   * c. not recommended due to cross-reactivity.
   d. not recommended because it is too low in fat.

9. Of the following foods, the one most likely to *not* contain eggs is
   a. root beer.
   * b. beef stew.
   c. tartar sauce.
   d. marshmallows.

10. The most common food allergens are found in foods having a high
   a. simple carbohydrate content.
   b. animal protein content.
   * c. plant or marine protein content.
   d. saturated fat content.

11. The diagnosis of food allergy by immunological function is most accurate when done by
   * a. the skin-prick test, ELISA, or RAST.
   b. cytotoxic testing or ELISA.
   c. sublingual testing, RAST, or the skin-prick test.
   d. ELISA, RAST, or neutralization testing.

12. When symptoms are subjective or when multiple food allergies are suspected, an effective method of diagnosis is the
   a. food challenge.
   b. single-blind food challenge.
   * c. double-blind food challenge.
   d. rotation diet.

13. Food allergies that are most likely to resolve with age are those that first manifest during the
   a. first year of life.
   * b. first 3 years of life.
   c. first 10 years of life.
   d. first 15 years of life.

14. For infants, the most common food allergen is found in
   a. cereal.
   * b. cow's milk.
   c. fruit.
   d. vegetable protein.

15. For the infant of atopic parents, the risk of food allergies may be reduced if the infant receives
   * a. only breast milk for the first 6 months.
   b. only breast milk and cereal for the first 6 months.
   c. cereal between breast milk feedings.
   d. diluted cereal and formula for the first 6 months.

16. Documented evidence shows that allergic reactions do occur with
   * a. cow's milk, egg, wheat, and fish.
   b. chocolate, fish, peanuts, and egg.
   c. strawberry, cow's milk, soy, and peanuts.
   d. soy, peanuts, cow's milk, and chocolate.

NUTRITIONAL CARE IN DISEASES OF THE NERVOUS SYSTEM

OVERVIEW

The purpose of this chapter is to provide students with a background on the many conditions affecting the nervous system which can affect nutritional status and/or be managed with nutritional intervention. The chapter begins with a description of the swallowing process and recommendations for the management of dysphagia. Additional feeding problems are also described. A variety of neurological conditions are then presented with the corresponding nutritional concerns and therapies for each.

LEARNING OBJECTIVES

This chapter will prepare the learner to be able to

1. Identify the three phases of swallowing.
2. Describe dysphagia and its consequences.
3. State the nutritional intervention strategies used to manage dysphagia.
4. Identify additional problems with self-feeding in the neurologically impaired individual.
5. State the nutritional concerns associated with stroke.
6. Describe the principles of nutritional care in multiple sclerosis.
7. Describe the principles of nutritional care in amyotrophic lateral sclerosis.
8. State the nutritional concerns associated with Alzheimer's disease.
9. State the nutritional considerations for the patient with Parkinson's disease.
10. Describe the principles of nutritional management of epilepsy.
11. Identify the neuropathies that can result from nutritional causes.
12. State the nutritional concerns associated with migraine headache.
13. Explain the nutritional implications of spinal cord injury.

CHAPTER OUTLINE ─────────────────

NOTES, TERMS, & TRANSPARENCY MASTERS

Figure 39-1 is a drawing of the spinal cord lying within the vertebral canal. The spinal nerves and the vertabrae are numbered.

Table 39-1 lists the sensory nerve roots and the area innervated.

Table 39-2 lists the motor nerve roots and the muscle action.

I. Neurologic Diseases: Feeding Concerns

Table 39-3 is a summary of the common disorders associated with neurological diseases. The sites in the brain, the specific impairments, and the results are included.

   A. Dysphagia

Figure 39-2 is a set of drawings showing the swallowing process, including the oral phase, pharyngeal phase, and esophageal phase.

Figure 39-3 is a drawing of the anterior mouth showing where food can become lodged in the sulcus area between the teeth and cheek.

Table 39-4 provides guidelines for planning a diet that is appropriate for the dysphagic patient.

dysphagia, oral phase, pharyngeal phase, esophageal phase

      1. Nutritional care
         a. Fluids

Key concept: Liquids can be thickened to achieve the desired consistency. Appropriate thickening agents include nonfat dried milk solids, cornstarch, fruit or potato flakes, and modular carbohydrate supplements.

         b. Textures

Table 39-5 is a description of a diet for the patient requiring easy chewing and swallowing.

   B. Other self-feeding problems

Figure 39-4 is a set of photographs that illustrates the range of normal vision and the range of vision in a person with hemianopsia.

limb weakness, paralysis, hemiparesis, hemi-anopsia, apraxia, dementia

II. Neurological Disease and Nutritional Implications
   A. Adrenomyeloneuropathy

adrenomyeloneuropathy, oligodendrocyte transplantation

   B. Stroke
      1. Description and etiology

stroke, focal, global, trans-ischemic attack, TIA

      2. Nutritional concerns

warfarin

C. Multiple sclerosis

1. Pathophysiology

2. Treatment

3. Nutritional care

D. Amyotrophic lateral sclerosis

1. Description and etiology
2. Clinical manifestations
3. Assessment
4. Early nutritional care
5. Late-stage nutritional care
6. Enteral feeding
7. Other nutritional concerns
    a. Oral secretions
    b. Constipation

E. Alzheimer's disease

1. Etiology
2. Treatment

3. Nutritional concerns

F. Parkinson's disease

1. Etiology and treatment

2. Nutritional care
    a. Modified protein diet

multiple sclerosis (MS)

Figure 39-5 is a graph showing the progression of decreasing function over time in MS.

adrenocorticotropic hormone, ACTH, pred- nisolone, methotrexate

Figure 39-6 is a schematic drawing of the areas of the body exhibiting neurological deficits in multiple sclerosis.
paresthesia, ataxia, dysarthria, dysphagia, neurogenic bladder

amyotrophic lateral sclerosis (ALS), Lou Gehrig's disease

bulbar ALS, fasciculations, spinal ALS

percutaneous endoscopic gastrostomy (PEG)

Valsalva maneuver, dihydroxphenylisatin

Alzheimer's disease (AD), primary degenera- tive dementia of senile onset, dysnomia

cholinesterase inhibitors, Tacrine, Alzheimer's Disease Assessment Scale, Clinical Global Impression of Change Scale, activities of daily living (ADLs)

Table 39-6 is a checklist that can be used to assess the feeding difficulties for a patient with Alzheimer's disease.

Parkinson's disease (PD)

See **Focus On:** "Neurotransmitters and Their Precursors."
dopamine, Levodopa, deprenyl

Table 39-7 is a sample menu plan for dietary con- trol of protein redistribution in L-dopa therapy.

G. Epilepsy

   1. Nutrient–drug interactions

   2. Ketogenic diet

H. Polyneuropathy
   1. Nutritional neuropathies

   2. Guillain-Barré syndrome

     a. Treatment
I. Migraine headache
   1. Etiology
   2. Nutritional concerns
   3. Pharmacology

J. Myasthenia gravis

   1. Treatment

K. Central nervous system (CNS) tumor
   1. Pathophysiology

   2. Treatment

L. Myotonic dystrophy

M. Neurotrauma
   1. Nutritional implications
   2. Resting energy expenditure
N. Spinal cord injury

   1. Nutritional implications

O. Permanently unconscious patients

---

epilepsy

phenobarbital, phenytoin, primidone

Table 39-8 is a sample diet and nutrient distribution in a ketogenic diet that uses MCT oil.
ketogenic diet, akinetic, myoclonic, petit mal, psychomotor, temporal lobe, seizures, medium-chain triglyceride-based ketogenic diet

nutritional neuropathies, dry beriberi, alcoholic neuropathy

Guillain-Barré syndrome (GBS), Landry's paralysis, Landry-Guillain-Barré syndrome, acute infectious polyneuritis, acute idiopathic polyneuritis

migraine headache

Imitrex, propanolol, diltiazem

myasthenia gravis (MG)

thymectomy, plasmapheresis, azathioprine (Imuran), cyclosporine

Figure 39-7 (Transparency) is a schematic drawing of the areas of the brain and their corresponding neurological functions.

sterotaxis, open craniotomy, decompressive laminectomy

myotonic dystrophy, Keshan disease

neurotrauma, closed head injury (CHI)

Figure 39-8 is a diagram of the spinal cord indicating the sequelae of spinal cord injury and rehabilitation challenge.
acute spinal cord injury (SCI)

persistently vegetative state (PVS)

CASE STUDY INSIGHTS

1. What recommendations would you make for his tube feedings, including content, protein, flush, and total calories?

It should be determined if 185 lbs is his current weight or his preinjury weight. His current weight and protein status should be assessed and his needs determined. The quality and quantity of the formula in use can then be evaluated. He is expected to be hypermetabolic and hypercatabolic as a result of this injury.

2. What lab data do you need to monitor and why?

The lab data to be monitored include nitrogen balance, serum electrolytes, blood gases, serum glucose, and serum transferrin. These factors will be affected by the metabolic response to the injury and the effects of various medications.

3. With corticosteroids being used, what side effects would you anticipate?

Corticosteroid therapy can result in abnormalities in carbohydrate and protein metabolism, as well as fluid and electrolyte imbalances.

4. When he is ready to progress to an oral diet, what type and content of diet would you recommend?

This depends on many factors that are assessed at the time of the transition to an oral diet. Some important considerations are motor skills, state of consciousness, and nutritional status.

SUGGESTED TEST QUESTIONS

1. For the patient experiencing difficulty swallowing, the foods easiest to swallow are
    a. thin liquids.
    b. room-temperature cream soups.
    c. lukewarm cooked cereals diluted with milk.
    * d. warm, textured foods with sauce or gravy.

2. When a patients is treated with the oral anticoagulant warfarin following stroke, it is recommended that dietary intake be limited for
    a. protein.
    * b. vitamin K.
    c. vitamin C.
    d. zinc.

3. Multiple sclerosis can result in neurogenic bladder and bowel problems that can cause diarrhea and constipation. When diarrhea is persistent, the best diet may be
    * a. high in fiber with adequate fluids.
    b. an elemental diet.
    c. bland and low in fiber.
    d. low in fat.

4. For the patient with ALS with bulbar involvement, the recommended position for feeding is
    a. supine.
    b. reclining .
    c. sitting bolt upright with neck hyperextended.
    * d. sitting bolt upright with head in chin-down position.

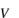

5. When urinary incontinence associated with a neurogenic bladder is present, it may be helpful to provide fluids
   a. only in the early morning hours.
   b. only in the evening hours.
 * c. evenly throughout the day and limited before bedtime.
   d. only at breakfast and lunch.

6. The greatest amount of coordination and control is needed for swallowing
   a. solid foods.
 * b. liquids of thin consistency.
   c. soft foods with a high percentage of water.
   d. thick, viscous liquids.

7. The best results from medical nutritional therapy in dysphagia associated with ALS can be achieved by
   a. nasogastric tube feeding.
 * b. percutaneous endoscopic gastrostomy.
   c. parenteral nutrition.
   d. peripheral nutrition.

8. Because of potential drug–nutrient interactions, patients with Parkinson's disease may benefit from being given the RDA for protein
 * a. primarily at the evening meal.
   b. primarily at breakfast.
   c. evenly throughout the day.
   d. primarily at the noon meal.

9. The effect of pyridoxine supplementation in Parkinson's disease is that it
   a. has no effect on levodopa.
 * b. reduces the effectiveness of levodopa.
   c. increases the effectiveness of levodopa.
   d. blocks the function of levodopa.

10. Phenobarbital used for anticonvulsant therapy may interfere with intestinal absorption of calcium because it
 * a. increases metabolism of vitamin D in the liver.
   b. blocks absorption of vitamin D in the intestinal mucosa.
   c. induces diarrhea and loss of electrolytes.
   d. damages the mucosal cells lining the intestinal wall.

11. The patient with nutritional neuropathy will most likely experience muscle wasting
   a. of the arms.
 * b. of the legs.
   c. of the proximal muscles.
   d. throughout the body.

12. Nutritional neuropathy is most effectively treated by a balanced diet supplemented with
 * a. B-complex vitamins.
   b. the fat-soluble vitamins.
   c. trace minerals.
   d. vitamins A and D.

13. Parenteral nutrition is *not* the preferred method of nutritional support for a patient with Guillian-Barré syndrome because
   a. the risk of sepsis is great.
 * b. the gastrointestinal tract is usually not affected.
   c. peripheral nutrition is the preferred method.
   d. hyperalimentation is not necessary.

14. The nutritional requirements and metabolic activity of a patient with a closed head injury are
   a. minor.
   b. slightly greater than those of a patient with a long bone fracture.
 * c. second only to those of a major burn.
   d. similar to those of a patient having minor surgery.

15. The dietary intake of a dysphagic patient may be improved when the diet includes
 * a. very warm or well-chilled foods with texture.
   b. bland, lukewarm foods.
   c. dry foods without sauces or gravies.
   d. foods that need to be washed down with liquids.

CHAPTER

NUTRITIONAL CARE IN RHEUMATIC DISEASES

OVERVIEW

The purpose of this chapter is to provide students with an understanding of the rheumatic diseases, arthritis and gout. The inflammatory response exhibited in arthritis is explained. Both rheumatoid and degenerative arthritis are described. The nutritional care for both conditions is presented, with emphasis on rheumatoid arthritis. Consideration is given for the side effects of pharmacological therapies used in arthritis. The condition of gout is described and the use of a low-purine diet is explained.

LEARNING OBJECTIVES

This chapter will prepare the learner to be able to

1. Explain the inflammatory process associated with arthritis.
2. Describe rheumatoid arthritis.
3. Identify the nutritional concerns for the patient with rheumatoid arthritis.
4. State the principles of nutritional management of rheumatoid arthritis.
5. Identify the nutritional care recommended for degenerative arthritis.
6. Explain the pathophysiology of gout.
7. State the recommended therapy for gout.
8. Explain the low-purine diet used in the treatment of gout.
9. List the unproven remedies for arthritis.

CHAPTER OUTLINE ──────────────── NOTES, TERMS, & TRANSPARENCY MASTERS

I. Inflammation in Arthritic Disease

Key concept: Arthritis is an autoimmune disease in which the body develops antibodies that respond to otherwise normal body components. An inflammatory response ensues.

prostaglandins, leukotrienes, nonsteroidal anti-inflammatory drugs (NSAIDs)

249

II. Rheumatoid Arthritis

Figure 40-1 is a photograph of the hands of an individual with advanced rheumatoid arthritis.
rheumatoid arthritis (RA)

A. Nutritional care

xerostomia

    1. Diet composition
        a. Energy
        b. Protein
        c. Lipids
        d. Minerals and vitamins

Key concept: The textbook points out that nutrition cures only malnutrition, suggesting that the use of supplemental nutrients should be limited to those actually needed to correct a deficiency.

B. Diet modifications for disease sequelae
    1. Sjögren's syndrome

Sjögren's syndrome

    2. Temporomandibular joint syndrome (TMJ)

temporomandibular joint syndrome (TMJ)

    3. Articular manifestations

C. Pharmacological therapy

Key concept: Drug therapy is the treatment of choice for rheumatoid arthritis. The seven primary classes of drugs are salicylates, nonsteroidal anti-inflammatory drugs (NSAIDs), antimalarial agents, gold salts, D-penicillamine, steroids, and immunosuppressive agents.
Table 40-1 lists the side effects associated with various arthritis medications.
salicylates, nonsteroidal anti-inflammatory drugs (NSAIDs), corticosteroids, Cushinoid symptoms, prednisone, antimalarial agents, gold salts, methyltrexate, cyclosporine, D-penicillamine, steroids, immunosuppressive agents

D. Other treatment

aphoresis

III. Osteoarthritis (Degenerative Arthritis)

osteoarthritis, degenerative arthritis, degenerative joint disease (DJD)

A. Nutritional care
B. Pharmacological therapy

IV. Gout

Figure 40-2 is a photograph of the ear of an individual with gout. There are tophi evident in the picture.
gout, uric acid, tophi

A. Nutritional care 1. Purines	**Table 40-2** lists foods grouped according to their purine content, ranging from high (100–1000 mg per 100 g of food) to negligible purine. **acute stage, interval stage**
a. Low-purine diet	**Table 40-3 (Transparency)** is a summary of the nutritional care principles for management of gout.
2. Alcohol B. Pharmacological therapy	**urate eliminants, probenecid (Benemid), sulfinpyrazone, allopurinol, colchicine, indomethacin, phenylbutazone**
V. Other Collagen Disorders	**systemic lupus erythematosus (SLE)**
VI. Unproven Remedies for Arthritis	

CASE STUDY INSIGHTS

1. How would you discretely advise him that these trends are not likely to be useful and may actually cause some harm?

This provides an opportunity for the instructor to discuss food faddism, as well as the need for developing sensitivity to the patient.

2. He has read in the newspaper that use of vitamin E and other antioxidants are useful in alleviating his condition, but you have no scientific articles to prove this. How would you discuss these topics with him?

The use of vitamin E and other antioxidants can be of potential benefit in conditions other than arthritis. It should be determined what dose was suggested in the newspaper article and what references or experts are quoted in the article. The use of a vitamin and mineral supplement that provides no more than 100% of the RDA would be acceptable.

3. From his diet history, it appears that Sam eats little at breakfast and has a heavy, high-fat lunch. He eats no fish, few fruits and vegetables, and drinks a highball before dinner. What suggestions do you have to improve his diet?

A diet based on the dietary guidelines is recommended. Suggest that he begin eating a light, well-balanced breakfast and cut back on his fat intake at lunch. He should try to eat three to five servings of vegetables and two to four servings of fruit per day. One alcoholic beverage per day may be acceptable if he is not overweight.

4. Sam does not mention being overweight. How would you bring up the subject, and what steps would you recommend for him?

Sam needs to be told about the relationship between his body weight and his condition. He may be limited in his ability to increase his level of activity. He should be encouraged to attain and maintain ideal body weight by eating a well-balanced diet appropriate to his energy needs.

SUGGESTED TEST QUESTIONS

1. The nutritional assessment of a patient with rheumatoid arthritis should include the
    a. impact of the disease on food preparation.
    b. impact of the disease on self-feeding.
    c. nutritional side effects of medications.
    *   d. all of the above.

2. Current research has suggested but not confirmed that lipids playing a role in the inflammatory process may include
    a. polyunsaturated fatty acids.
    b. monounsaturated fatty acids.
    *   c. omega-3 and omega-6 fatty acids.
    d. medium-chain triglycerides.

3. For the patients with rheumatoid arthritis who are treated with aspirin, side effects can be minimized by taking the medication
    a. only when the disease is active.
    *   b. with milk, food, or antacids.
    c. on an empty stomach and taking mineral supplements.
    d. with citrus juices and increasing green leafy vegetables in the diet.

4. The primary nutritional goal for the patient with osteoarthritis should be to
    *   a. achieve and maintain normal weight.
    b. increase fiber intake to prevent constipation.
    c. increase omega-3 oils in the diet.
    d. decrease sodium intake to reduce edema.

5. The dietary recommendation for the patient with gout during the acute stage is a
    a. high-purine diet with decreased fluid intake.
    *   b. low-purine diet with increased fluids.
    c. high-fat, low-carbohydrate diet.
    d. low-pyrimidine diet with decreased carbohydrates.

6. Foods having a high-purine content include
    a. enriched white bread, rice, and tomatoes.
    b. cheese, chocolate, butter, and coffee.
    c. fruit, ice cream, pasta, and nuts.
    *   d. herring, kidney, sardines, and consommé.

7. When an arthritic patient is receiving intensive daily physical therapy, energy needs are based on his basal energy expenditure multiplied by a factor of
    a. 2.
    b. 2.5.
    *   c. 1.3.
    d. 1.8.

8. Chronic ingestion of aspirin by the patient with arthritis may result in gastric mucosal injury and
    a. decreased urinary excretion of vitamin C.
    *   b. increased urinary excretion of vitamin C.
    c. increased urinary excretion of calcium.
    d. decreased urinary excretion of potassium.

9. The dietary recommendation for the patient with gout is a
    *   a. high-carbohydrate, moderate-protein, low-fat diet.
    b. high-carbohydrate, high-protein, high-fat diet.
    c. low-protein, low-fat, high-carbohydrate diet.
    d. high-protein, high-fat, low-carbohydrate diet.

10. When assessing the nutritional status of a patient with arthritis, the most reliable parameter is
    a. serum albumin.
    *   b. weight change.
    c. triceps skinfold.
    d. serum transferrin.

11. The plasma copper levels seen in rheumatoid arthritis have been shown to correlate with
    a. dietary intake of copper.
    b. type of medication.
    *   c. degree of joint inflammation.
    d. gastrointestinal symptoms such as malabsorption and diarrhea.

12. In cases of severe or advanced gout, the purine content of the daily diet is restricted to about
*   a.   100–150 mg.
    b.   200–250 mg.
    c.   300–350 mg.
    d.   400–450 mg.

13. The first line of drug therapy for controlling the inflammatory process seen in arthritis is
    a.   corticosteroids.
*   b.   salicylates.
    c.   gold salts.
    d.   methyltrexate.

14. The recommendation for vitamin and mineral supplementation in the patient with arthritis is
*   a.   to not exceed the RDA.
    b.   to limit to 75% of the RDA.
    c.   to increase to 200% of the RDA.
    d.   unable to be determined accurately.

15. Sjögren's syndrome is characterized by
    a.   excessive sweating and salivation.
    b.   temporomandibular joint symptoms.
*   c.   diminished production of tears and saliva.
    d.   diminished production of hydrochloric acid in the stomach.

NUTRITIONAL CARE IN METABOLIC DISORDERS

OVERVIEW

The purpose of this chapter is to provide students with the basic principles of nutritional management of inborn errors of metabolism. A significant portion of the chapter is devoted to hyperphenylalaninemias. The pathophysiology of this group of amino acid disorders is described, including the diagnostic procedures and the prognosis of the conditions. The nutritional management of the diet in phenylketonuria (PKU) is presented with sample calculations. Other conditions included in the chapter are organic acid disorders, urea cycle defects, maple syrup urine disease, galactosemia, glycogen storage disease, and disorders of fatty acid oxidation.

LEARNING OBJECTIVES

This chapter will prepare the learner to be able to

1. Define inborn error of metabolism.
2. State the goals for nutritional care in inborn errors of metabolism.
3. Explain the metabolic defect seen in classic phenylketonuria.
4. State the principles of nutritional management of hyperphenylalaninemia.
5. Identify foods containing phenylalanine and medical foods with altered phenylalanine content.
6. Calculate the dietary prescription for an infant with phenylketonuria.
7. Identify appropriate educational goals for the child with an inborn error of metabolism.
8. State the nutritional concerns for the adult with phenylketonuria including the pregnant woman.
9. State the recommended nutrition intervention for the common organic acid disorders.
10. Describe the defects that can occur in the urea cycle and the conditions that result.
11. State the principles of nutritional management of maple syrup urine disease.
12. State the principles of nutritional management of galactosemia.
13. State the recommended nutritional management of disorders of fatty acid oxidation.
14. State the principles of nutritional management of glycogen storage disease.

CHAPTER OUTLINE	NOTES, TERMS, & TRANSPARENCY MASTERS
I. Goals of Nutritional Care	See **Focus On:** "PKU Time Line."
II. Amino Acid Disorders and Their Management	**Table 41-1** lists the amino acid requirements for infants and children (in mg/kg body weight) at ages ranging from birth to 10 years.
A. Hyperphenylalaninemias	**Table 41-2** lists the metabolic disorders that respond to dietary treatment. The disorders are listed by category with the specific enzyme defect, incidence, clinical and biochemical features, and dietary treatment indicated. **Figure 41-1 (Transparency)** is a schematic illustration of the metabolic defects seen in hyperphenylalaninemias. **hyperphenylalaninemia, phenylketonuria (PKU), phenylalanine hydroxylase, dihydropteridine reductase (DHPR) deficiency, biopterin (BH$_4$)**
1. Diagnosis and outcome	**Guthrie bacterial inhibition assay, phenylpyruvic acid, *o*-hydroxyphenylacetic acid**
2. Nutritional care for infants and children a. Formula	**Table 41-3** lists dietary products that are available for the management of inborn errors of metabolism. The conditions listed include PKU, tyrosinemia, and MSUD. **Table 41-4** demonstrates the method for calculating a low-protein phenylalanine-restricted diet. **Table 41-5** is a comparison of nutrient intakes of infants without a metabolic defect and those with PKU, MUSD, urea cycle disorders, and organic acid disorders.
b. Low-phenylalanine foods	**Table 41-6** lists the approximate phenylalanine, tyrosine, fat, protein, and energy content of foods by food group. **Table 41-7** is a comparison of the energy and protein content of foods and the low-protein complement. See **Clinical Insight:** "Sources of Low-Protein Foods." **Table 41-8** compares the phenylalanine content of the foods on a PKU menu and a regular menu. **Phenyl-free**
c. Blood phenylalanine control	**Figure 41-2** is a sample PKU food record for foods eaten, amounts, and phenylalanine content.

d. Education on therapy management

Table 41-9 summarizes the age-appropriate tasks for planning the educational needs of a child with PKU.

e. Psychosocial development

Figure 41-3 is a photograph of a child learning to manage her own low-phenylalanine diet.

3. Nutritional care in maternal phenylketonuria

Table 41-10 summarizes the frequency of abnormalities seen in infants of mothers with PKU. The results are categorized by maternal phenylalanine levels.

Key concept: If a woman with PKU becomes pregnant, her prepregnancy management of phenylalanine levels may decrease the risk to the fetus. However, during pregnancy, metabolic control is imperative but may not be easy to accomplish given the changing physiology of pregnancy and nutritional needs of the mother.

4. Nutritional care for adults with phenylketonuria

B. Organic acid disorders

Figure 41-4 is a schematic drawing of the metabolic defect seen in organic acidemias and maple syrup urine disease.

L-carnitine, carnitine deficiency, propionic acidemia, methylmalonic acidemia, methylmalonyl CoA mutase apoenzyme

C. Urea cycle defects

Figure 41-5 is a schematic drawing of the metabolic defect seen in disorders of the urea cycle.

ornithine transcarbamylase deficiency (OTC), ornithine, carbamyl phosphate, citrulline, hyperammonemia, urinary orotic acid, argininosuccinic acid, citrullinemia, argininosuccinic acid synthetase, argininosuccinic aciduria (ASA), carbamyl phosphate synthetase (CPS) deficiency

D. Protein-restricted diets

Table 41-11 provides a step-by-step method for developing a low-protein food pattern.

E. Maple syrup urine disease

Table 41-12 lists the approximate isoleucine, leucine, valine, protein, fat, and energy content of foods by food group.

maple syrup urine disease (MUSD), branched-chain ketoaciduria

III. Disorder of Carbohydrate Metabolism
   A. Galactosemia

Figure 41-6 (Transparency) is a schematic drawing of the metabolic defect in galactosemia.
Table 41-13 is a list of foods that contain galactose and those not containing galactose.
galactosemia, galactokinase deficiency, galactose 1-phosphate uridyl transferase deficiency, classic galactosemia

IV. Disorders of Fatty Acid Oxidation

long-chain acyl-CoA dehydrogenase deficiency (LCAD), medium-chain acyl-CoA dehydrogenase deficiency (MCAD)

V. Glycogen Storage Diseases

glycogen storage disease type Ia (GSD Ia), amylo 1,6-glucosidase deficiency (GSD III), debrancher enzyme defect

   A. Other disorders

VI. Nutritional Care Management

Table 41-14 is a set of intervention objectives for use by the nutrition care provider involved in treatment of metabolic disorders.

CASE STUDY INSIGHTS

1. What is the expected energy need for this infant with phenylketonuria?

   Table 41-1 shows that the recommended energy intake for this infant is 108 kcal/kg body weight. Based on a weight of 3.6 kg given in the case description, he should be getting about 390 kcal.

2. What baseline formula would you calculate for this infant to provide phenylalanine at 60 mg/kg, formula at 20 kcal/oz, and protein and energy intakes at recommended levels?

   In preparing a baseline formula in PKU, an infant formula is often used, such as Similac, which has 20 kcal/oz, as specified in the case study. In 100 mL of Similac, there are 71 mg of phenylalanine, 1.45 g of protein, and 68 kcal. To meet the requirement for 60 mg of phenylalanine per kg of body weight, this infant needs 300 mL of Similac (3 x 71 mg = 213 mg). This provides 4.35 g of protein and 204 kcal. If using the RDA for protein and energy, the requirements are 7.9 g of protein and 390 kcal. (Note that some references suggest 115 kcal/kg and 3.3 g protein/kg for a PKU infant.) The remaining calories (186 kcal) can be provided by adding a phenylalanine-modified supplement. If using Phenex-1 (Ross), 39 g would provide 187 kcal and 5.85 g of protein. The total protein from both Similac and Phenex-1 would thus be 10.2 g. This amount equals 2.8 g protein/kg, which should not be a problem if phenylalanine is limited and fluid needs are met. Similac and Phenex-1 should be mixed together with water added to make a total of 504 mL. During the first 10 days of life, fluid requirements are 125–150 mL/kg.

3. What are the growth expectations for his infant?

   This infant has been identified as having PKU at birth, and nutritional therapy has been initiated. His prognosis is very good at this time. He can attain his full potential for growth, development, and IQ provided that biochemical equilibrium is maintained.

4. What steps would you take if the plasma phenylalanine concentration rose above 6 mg/dL on subsequent measurements?

The requirement for phenylalanine is expected to remain the same through the first 6 months of life. After that time, requirements begin to decrease. If this infant demonstrates an increase in blood phenylalanine concentration, the diet and the mother's compliance with the diet should be reviewed.

SUGGESTED TEST QUESTIONS

1. Dietary management for a newborn diagnosed with phenylketonuria must be continued
   a. until she is eating solid foods.
   b. until she is at least 10 years old.
   c. until she has completed the growth spurt of adolescence.
   * d. for the rest of her life.

2. Nutritional intervention for disorders of amino acid metabolism is most often based on
   a. supplementing the enzymatic cofactor.
   b. supplementing the amount of product.
   * c. substrate restriction.
   d. amino acid therapy.

3. A reliable and easily measured index of well-being and nutritional adequacy is
   a. the nitrogen balance study.
   * b. weight gain.
   c. calorie and protein intake.
   d. head circumference.

4. The defect seen in classic phenylketonuria is the inability to metabolize phenylalanine to
   * a. tyrosine.
   b. alanine.
   c. glycine.
   d. threonine.

5. A nutritional formula with modified phenylalanine that can be used in a restricted-phenylalanine diet for an infant is
   a. AminAid.
   * b. Lofenalac.
   c. Sustacal.
   d. Jevity.

6. The desirable range for blood phenylalanine in a child with PKU is
   * a. 2–6 mg/dL.
   b. 5–15 mg/dL.
   c. 7–17 mg/dL.
   d. 10–20 mg/dL.

7. The current recommendation from most PKU treatment centers is that the restricted-phenylalanine diet be continued
   a. until the child is 6 years of age.
   b. until the child is 13 years of age.
   c. into early adulthood.
   * d. for life.

8. The metabolic result of defects in the urea cycle is an accumulation of
   * a. ammonia in the blood.
   b. purines in the blood.
   c. ketoacids in the blood.
   d. ketone bodies.

9. Maple syrup urine disease results from an abnormality in the metabolism of
   a. aromatic amino acids.
   * b. branched-chained amino acids.
   c. essential amino acids.
   d. nonessential amino acids.

10. In galactosemia, high levels of galactose accumulate in the blood because of a defect in the conversion of
    a. glucose to galactose.
    * b. galactose to glucose.
    c. glycogen to glucose.
    d. galactose to lactose.

11. Nutritional management of galactosemia requires
    a. medication that converts galactose to glucose.
  * b. life-long galactose restriction.
    c. galactose supplementation.
    d. a low-lactose diet.

12. Glycogen storage disease results in impaired
    a. glycolysis.
    b. gluconeogenesis.
    c. fatty acid oxidation.
  * d. glycogenesis and glycogenolysis.

13. The nutritional management of glycogen storage disease includes
  * a. oral administration of raw cornstarch.
    b. small, frequent high-protein meals.
    c. severe restriction of all carbohydrates.
    d. three well-balanced meals a day.

14. The initial daily phenylalanine intake for a infant with PKU is recommended to be
    a. 10 mg/kg.
    b. 40 mg/kg.
  * c. 70 mg/kg.
    d. 100 mg/kg.

15. The infant of a woman with PKU who becomes pregnant will
    a. not be affected by the condition.
  * b. have a greater risk of cardiac defects and mental retardation.
    c. always have PKU.
    d. have an elevated blood phenylalanine level at birth that returns to normal within a week.

Transparency Masters

Chapter	Transparency Number	Description
Chapter 3	1	Structure of glucose and fructose
	2	Glycogenesis, glycogenolysis, and glycolysis
	3	The Cori and alanine cycles
Chapter 4	4	18-Carbon fatty acids
	5	Structure of a triglyceride or triacylglycerol
Chapter 5	6	Formation of a dipeptide
	7	Transamination and deamination
Chapter 6	8	The pathway by which dietary vitamin A reaches target cells of an organ
	9	Retinol equivalents (RE)
	10	The metabolism and functions of vitamin D.
	11	Vitamin D terminology and equivalents
Chapter 7	12	Schematic outline of iron metabolism in adults
	13	A model for zinc absorption showing the relationship between metallothionein and cysteine-rich intestinal protein (CRIP)
Chapter 8	14	Distribution of body water as percentage of body weight
	15	Generation of $NaHCO_3$ and clearance of H^+ by the three buffer systems that function in the kidney
Chapter 14	16	Number of persons aged 65 and older from 1900 to 2030
Chapter 15	17	A comparison of the average intake of energy from protein, carbohydrate, and fat for people in the United States in 1977 and 1985
Chapter 17	18	Optimal nutritional status as a balance between nutrient intake and nutrient requirements
Chapter 18	19	Examples of drugs that may cause loss of appetite
	20	Examples of medications that alter or diminish taste perception
	21	Some commonly used drugs that increase appetite
	22	Drugs that inhibit the action of the oxidases
Chapter 19	23	Nutritional screening information
Chapter 20	24	Diagram of enteral feeding tube placement
	25	Monitoring the enterally tube-fed patient
	26	Venous access sites from which the superior vena cava may be cannulated

(continued)

261

Chapter	Transparency Number	Description
Chapter 21	27	Spectrum of eating disorders
Chapter 25	28	Common drugs that increase calcium loss
Chapter 26	29	Formation of dental caries
	30	Factors affecting food cariogenicity
	31	Caries prevention guidelines
Chapter 28	32	High-fiber diet
	33	Possible gas-forming foods
	34	Irritable bowel syndrome
	35	Mechanism by which low-fiber, low-bulk diets might generate diverticula
Chapter 29	36	Normal liver; liver with hepatic damage; and cirrhotic liver
	37	Amino acids commonly altered in liver disease
	38	Relationship of organs of the upper abdomen
Chapter 31	39	The action of insulin on carbohydrate, protein, and fat metabolism
	40	Nutrition assessment
Chapter 33	41	Sodium-containing additives
	42	Food labeling claims for sodium
Chapter 34	43	Adverse effects of lung disease on nutritional status
Chapter 35	44	The nephron
	45	Renin-angiotensin mechanism
	46	Some causes of acute renal failure
	47	Recommended dietary allowances for acute renal failure
Chapter 38	48	Most common allergens by age group
Chapter 39	49	Areas of the brain and neurologic function
Chapter 40	50	Summary of nutritional care for gout
Chapter 41	51	Hyperphenylalaninemias
	52	Schematic metabolism of galactose in galactosemia

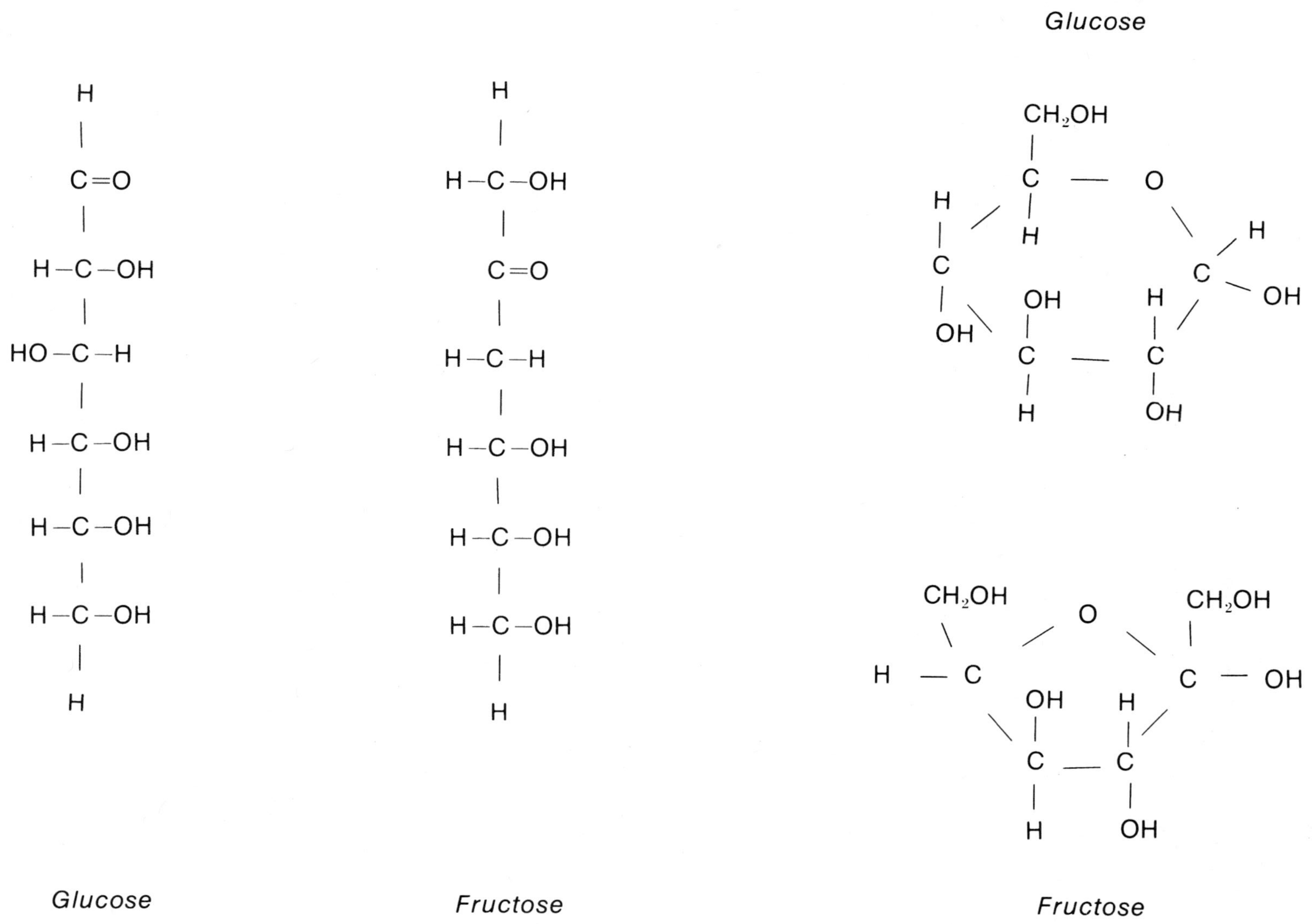

Glucose

Fructose

Fructose

Glucose

Figure 3-2 Structure of glucose and fructose.

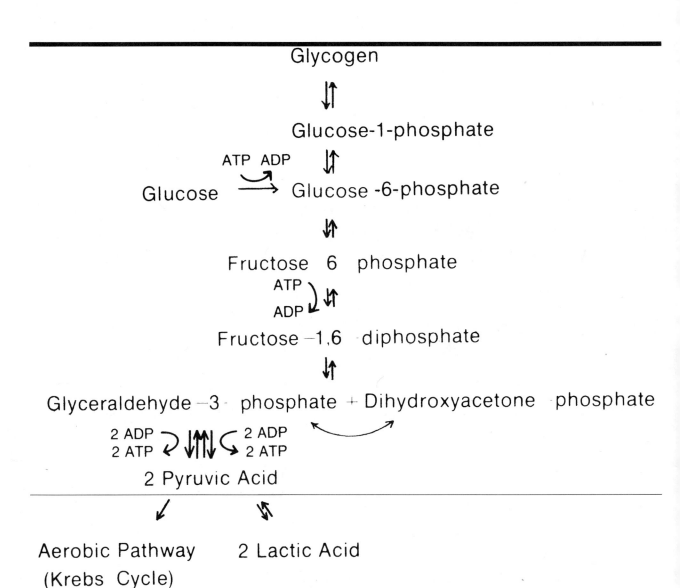

Figure 3-5   Glycogenesis, glycogenolysis, and glycolysis.

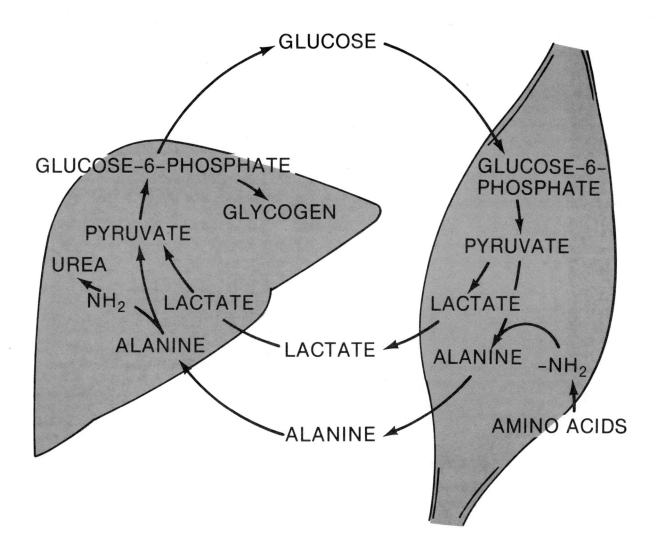

Figure 3-6 The Cori and alanine cycles.
The Cori cycle rids the muscle of lactic acid, and the alanine cycle represents the major
pathway by which the amino groups from muscle amino acids are conveyed to the liver
for conversion to urea.

$$CH_3(CH_2)_{16}COOH$$

$$CH_3(CH_2)_7CH=CH(CH_2)_7COOH$$

$$CH_3(CH_2)_4CH=CHCH_2CH=CH(CH_2)_7COOH$$

$$CH_3CH_2CH=CHCH_2CH=CH-CH_2-CH=CH(CH_2)_7COOH$$

Figure 4-1   18-Carbon fatty acids.

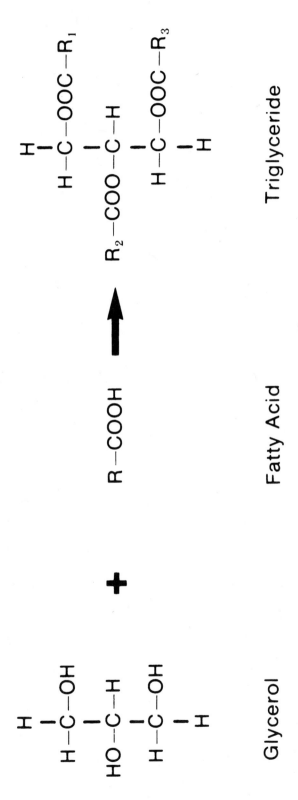

Figure 4-4   Structure of a triglyceride or triacylglycerol.

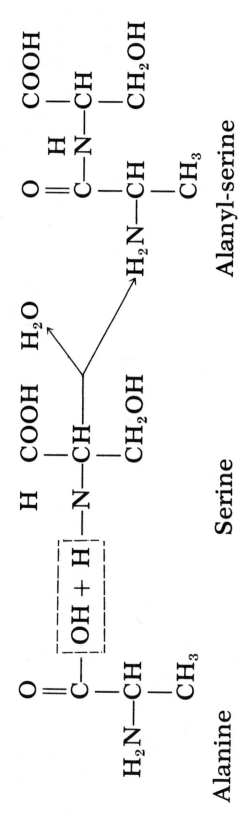

Figure 5-2 Formation of a dipeptide.

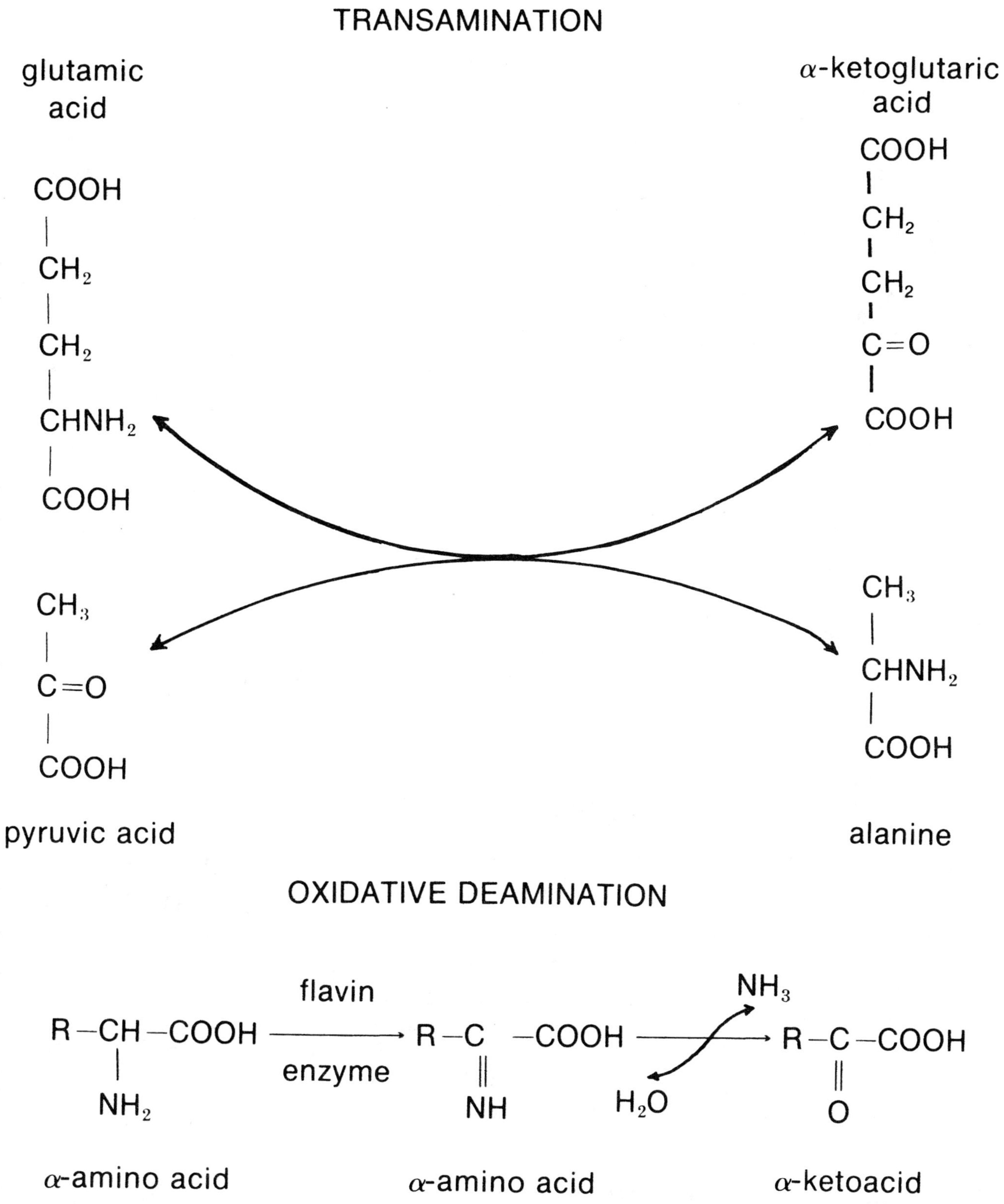

TRANSAMINATION

glutamic
acid

α-ketoglutaric
acid

$$COOH$$
$$|$$
$$CH_2$$
$$|$$
$$CH_2$$
$$|$$
$$CHNH_2$$
$$|$$
$$COOH$$

$$COOH$$
$$|$$
$$CH_2$$
$$|$$
$$CH_2$$
$$|$$
$$C=O$$
$$|$$
$$COOH$$

$$CH_3$$
$$|$$
$$C=O$$
$$|$$
$$COOH$$

$$CH_3$$
$$|$$
$$CHNH_2$$
$$|$$
$$COOH$$

pyruvic acid

alanine

OXIDATIVE DEAMINATION

$$R-CH-COOH \longrightarrow R-C-COOH \longrightarrow R-C-COOH$$

flavin / enzyme

NH_2 NH   O

NH_3, H_2O

α-amino acid   α-amino acid   α-ketoacid

Figure 5-4 Transamination and deamination.

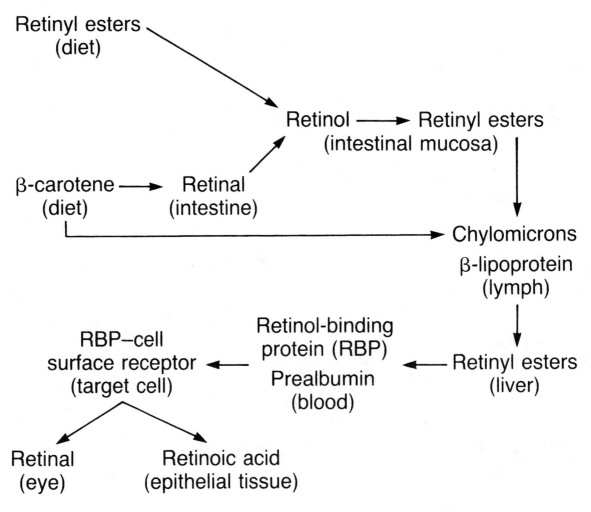

Figure 6-1 The pathway by which dietary vitamin A reaches target cells of an organ.

TABLE 6–1.
RETINOL EQUIVALENTS (RE)

1 retinol equivalent = 1 μg retinol

= 6 μg β-carotene

= 12 μg other provitamin A carotenoids

= 3.33 IU vitamin A activity from retinol

= 10 IU vitamin A activity from β-carotene

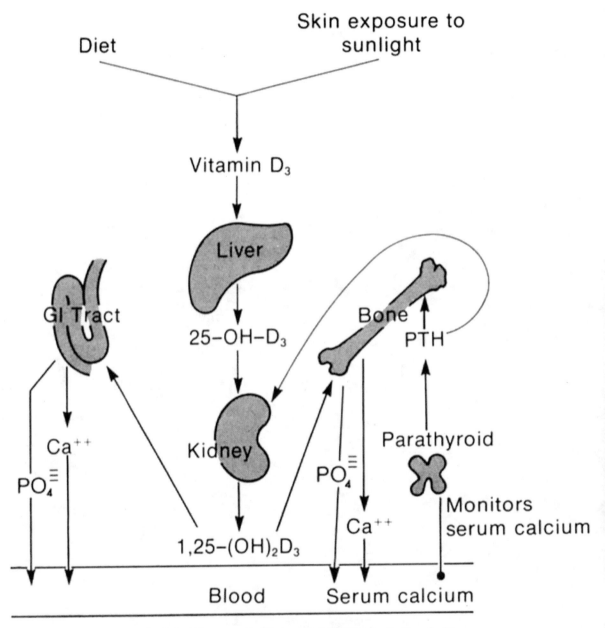

Figure 6-3 The metabolism and functions of vitamin D.
Vitamin D₃ (cholecalciferol) is changed to its biologically active forms, 25-OHD₃ and 1,25-(OH)₂D₃. 1,25-(OH)₂D₃ acts on the intestine to increase calcium and phosphate absorption and on the bones to increase calcium and phosphate resorption.

TABLE 6 – 5.
VITAMIN D TERMINOLOGY AND EQUIVALENTS
TERMINOLOGY

7-Dehydrocholesterol (vitamin D_3 precursor)	Ergosterol (vitamin D_2 precursor)
(Source: animal epidermis)	(Source: plant tissue)
Vitamin D_3 25-hydroxycholecalciferol Cholecalciferol $25(OH)D_3$ (Source: precursor irradiation)	Vitamin D_2 25-hydroxyergocalciferol Ergocalciferol $25(OH)D_2$ (Source: precursor irradiation)
Vitamin D_3 (active form)* 1,25-dihydroxycholecalciferol Calcitriol $1,25(OH)_2D_3$ (Source: kidney activation)	Vitamin D_2 (active form)* 1,25-dihydroxyergocalciferol Ercalcitriol $1,25(OH)_2D_2$ (Source: kidney activation)

EQUIVALENTS

1 International Unit (IU) = 0.025 μg of cholecalciferol (vitamin D_3)

1 μg cholecalciferol (vitamin D_3) = 40 IU vitamin D

* *Vitamin D_3 usually used to denote both active forms.*

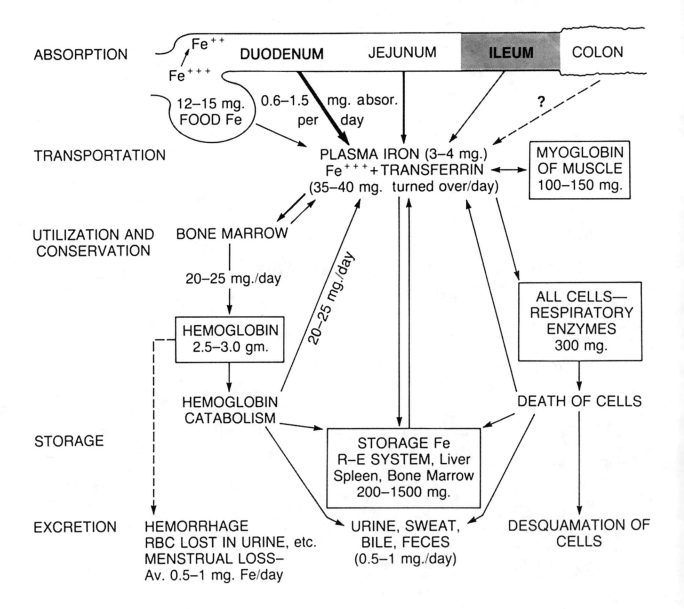

Figure 7-4 Schematic outline of iron metabolism in adults.
Most iron is absorbed from the duodenum and jejunum, after which it is transported as plasma iron or bound to transferrin.

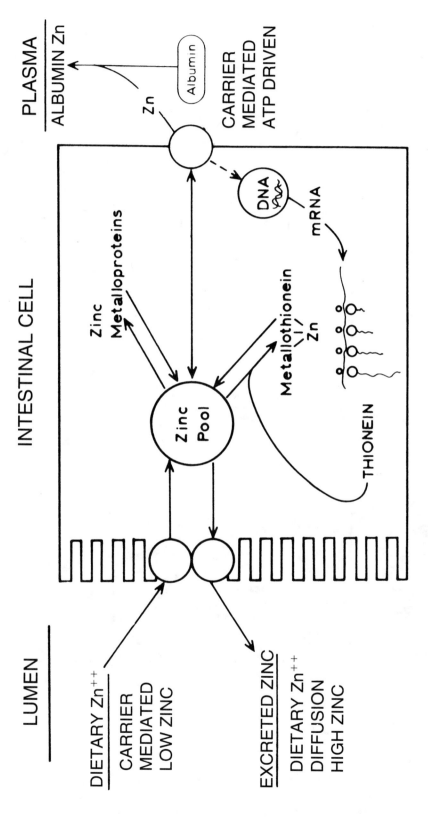

Figure 7-6 A model for zinc absorption showing the relationship between metallothionein and cysteine-rich intestinal protein (CRIP).

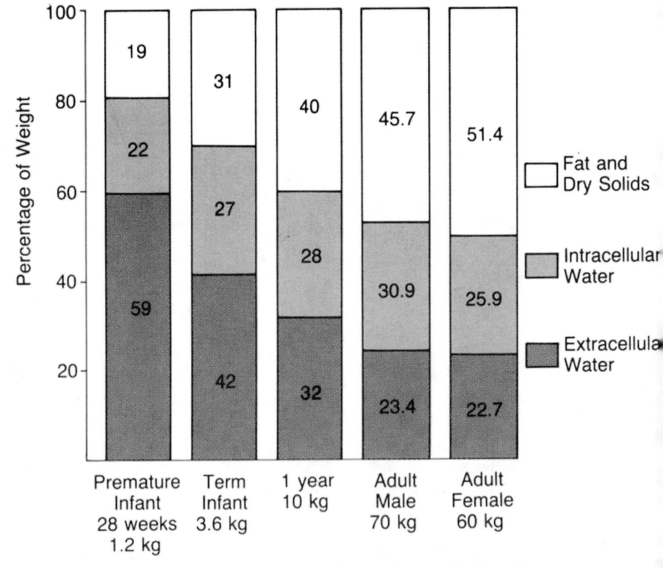

Figure 8-1 Distribution of body water as percentage of body weight.
(Data from Forman, S.J., et al.: Body composition of reference children, birth to age ten years.
Am J Clin Nutr 35:1169, 1982; and Moore, F.D., et al.: Body Cell Mass and Its Supporting
Environment. Philadelphia, W.B.Saunders, 1963.)

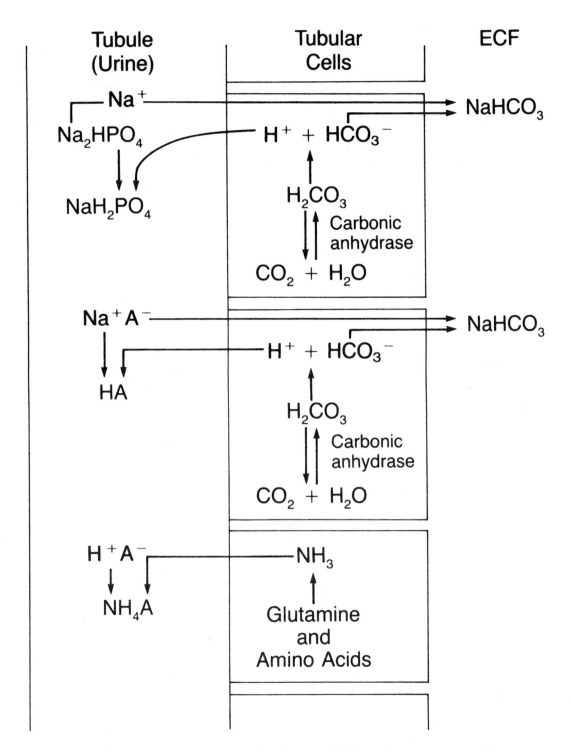

Figure 8-3 Generation of $NaHCO_3$ and clearance of H^+ by the three buffer systems that function in the kidney. (ECF = extracellular fluid; HA = any acid in the body.)

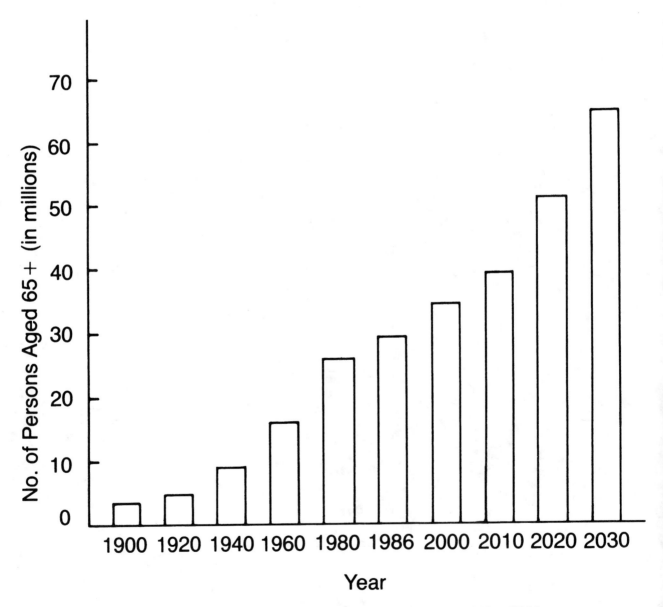

**Figure 14-1 Number of persons aged 65 and older from 1900 to 2030.
Increments in years on horizontal scale are uneven. (Data from US Bureau of the Census.)**

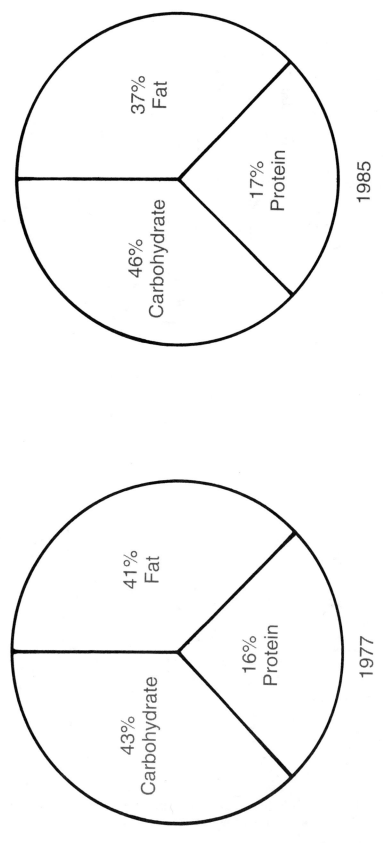

Figure 15-2 A Comparison of the average intake of energy from protein, carbohydrate, and fat for people in the United States in 1977 and 1985.

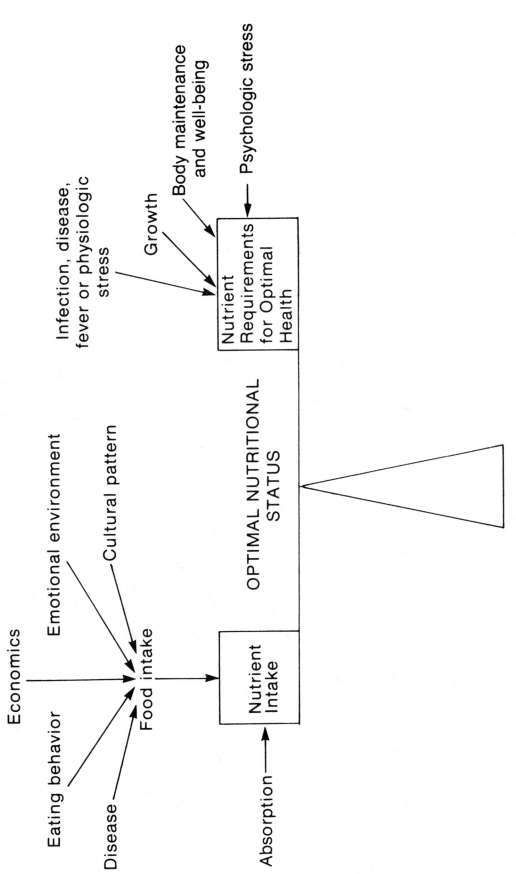

Figure 17-1 Optimal nutritional status as a balance between nutrient intake and nutrient requirements.

TABLE 18–1.
EXAMPLES OF DRUGS THAT MAY CAUSE LOSS OF APPETITE

Sulfasalazine (Azulfidine)	Diabinese
Colchicine	Furosemide (Lasix)
Temazepam (Restoril)	Hydrochlorothiazide (Hydrouril)
Tylenol with Codeine	Hydralazine (Apresoline)
Tamoxifen	Fluphenazine (Prolixin)
Digitalis	Carbamazepine (Tegretol)
Amphogel	

TABLE 18–2.
EXAMPLES OF MEDICATIONS THAT ALTER OR DIMINISH TASTE PERCEPTION

Acetyl sulfasalicylic acid

Amphetamines

Amylocaine

Benzocaine

Clofibrate

Dinitrophenol

5-Fluorouracil

Flurazepam (Dalmane)

Griseofulvin

Lidocaine

Lithium carbonate

Meprobamate

Methicillin sodium

Methylthiouracil

D-Penicillamine

Phenindione

Phenytoin

Probucol

Triazolam (Halcion)

TABLE 18–3.
SOME COMMONLY USED DRUGS THAT INCREASE APPETITE

Antihistamines
Cycloheptadine hydrochloride (Periactin)

Psychotropic Drugs
Chlordiazepoxide hydrochloride (Librium)
Diazepam (Valium)
Chlorpromazine hydrochloride (Thorazine)
Meprobamate (Equanil)
Amitriptyline hydrochloride (Elavil)
Trifluoperazine

Corticosteroids
Cortisone
Prednisone

TABLE 18–4.
DRUGS THAT INHIBIT THE ACTION OF THE OXIDASES

Antidepressants
 Phenelzine sulfate (Nardil)
 Tranylcypromine sulfate
 Isocarboxazid (Marplan)
 Moclobemide (Aurorix)

Antimicrobial
 Furazolidone (Furoxone)

Antineoplastics
 Procarbazine (Matulane)
 Isoniazid (INH)

TABLE 19-1.
NUTRITIONAL SCREENING INFORMATION

Age

Height

Usual weight

Ideal weight

Present weight

Percentage weight change from the ideal or usual weight

Change in appetite

Dysphagia or difficulty with chewing

Presence of nausea, vomiting, or diarrhea

Serum albumin

Hemoglobin and hematocrit

Total lymphocyte count

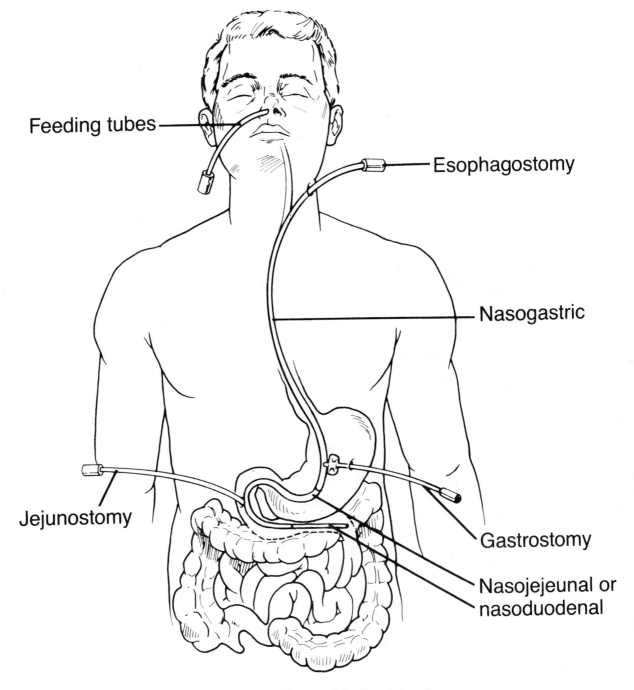

Feeding tubes

Esophagostomy

Nasogastric

Jejunostomy

Gastrostomy

Nasojejeunal or
nasoduodenal

Figure 20-1 Diagram of enteral feeding tube placement.

TABLE 20-4.
MONITORING THE ENTERALLY TUBE-FED PATIENT

Weight (at least 3 times/week)

Signs of edema (daily)

Signs of dehydration (daily)

Fluid intake and output (daily)

Calorie, protein, fat, carbohydrate, vitamin, and mineral intake (at least 2 times/week)

Nitrogen balance (24-hr urine urea nitrogen) (weekly)

Gastric residuals (every 4 hours)

Stool output and consistency (daily)

Urine glucose (every 6 hours until maximum feeding rate established, then daily for persons with diabetes)

Serum electrolytes, blood urea nitrogen (BUN), creatinine, and blood count (2-3 times weekly)

Chemistry profile including serum total protein, albumin, prealbumin, calcium, magnesium, phosphorus, and liver function tests (weekly)

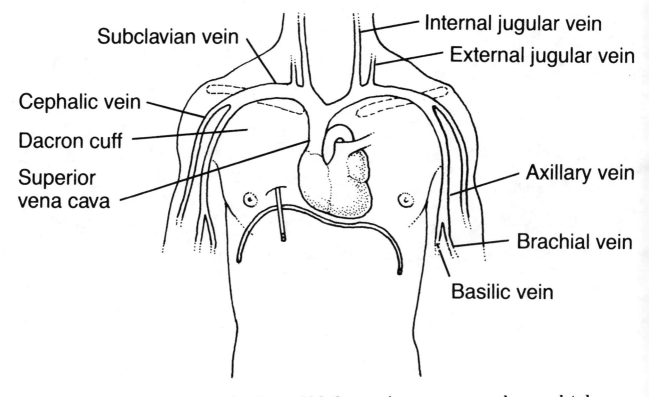

Figure 20-3 - Venous access sites from which the superior vena cava may be cannulated.

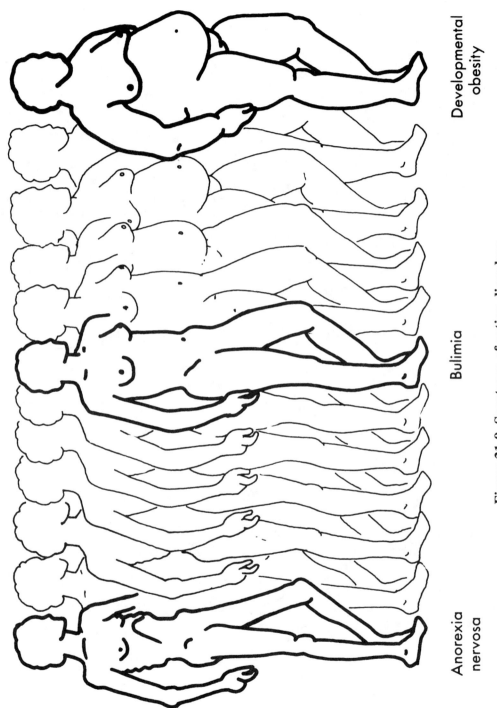

Anorexia
nervosa

Bulimia

Developmental
obesity

Figure 21-9 Spectrum of eating disorders.
(From Mahan, L.K., and Rees, J.M.: Nutrition in Adolescence. St. Louis, CV Mosby, 1984, p. 105.)

TABLE 25–1.
COMMON DRUGS THAT INCREASE CALCIUM LOSS

Phenytoin (Dilantin)

Phenobarbital

Thyroid hormone

Corticosteroids

Methotrexate

Cyclosporin

Lithium

Tetracycline

Aluminum-containing antacids

Heparin

Phenothiazine derivatives

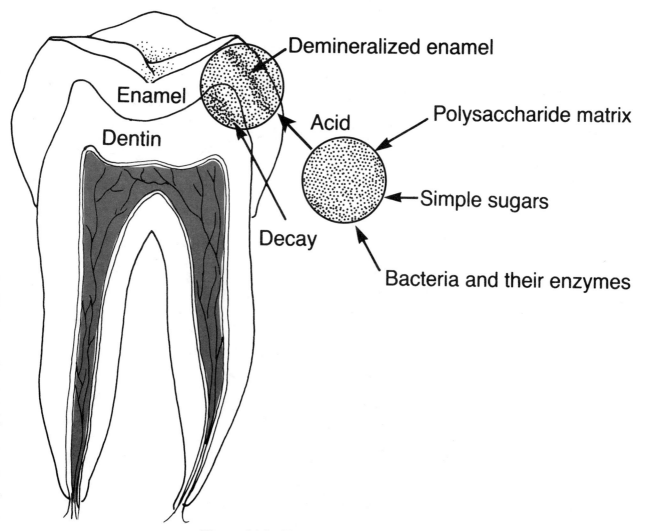

Figure 26-2 - Formation of dental caries.

TABLE 26-2.
FACTORS AFFECTING FOOD CARIOGENICITY

Factors Affecting Food Cariogenicity	Examples of High Cariogenicity
Frequency of consumption of fermentable carbohydrates	Consuming sweetened beverages 6× daily
Food form: liquid, solid, slowly dissolving	Caramel candy or syrup
Sequence of eating foods	Eating cookie at end of meal
Combination of foods	Crackers with jelly
Nutrient composition of foods and beverages	Sweetened Kool-Aid

TABLE 26–5.
CARIES PREVENTION GUIDELINES

Brush at least twice daily, preferably after meals

Rinse mouth after meals and snacks when brushing is not possible

Chew sugarless gum for 15–20 minutes after meals and snacks

Floss twice daily

Use fluoridated toothpastes

Pair cariogenic foods with cariostatic foods

Snack on cariostatic foods such as cheese, nuts, popcorn, and vegetables

Limit between-meal eating and drinking of fermentable carbohydrates

T A B L E   28–2.
HIGH-FIBER DIET*

1. Include ¼ to ½ cup of wheat bran daily.
2. Increase consumption of whole-grain breads, cereals, flours, and other whole-grain products.
3. Increase consumption of vegetables and fruits, especially those with edible skins, seeds, and hulls.
4. Choose enough servings from the food groups described in Table 3–5 to provide at least 25 g of dietary fiber.
5. Increase consumption of water to 2 qt (64 oz) daily.

* Provides 25 to 50 g/day of dietary fiber.

TABLE 28–4.
POSSIBLE GAS-FORMING FOODS

VEGETABLES

Beans, kidney	Onions
Beans, lima	Peas, split or black-eyed
Beans, navy	Peppers, green
Broccoli	Pimentos
Brussels sprouts	Radishes
Cabbage	Rutabagas
Cauliflower	Sauerkraut
Corn	Scallions
Cucumbers	Shallots
Kohlrabi	Soybeans
Leeks	Turnips
Lentils	

FRUIT

Apples (raw)	Cantaloupe
Apple juice	Honeydew melon
Avocados	Watermelon

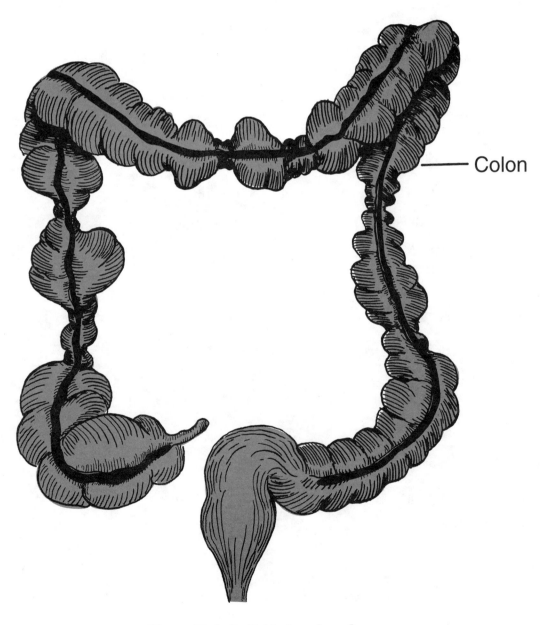

Colon

Figure 28-4 - Irritable bowel syndrome.

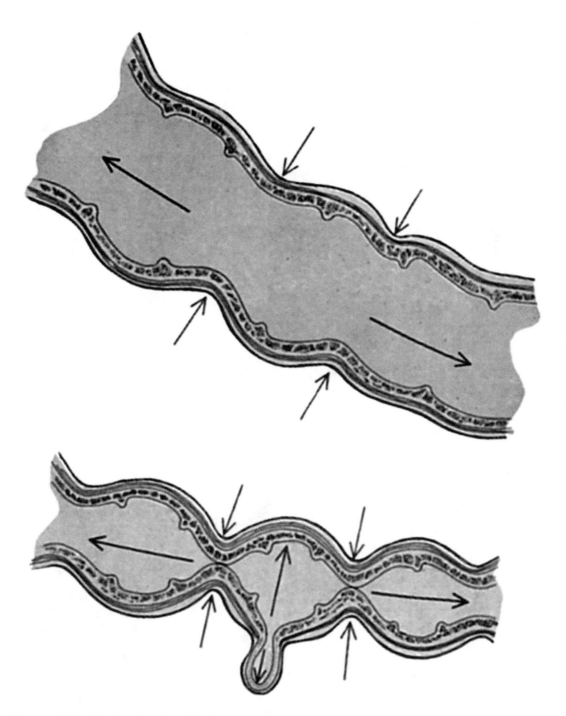

Figure 28-5 Mechanism by which low-fiber, low-bulk diets might generate diverticula.
Where the colon contents are bulky (top), muscular contractions exert pressure longitudinally.
If the lumen is smaller (bottom), contractions can produce occlusion and exert pressure against
colon wall, which may produce a diverticular "blow-out."

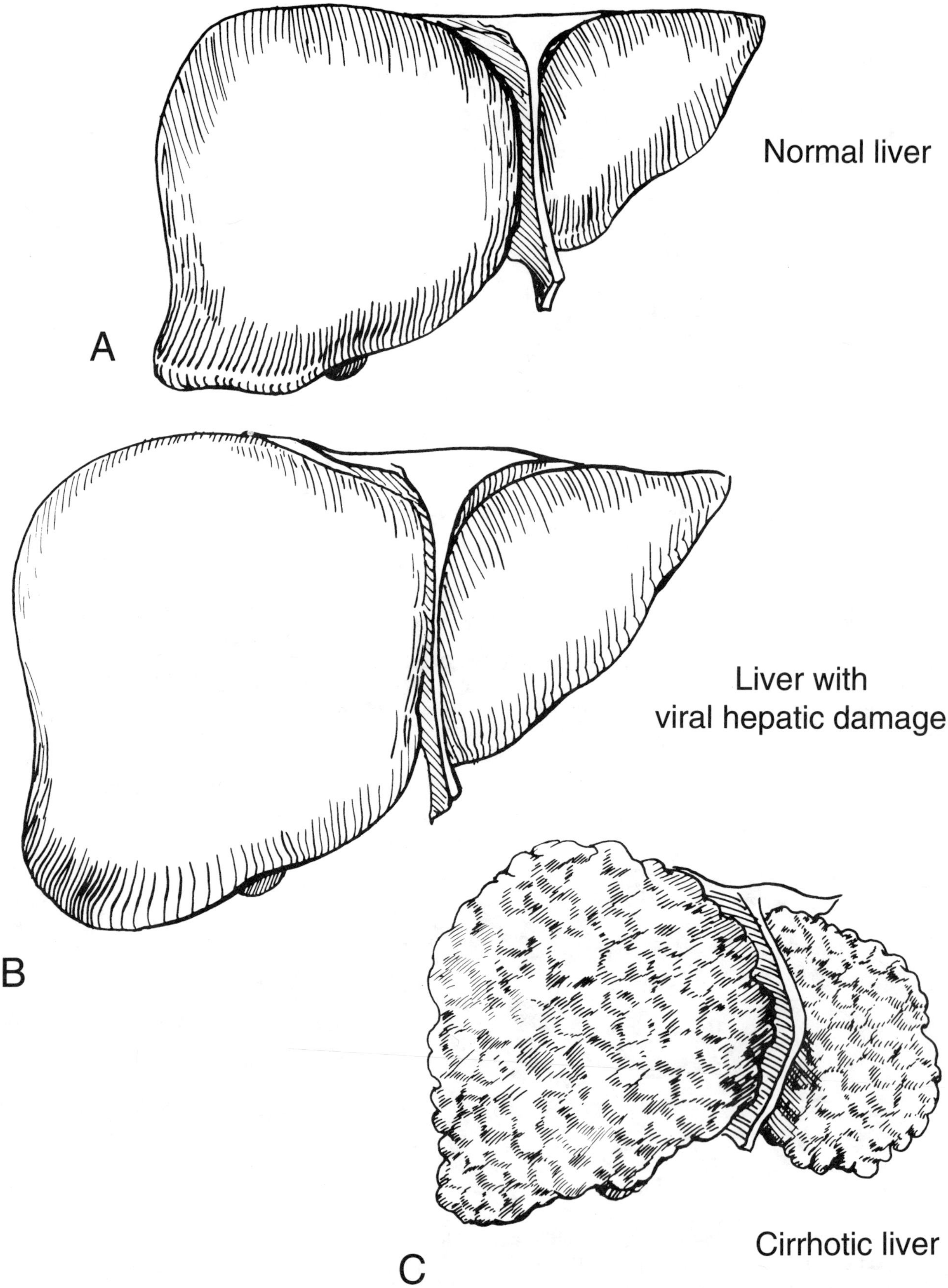

Normal liver

Liver with
viral hepatic damage

Cirrhotic liver

Figure 29-1 (A) Normal liver; (B) liver with viral hepatic damage; and (C) cirrhotic liver.

TABLE 29–1.
AMINO ACIDS COMMONLY ALTERED IN LIVER DISEASE

Aromatic amino acids (AAA)

Tyrosine

Phenylalanine*

Free tryptophan*

Branched-chain amino acids (BCAA)

Valine*

Leucine*

Isoleucine*

Ammoniogenic amino acids

Glycine

Serine

Threonine*

Glutamine

Histidine*

Lysine*

Asparagine

Methionine*

* Denotes essential amino acids.

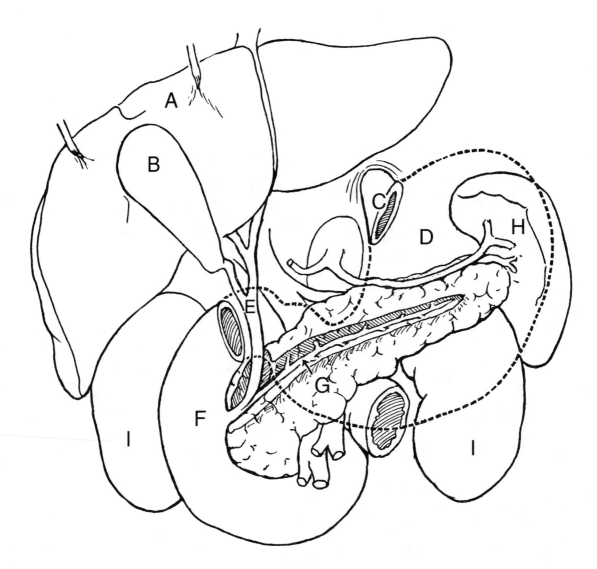

Figure 29-4 Schematic drawing showing relationship of organs of the upper abdomen.
(A) liver (retracted upward); (B) gallbladder; (C) esophageal opening of the stomach;
(D) stomach (shown in dotted outline); (E) common bile duct; (F) duodenum; (G) pancreas and
pancreatic duct; (H) spleen; (I) kidneys.

TABLE 31–4.
THE ACTION OF INSULIN ON CARBOHYDRATE, PROTEIN, AND FAT METABOLISM

EFFECT	CARBOHYDRATE	PROTEIN	FAT
Anticatabolic (prevent breakdown)	Decreases breakdown and release of glucose from glycogen in the liver	Inhibits protein degradation; diminishes gluconeogenesis	Inhibits lipolysis; prevents excessive production of ketones and ketoacidosis
Anabolic (promote storage)	Facilitates conversion of glucose to glycogen for storage in liver and muscle	Stimulates protein synthesis	Facilitates conversion of pyruvate to free fatty acids stimulating lipogenesis
Transport	Activates transport system of glucose into muscle and adipose cells	Lowers blood amino acids in parallel with blood glucose	Activates lipoprotein lipase, facilitating transport of triglycerides into adipose tissue

TABLE 31-19.
NUTRITION ASSESSMENT

- Minimal referral data: treatment regimen; medical history; medications; laboratory data (glycated hemoglobin, cholesterol and fractionations, blood pressure, renal function if applicable); physician goals; clearance for exercise
- Clinical data: exercise history; psychosocial and economic issues; blood glucose monitoring; knowledge; skill level; attitudes; motivation
- Nutrition history: current eating habits with beginning modifications

T A B L E   3 3 – 6.
SODIUM-CONTAINING ADDITIVES

NAME	FOODS LIKELY TO CONTAIN
Disodium phosphate	Cereals, cheeses, ice cream, bottled drinks
Monosodium glutamate	Accent (a flavor enhancer), meats, condiments, pickles, soups, candy, baked goods
Sodium alginate	Ice cream, chocolate milk
Sodium benzoate	Fruit juices
Sodium hydroxide	Pretzels, sour cream, cocoa products, canned peas
Sodium propionate	Breads
Sodium sulfite	Dried fruits, cut salad greens
Sodium pectinate	Syrups and toppings, ice cream, sherbet, salad dressings, jams and jellies
Sodium caseinate	Ice cream and other frozen products
Sodium bicarbonate	Baking powder, tomato soup, self-rising flour, sherbets, confections

TABLE 33-9.
FOOD LABELING CLAIMS FOR SODIUM

Sodium free:	Less than 5 mg per standard serving; cannot contain any sodium chloride
Very low sodium:	35 mg or less per standard serving
Low sodium:	140 mg or less per standard serving
Reduced sodium:	At least 25% less sodium per standard serving than in the regular food
Light in sodium:	50% less sodium per standard serving than in the regular food
Unsalted, Without added salt, or No salt added:	No salt added during processing and the product it resembles is normally processed with salt
Lightly salted:	50% less added sodium than is normally added; product must state not a low sodium food if that criteria is not met

TABLE 34–1.
ADVERSE EFFECTS OF LUNG DISEASE ON NUTRITIONAL STATUS

Increased Energy Expenditure
  Increased work of breathing
  Chronic infection
  Medical treatments (e.g., bronchodilators, chest physical therapy)
Reduced Intake
  Fluid restriction
  Shortness of breath
  Decreased oxygen saturation when eating
  Anorexia due to chronic disease
  Gastrointestinal distress and vomiting
Additional Limitations
  Difficulty in preparing food due to fatigue
  Lack of financial resources
  Impaired feeding skills (for infants and children)
  Altered metabolism

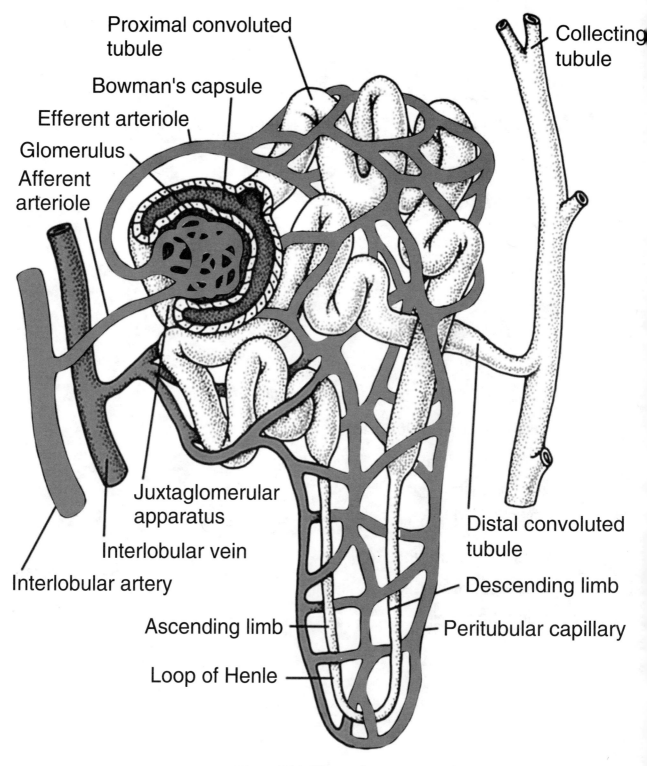

Proximal convoluted tubule

Bowman's capsule

Efferent arteriole

Glomerulus

Afferent arteriole

Collecting tubule

Juxtaglomerular apparatus

Interlobular vein

Interlobular artery

Distal convoluted tubule

Descending limb

Ascending limb

Peritubular capillary

Loop of Henle

Figure 35-1 The nephron.

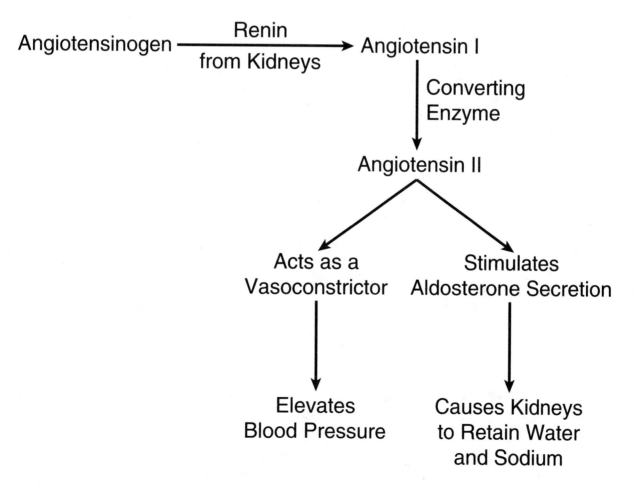

Figure 35-2 Renin-angiotensin mechanism.

TABLE 35-1.
SOME CAUSES OF ACUTE RENAL FAILURE

Prerenal
  Severe dehydration
  Circulatory collapse
Intrinsic
  Acute tubular necrosis
    Trauma, surgery
    Septicemia
  Nephrotoxicity
    Antibiotics, contrast agents, and other drugs
  Vascular disorders
    Bilateral renal infarction
  Acute glomerulonephritis of any cause
    Poststreptococcal infection
    Systemic lupus erythematosus
Postrenal Obstruction
  Benign prostatic hypertrophy
  Carcinoma of the bladder or prostate
  Ureterovesical stricture

TABLE 35-3.
RECOMMENDED DIETARY ALLOWANCES FOR ACUTE RENAL FAILURE

NUTRIENT	AMOUNT
Protein	0.6 to 0.8 g/kg IBW, increasing as GFR returns to normal. 60% should be HBV protein.
Energy	45–55 kcal/kg body weight.
Potassium	30–50 mEq/day in oliguric phase (depending on urinary output, dialysis and serum K^+ level); replace losses in diuretic phase.
Sodium	20–40 mEq/day in oliguric phase (depending on urinary output, edema, dialysis and serum Na^+ level); replace losses in diuretic phase.
Fluid	Replace output from the previous day (vomitus, diarrhea, urine) plus 500 ml.
Phosphorus	Limit as needed

GFR = glomerular filtration rate; HBV = high biologic value; IBW = ideal body weight.

TABLE 38–3.
MOST COMMON ALLERGENS BY AGE GROUP

INFANTS/CHILDREN	ADULTS
Egg	Fish
Fish	Nuts
Milk	Peanuts
Peanuts	Shellfish
Soy	Soy
Wheat	

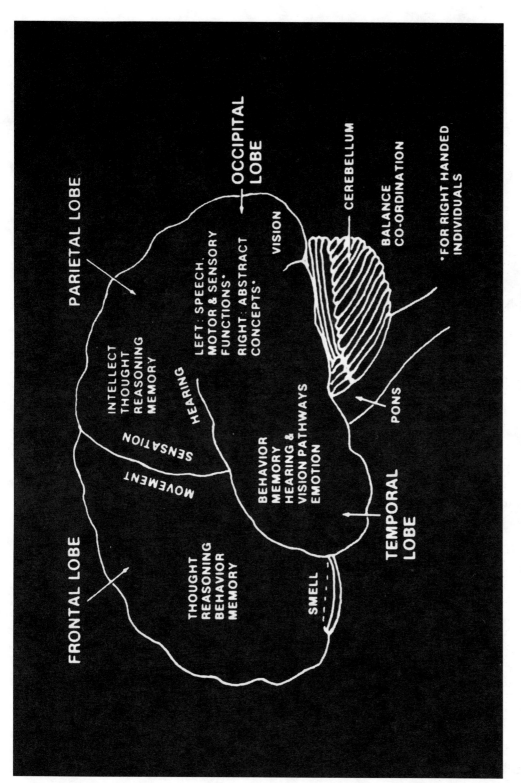

Figure 39-7 Areas of the brain and neurologic function.

TABLE 40-3.
SUMMARY OF NUTRITIONAL CARE FOR GOUT

1. Moderation of foods high in purines as shown in Table 40-2.
2. Moderate protein intake with large proportion of protein coming from low fat dairy products.
3. Liberal carbohydrate intake (at least 50% of total daily kcal).
4. Fat intake of about 30% total kcal.`
5. Maintenance of, or gradual reduction to, ideal body weight.
6. Restriction or elimination of alcohol.
7. Liberal fluid intake to keep urine dilute.

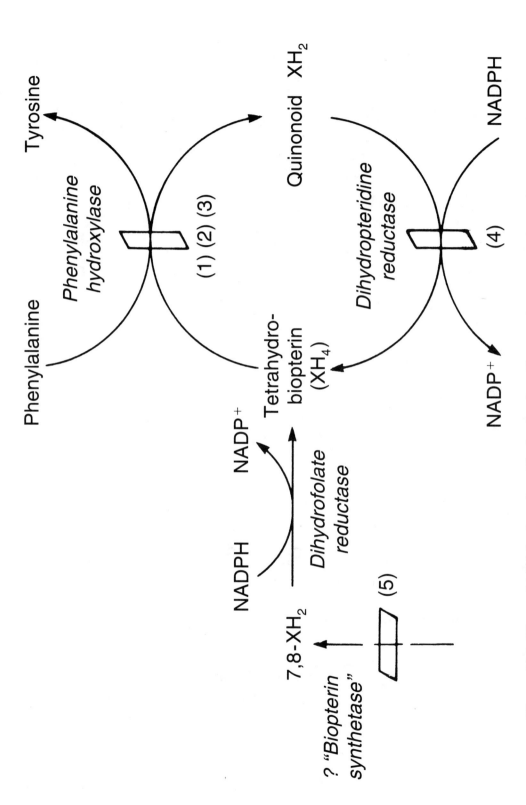

Figure 41-1 Hyperphenylalaninemias: (1) classic phenylketonuria, (2) atypical phenylketonuria, (3) benign hyperphenylalaninemia, (4) dihydropteridine reductase deficiency, and (5) biopterin synthetase deficiency.

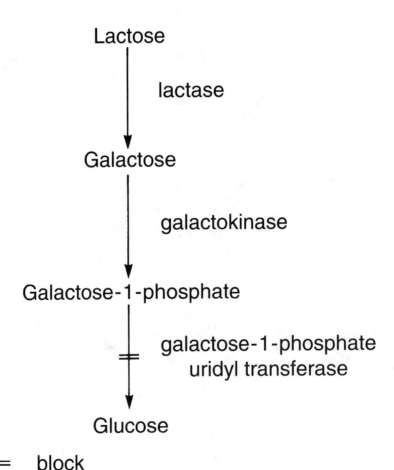

= block

Figure 41-6 Schematic metabolism of galactose in galactosemia

HANDOUTS

Chapter	Handout Number	Description
Chapter 1	1	The digestive system
	2	Sites of secretion and absorption in the gastrointestinal tract
Chapter 7	3	Daily calcium intake for males and females in the United States
	4	Daily magnesium intake for males and females in the United States
	5	The absorbed iron requirement in males and females for various ages
Chapter 9	6	Transfer across the placental membrane
Chapter 11	7	Classification of newborns based on maturity and intrauterine growth
Chapter 16	8	The Food Guide Pyramid
	9	The traditional healthy Mediterranean diet pyramid
	10	"Nutrition Facts" on new food labels
Chapter 21	11	Gastric surgeries for obesity
Chapter 22	12	Pathways of energy production
Chapter 23	13	Development of atherosclerosis; coronary arteries
Chapter 26	14	Anatomy of a tooth
Chapter 27	15	Gastric surgical procedures
	16	The stomach and duodenum with eroded lesions; gastric ulcer; duodenal ulcer
Chapter 30	17	Physiologic and metabolic changes immediately after an injury or burn
	18	The involvement of cytokines in response to injury
Chapter 31	19	Worksheet for Nutrition Assessment and implementation of a meal or food plan
Chapter 35	20	Simple menu plan for dialysis patient

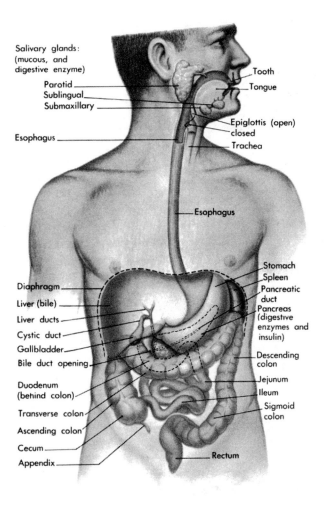

Figure 1-1 The digestive system.

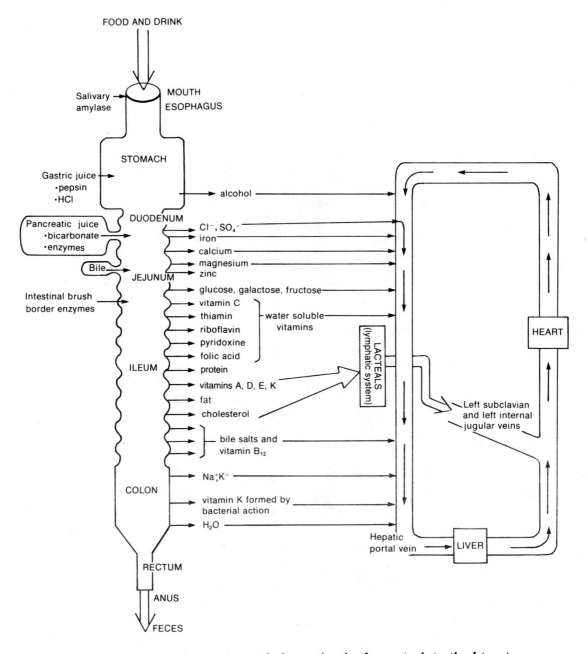

Figure 1-7 Sites of secretion and absorption in the gastrointestinal tract.

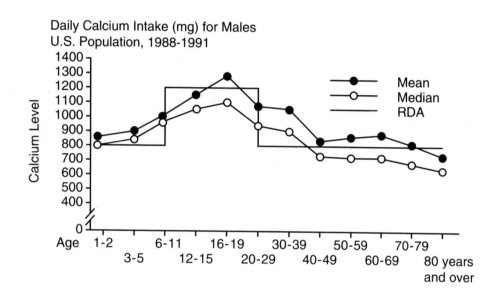

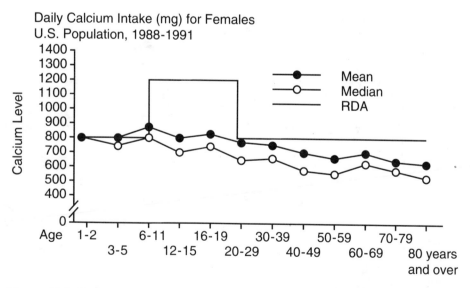

Figure 7-1 Daily calcium intake for males and females in the United States.
(Data from Alaimo, K., et al., 1994, which summarizes some information obtained in Phase I of
the Third National Health and Examination Survey.)

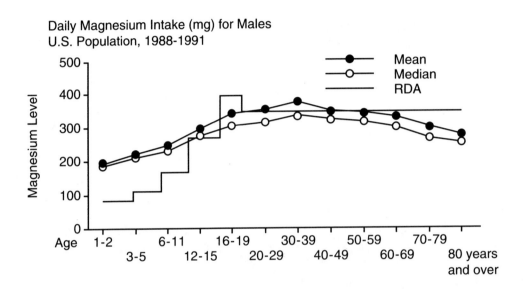

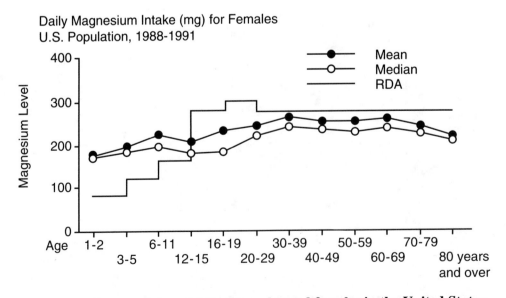

**Figure 7-3 Daily magnesium intake for males and females in the United States.
(Data from Alaimo, K., et al., 1994, which summarizes some information obtained in Phase I of
the Third National Health and Examination Survey.)**

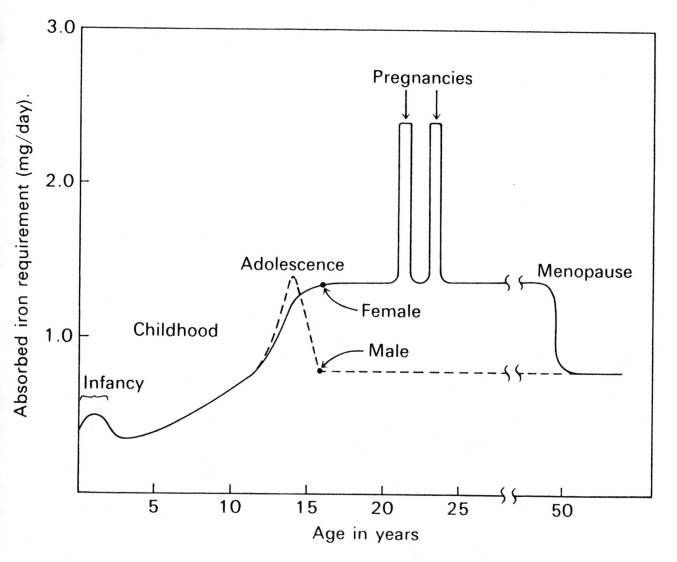

Figure 7-5 The absorbed iron requirement in males and females of various ages. The greatest requirement in relation to food intake occurs during infancy. During childhood, requirements are the same for both sexes. During the adolescent growth spurt, there is an increase in iron needs—more in the male than in the female. Because of menstruation, the female's requirement remains high while the requirement for the male decreases after adolescence.
(From Wintrobe, M. S., et al.: Clinical Hematology, 7th ed. Philadelphia, Lea & Febiger, 1974.)

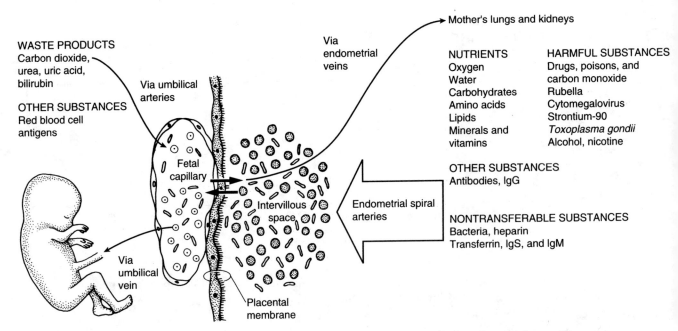

WASTE PRODUCTS
Carbon dioxide,
urea, uric acid,
bilirubin

OTHER SUBSTANCES
Red blood cell
antigens

Via umbilical
arteries

Via
endometrial
veins

Mother's lungs and kidneys

NUTRIENTS
Oxygen
Water
Carbohydrates
Amino acids
Lipids
Minerals and
vitamins

HARMFUL SUBSTANCES
Drugs, poisons, and
carbon monoxide
Rubella
Cytomegalovirus
Strontium-90
Toxoplasma gondii
Alcohol, nicotine

Fetal
capillary

Intervillous
space

Endometrial spiral
arteries

OTHER SUBSTANCES
Antibodies, IgG

NONTRANSFERABLE SUBSTANCES
Bacteria, heparin
Transferrin, IgS, and IgM

Via
umbilical
vein

Placental
membrane

**Figure 9-6 Diagrammatic illustration of transfer across the placental membrane.
(From Moore, K.L.: The Developing Human, 5th ed. Philadelphia, W.B. Saunders, 1993, p. 120.)**

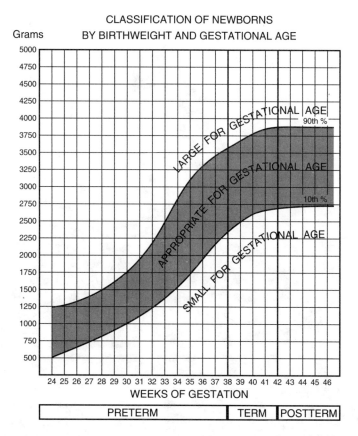

Figure 11-1 Classification of newborns based on maturity and intrauterine growth.
SGA = small for gestational age; AGA = appropriate for gestational age; LGA = large for gesta-
tional age. (From Battaglia, F.C., and Lubchenco, L.O.: A practical classification of newborn
infants by weight and gestational age. J. Pediatr 71:159, 1967.)

FOOD GUIDE PYRAMID

A Guide to Daily Food Choices

The Pyramid is an outline of what to eat each day. It's not a rigid prescription, but a general guide that lets you choose a healthful diet that's right for you. The Pyramid calls for eating a variety of foods to get the nutrients you need and at the same time the right amount of calories to maintain a healthy weight.

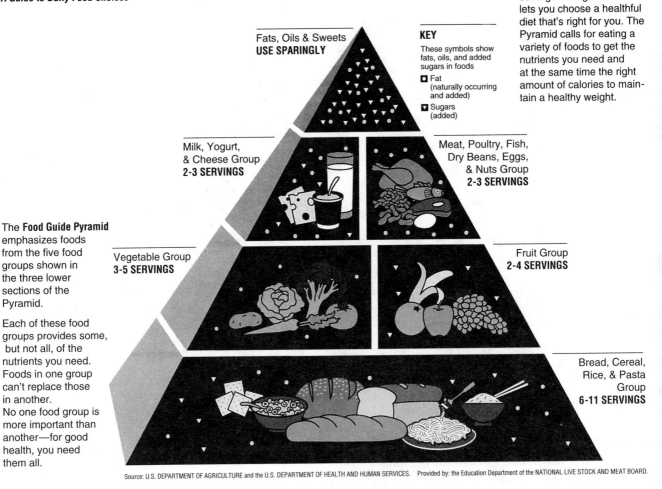

Fats, Oils & Sweets
USE SPARINGLY

KEY
These symbols show fats, oils, and added sugars in foods
◻ Fat (naturally occurring and added)
▼ Sugars (added)

Milk, Yogurt,
& Cheese Group
2-3 SERVINGS

Meat, Poultry, Fish,
Dry Beans, Eggs,
& Nuts Group
2-3 SERVINGS

The **Food Guide Pyramid** emphasizes foods from the five food groups shown in the three lower sections of the Pyramid.

Each of these food groups provides some, but not all, of the nutrients you need. Foods in one group can't replace those in another.
No one food group is more important than another—for good health, you need them all.

Vegetable Group
3-5 SERVINGS

Fruit Group
2-4 SERVINGS

Bread, Cereal,
Rice, & Pasta
Group
6-11 SERVINGS

Source: U.S. DEPARTMENT OF AGRICULTURE and the U.S. DEPARTMENT OF HEALTH AND HUMAN SERVICES.   Provided by: the Education Department of the NATIONAL LIVE STOCK AND MEAT BOARD.

Figure 16-1 The Food Guide Pyramid

The Traditional Healthy
MEDITERRANEAN Diet Pyramid.

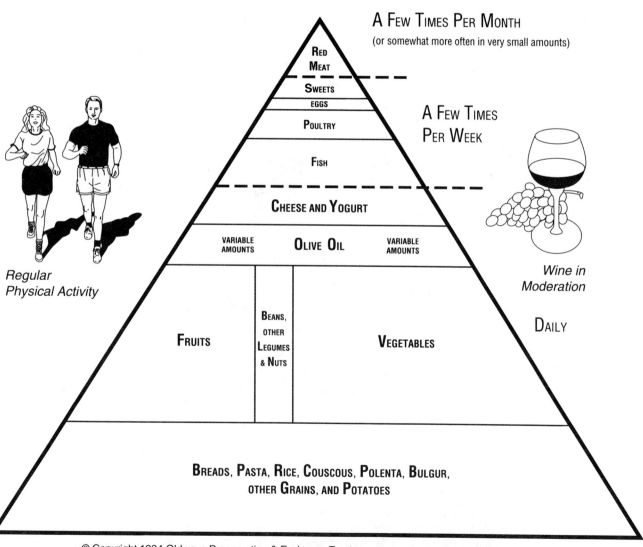

A FEW TIMES PER MONTH
(or somewhat more often in very small amounts)

RED MEAT

SWEETS

EGGS

POULTRY

A FEW TIMES PER WEEK

FISH

CHEESE AND YOGURT

VARIABLE AMOUNTS   OLIVE OIL   VARIABLE AMOUNTS

FRUITS

BEANS, OTHER LEGUMES & NUTS

VEGETABLES

DAILY

BREADS, PASTA, RICE, COUSCOUS, POLENTA, BULGUR, OTHER GRAINS, AND POTATOES

Regular Physical Activity

Wine in Moderation

Figure 16-2 The traditional healthy Mediterranean diet pyramid.

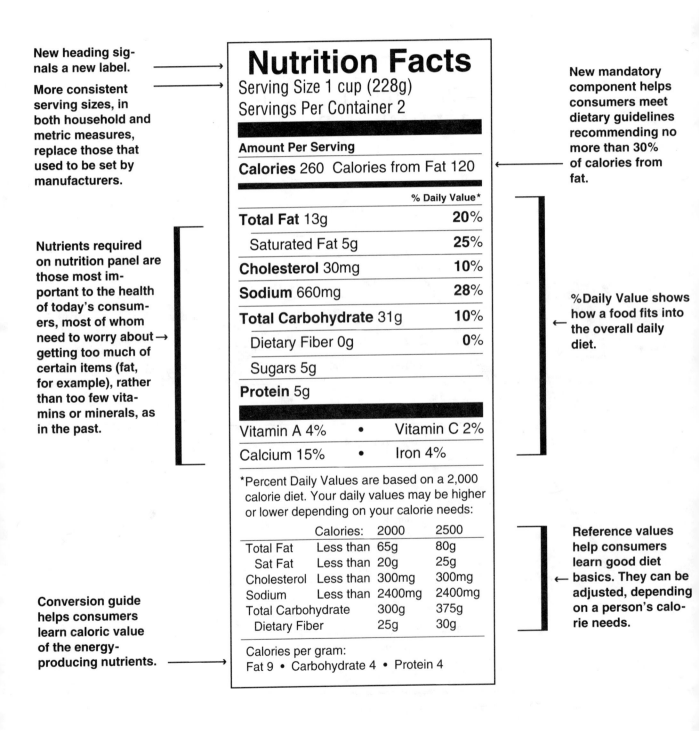

New heading sig-
nals a new label.

More consistent
serving sizes, in
both household and
metric measures,
replace those that
used to be set by
manufacturers.

Nutrients required
on nutrition panel are
those most im-
portant to the health
of today's consum-
ers, most of whom
need to worry about →
getting too much of
certain items (fat,
for example), rather
than too few vita-
mins or minerals, as
in the past.

Conversion guide
helps consumers
learn caloric value
of the energy-
producing nutrients.

New mandatory
component helps
consumers meet
dietary guidelines
recommending no
more than 30%
of calories from
fat.

%Daily Value shows
how a food fits into
the overall daily
diet.

Reference values
help consumers
learn good diet
basics. They can be
adjusted, depending
on a person's calo-
rie needs.

Nutrition Facts
Serving Size 1 cup (228g)
Servings Per Container 2

Amount Per Serving

Calories 260   Calories from Fat 120

	% Daily Value*
Total Fat 13g	**20**%
Saturated Fat 5g	**25**%
Cholesterol 30mg	**10**%
Sodium 660mg	**28**%
Total Carbohydrate 31g	**10**%
Dietary Fiber 0g	**0**%
Sugars 5g	
Protein 5g	

Vitamin A 4%	•	Vitamin C 2%	
Calcium 15%	•	Iron 4%	

*Percent Daily Values are based on a 2,000
calorie diet. Your daily values may be higher
or lower depending on your calorie needs:

		Calories:	2000	2500
Total Fat	Less than		65g	80g
Sat Fat	Less than		20g	25g
Cholesterol	Less than		300mg	300mg
Sodium	Less than		2400mg	2400mg
Total Carbohydrate			300g	375g
Dietary Fiber			25g	30g

Calories per gram:
Fat 9 • Carbohydrate 4 • Protein 4

Figure 16-3 "Nutrition Facts" on new food labels.

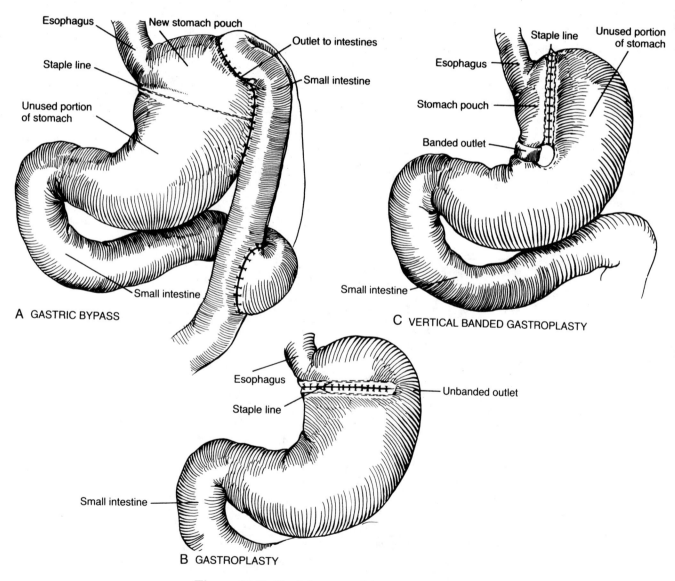

Esophagus

New stomach pouch

Outlet to intestines

Staple line

Small intestine

Unused portion
of stomach

Small intestine

A GASTRIC BYPASS

Staple line

Unused portion
of stomach

Esophagus

Stomach pouch

Banded outlet

Small intestine

C VERTICAL BANDED GASTROPLASTY

Esophagus

Unbanded outlet

Staple line

Small intestine

B GASTROPLASTY

Figure 21-7 Gastric surgeries for obesity.

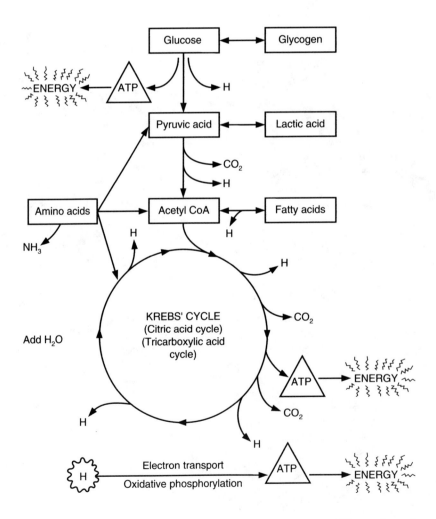

Figure 22-2 Pathways of energy production (H = hydrogen atoms; ATP = adenosine triphosphate.)

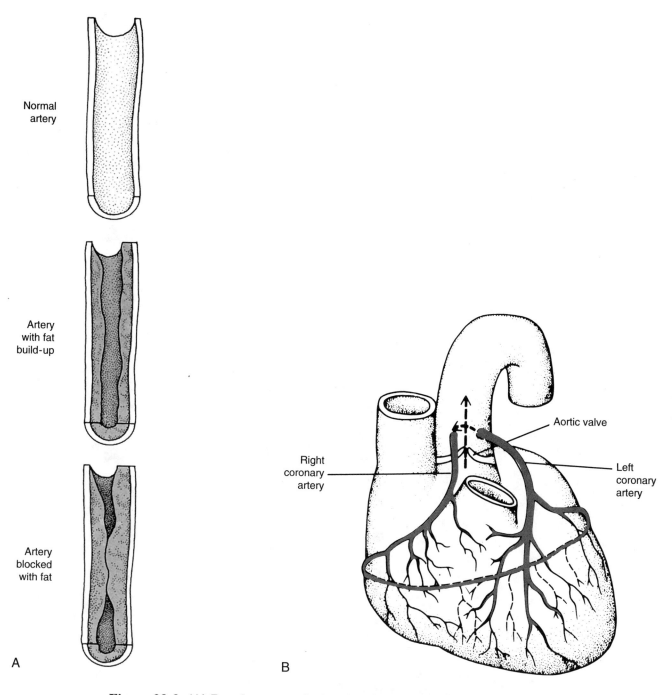

Normal
artery

Artery
with fat
build-up

Artery
blocked
with fat

A

B

Aortic valve

Right
coronary
artery

Left
coronary
artery

**Figure 23-3 (A) Development of atherosclerosis. (B) Coronary arteries
(B, from Guyton, A.C.: Textbook of Medical Physiology, 8th ed. Philadelphia: W.B. Saunders,
1991, p. 237.)**

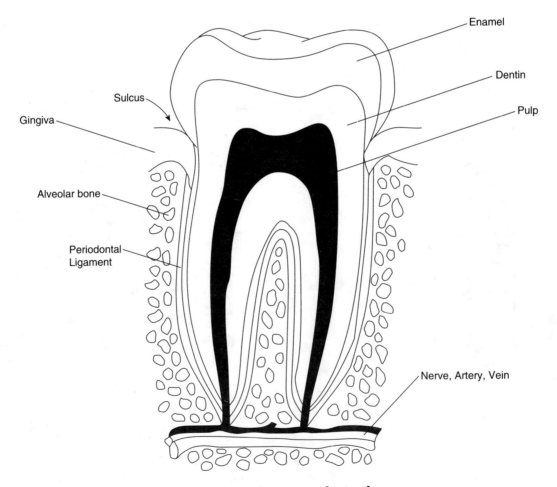

Figure 26-1 Anatomy of a tooth.

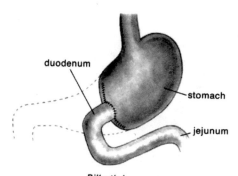

duodenum

stomach

jejunum

Billroth I
gastroduodenostomy

Less dumping than
with Billroth II.

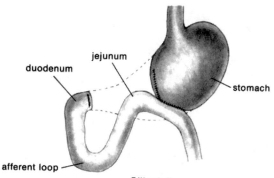

duodenum

jejunum

stomach

afferent loop

Billroth II
gastrojejunostomy

Sequelae such as steatorrhea, weight
loss, dumping, vomiting and bacterial
overgrowth occur more often with the
Billroth II procedure.

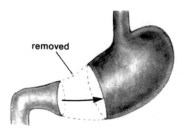

removed

Partial Gastric Resection

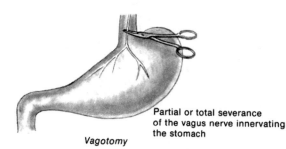

Partial or total severance
of the vagus nerve innervating
the stomach

Vagotomy

Depending on the extent of the
vagotomy, HCl secretion is reduced
and gastric emptying is slowed.
Dumping syndrome often follows
this surgery.

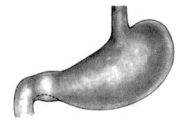

enlargement
of pyloric sphincter

Pyloroplasty

Duodenal reflux frequently
follows this surgery.

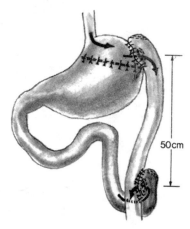

50cm

Roux-en-Y procedure

Figure 27-3 Gastric surgical procedures.

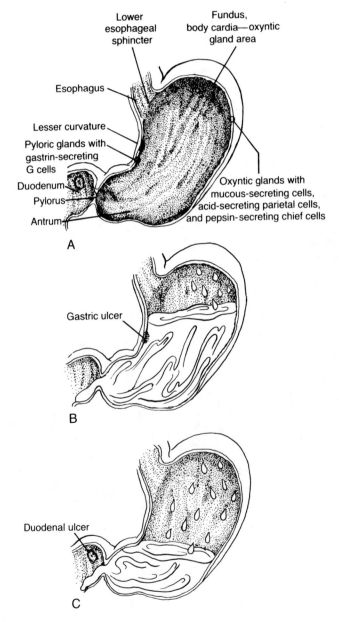

Figure 27-4 Diagram showing (A) the stomach and duodenum with eroded lesions; (B) gastric ulcer; and (C) duodenal ulcer.

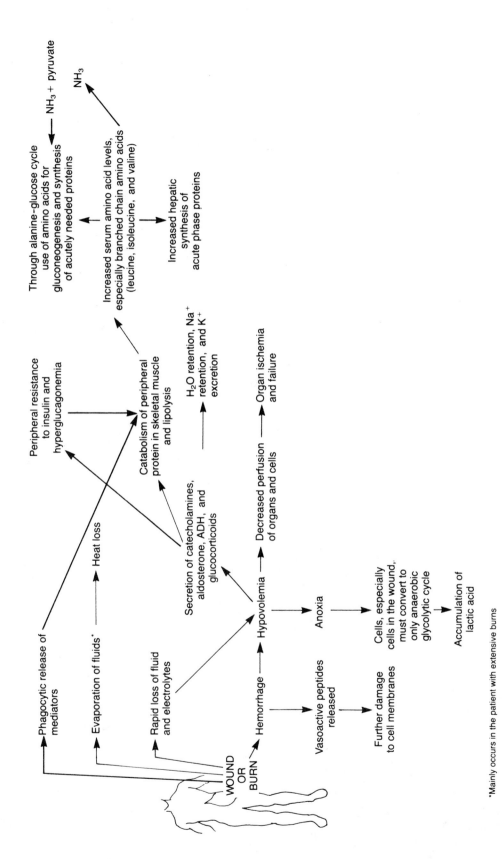

Figure 30-1 Physiologic and metabolic changes immediately after an injury or burn. The extent of these changes depends on the severity of the trauma.

*Mainly occurs in the patient with extensive burns

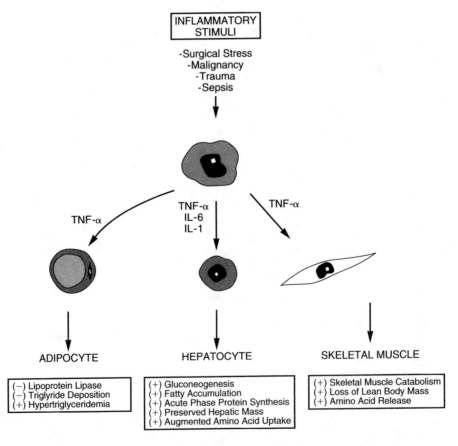

**Figure 30-2 The involvement of cytokines in response to injury response.
(From Espat, N.J., Moldawer, L.L., and Copeland, E.M.: Cytokines, inflammation and nutrition.
Support Line XVI(1):2, 1994. Reprinted by permission.)**

Food Group	Breakfast	Snack	Lunch	Snack	Dinner	Snack	Total Servings/ day	CHO (g)	Protein (g)	Fat (g)	Calories
	Breakfast	Snack	Lunch	Snack	Dinner	Snack					
Starch								15	3	1	80
Fruit								15			60
Milk								12	8	1	90
Vegetables								5	2		25
Meats/ Substitutes									7	5(3)	75(55)
Fats										5	45
Total											
Calories								X4=	X4=	X9=	Total=
Percent calories											

Meal/Snack/Time

*Calculations are based on medium-fat meats and skim/very low fat milk. If diet consists predominantly of low-fat meats, use the factor 3 g instead of 5 g fat; if predominantly high-fat meats, use 8 g fat. If low-fat (2%) milk is used, use 5 g fat; if whole milk is used, use 8 g fat.

Figure 31-3 Worksheet for Nutrition Assessment and implementation of a meal or food plan.

Simple Menu Plan for Dialysis Patient

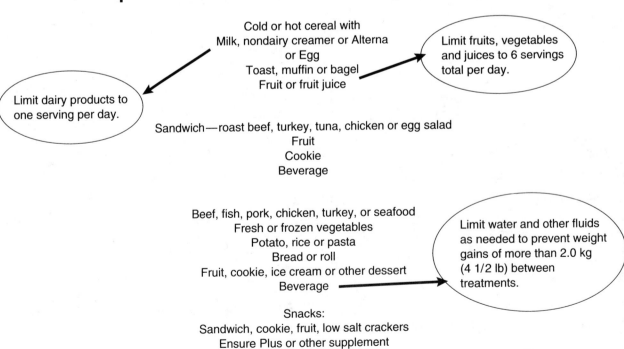

Cold or hot cereal with
Milk, nondairy creamer or Alterna
or Egg
Toast, muffin or bagel
Fruit or fruit juice

Limit fruits, vegetables and juices to 6 servings total per day.

Limit dairy products to one serving per day.

Sandwich—roast beef, turkey, tuna, chicken or egg salad
Fruit
Cookie
Beverage

Beef, fish, pork, chicken, turkey, or seafood
Fresh or frozen vegetables
Potato, rice or pasta
Bread or roll
Fruit, cookie, ice cream or other dessert
Beverage

Limit water and other fluids as needed to prevent weight gains of more than 2.0 kg (4 1/2 lb) between treatments.

Snacks:
Sandwich, cookie, fruit, low salt crackers
Ensure Plus or other supplement

Figure 35-6 Simple menu plan for dialysis patient.

HANDOUT FOR REACTIVE HYPOGLYCEMIA
(POSTPRANDIAL SYNDROME)

Hypoglycemia is a symptom of disordered carbohydrate metabolism. It is usually defined by a plasma glucose level below 50 mg/dl (blood glucose of 40 mg/dl or less) after a meal or glucose load, accompanied by typical symptoms of adrenergic neural activation. Accurate diagnosis of hypoglycemia should include measurement of plasma glucose at the time of symptoms (Palardy et al., 1989). The mixed meal tolerance test entails measurement of plasma or blood glucose at specific times after consumption of a meal containing 75 grams of carbohydrate combined with fat and protein that would be present in a normal meal.

The typical symptoms of sweating, weakness, hunger, tachycardia, and "inward trembling" are produced by a compensatory increase in sympathetic nervous system activity as the body attempts to increase hepatic glycogenolysis to offset the falling blood glucose level. Other nonspecific symptoms are headache, blurred vision, mental confusion, incoherent speech, bizarre behavior, or convulsions, which usually result from a slow and severe decline in blood glucose.

Fasting hypoglycemia is characterized by the development of hypoglycemic symptoms 6 or more hours after a meal. Although fasting hypoglycemia occurs rarely, there are several possible causes, some of which are hypersecretion of insulin due to an insulinoma (tumor of the pancreatic islet beta cells), other endocrine tumors, hypothyroidism, overadministration of insulin or sulfonylureas, and liver damage. The treatment for this type of hypoglycemia is to correct the underlying medical problem.

Hypoglycemia in the "fed" state, or *reactive postprandial hypoglycemia*, occurs 2 to 5 hours after the intake of food, especially of carbohydrates. Sensitive individuals are those with impaired glucose tolerance due to a delayed but excessive insulin response to glucose, or those with alimentary hypoglycemia resulting from dumping syndrome (see p. 604 in Chapter 27). The former is characterized by a delay in insulin secretion, with the peak response occurring between 90 and 180 minutes after a meal as opposed to a normal peak occurring between 30 and 60 minutes postprandially. The liver has already started taking up glucose at this time, so that maximal levels of serum glucose and serum insulin do not coincide. Thus, the late-arriving insulin causes an excessively large drop in serum glucose between 180 and 270 minutes after food intake, and hypoglycemia and symptoms result. The symptoms are relieved with carbohydrate intake.

The work-up for the patient who has hypoglycemic symptoms should include a dietary history to identify the content of the diet and the timing of symptoms. In addition, it should be determined how the symptoms are relieved and what triggers them. Symptoms of true hypoglycemia should be relieved by carbohydrate intake. An oral glucose tolerance test may or may not be useful in the diagnosis.

MANAGEMENT

Surgery is the preferred treatment when a tumor is established as the cause of fasting hypoglycemia. Some patients refuse to have an operation, and others with mild symptoms may prefer to try medical regimens including diet. The basic principles of the dietary treatment for hypoglycemia focus upon slowing the quick absorption and utilization of carbohydrates, which stimulate the islet cells of the pancreas to secrete insulin and move glucose from the blood. Because the glucose available after the absorption and metabolism of complex carbohydrate (starches), fiber, and protein is released into the blood stream evenly and more slowly causing less stimulation of insulin secretion, a diet rich in these components is recommended.

The diet for hypoglycemia is calculated in a procedure similar to that used to plan the diet for the person with diabetes, and the Exchange Lists for Meal Planning given in Appendix 55, pages 1163-73 can be used. A diet divided into five or six meals, with some protein and fiber in each meal in order to provide a less rapidly available source of glucose and slow down glucose absorption, helps to maintain blood glucose at a normal level.

The energy content of the diet is based upon the patient's normal requirements. If the person is overweight, there should be attention to reducing the level of body fatness. Excessive body fatness interferes with optimal insulin function. A moderate protein content of 70 to 130 g (12 to 20% of calories) is average, and a moderate carbohydrate content of 40 to 55% of calories is the usual range. The balance of kilocalories is allotted to fats. However, fat intake should be no more than 30% of kilocalories, because a high fat diet interferes with insulin use. Refined carbohydrates are avoided, and the intake of carbohydrates with fiber should be increased. Fruits, vegetables, breads, cereals, and potatoes should provide the carbohydrate in the diet.

Because alcohol can potentiate hypoglycemia by blocking gluconeogenesis, it should be omitted or restricted to one drink per day. Caffeine should also be omitted, as it affects blood glucose levels through epinephrine stimulation.